TECHNOLOGY
IN THE
HOSPITAL

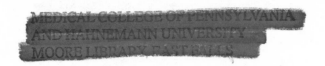
TECHNOLOGY
IN THE
HOSPITAL

Transforming Patient Care
in the
Early Twentieth Century

JOEL D. HOWELL

The Johns Hopkins University Press
Baltimore and London

© 1995 The Johns Hopkins University Press
All rights reserved. Published in 1995
Printed in the United States of America on acid-free paper
04 03 02 01 00 99 98 97 96 95   5 4 3 2 1

The Johns Hopkins University Press
2715 North Charles Street
Baltimore, Maryland 21218-4319
The Johns Hopkins Press Ltd., London

Library of Congress Cataloging-in-Publication Data will be found at the
back of this book.

A catalog record for this book is available from the British Library

ISBN 0-8018-5020-7

This book is dedicated to my father

CONTENTS

FIGURES

TABLES

PREFACE

Some time ago I started a comparative study of the use of medical technology in hospitals in England and the United States. This book discusses only the United States side of the story; the English side will be told in a forthcoming volume.

It would not have been possible to complete this book without the help of numerous colleagues who have listened, read, argued, agreed, and disagreed. They include Janet Golden, Kathryn Montgomery Hunter, Nancy Knight, Kenneth Ludmerer, Steven Peitzman, Martin Pernick, Maris Vinovskis, and John Harley Warner. Ellen Koch responded to several early drafts, read the entire manuscript, and made many useful suggestions. Keith Wailoo commented on the chapters having to do with blood counts, and David August added a surgical perspective to the discussion of appendicitis. Barbara Stafford helped me to think about the nature of images. Rosemary Stevens and Charles E. Rosenberg have given me inspiration as well as excellence to strive for. The comments of an anonymous reviewer for the Johns Hopkins University Press were extremely useful, as was the assistance of the editor for this volume, Jacqueline Wehmueller. Members of the basement crowd at Smith Hall at the University of Pennsylvania and the Division of General Medicine at the University of Michigan provided provocative responses to various chapters. In addition, the discussions that followed presentation of book chapters to seminars at Indiana University, the University of Pennsylvania, the University of Wisconsin, the Wellcome Institute for the History of Medicine, London, and Yale University gave many useful insights. While I did not always agree with what my colleagues had to say, their constant pressure to improve the message has made this a better book than it might otherwise have been.

I am grateful to the many archives that allowed me to use their material, and particularly to Adele Lerner at the Archives of the

New York Hospital-Cornell Medical Center and Caroline Morris at the Pennsylvania Hospital. Thanks are due also to the staffs of the College of Physicians of Philadelphia, the New York Academy of Medicine, and the National Library of Medicine. Taubman Medical Library at the University of Michigan was a welcome home, and the interlibrary loan department staff there deserves particular mention.

Writing history as a clinician in an academic medical setting has been made far easier than it might have been through the far-sighted support of three physician-mentors—Lester King, Alvan Tarlov, and William N. Kelley—and I appreciate their consistent encouragement to pursue what at times appeared to be an impossible career path. The Robert Wood Johnson Foundation, through its Clinical Scholars Program, allowed me the opportunity to obtain essential historical training at the University of Pennsylvania and directly supported some of the early research.

It would not have been possible to collect the data from patient records which forms the core of this book without generous financial assistance from a number of organizations, including the American College of Physicians, the American Council of Learned Societies, the National Endowment for the Humanities, and the Henry J. Kaiser Family Foundation, both as a grant recipient and as a Henry J. Kaiser Foundation Faculty Scholar in General Internal Medicine. I was a Charles E. Culpeper Foundation Fellow in Medical Humanities during the final phase of preparation. At the University of Michigan I have received support for this research from the Cancer Center and the Clinical Research Center and am grateful for the support of each of these organizations. I appreciate permission from Cornell University Press to reprint portions of chapter 4.

Chris Bass and Grace Brill helped to gather data from patient records, spending weeks filling out coding forms, going through big, dusty, dirty volumes in rooms that were sometimes hot and dim. Nonetheless, they maintained an amazingly high standard of accuracy and good cheer. Steven Grossbart started the data analysis and taught me a great deal about the realities of doing quantitative history. Peter Laipson found many popular press short stories from the early years of the twentieth century. Clare Weipert and Elizabeth

Gratch provided unstinting help in manuscript preparation. Elizabeth Dixon designed the graphic presentations.

Finally, I owe a special debt to Linda Samuelson, who has been supportive of this project from the start in many, many ways. Jonathan and Benjamin arrived too late to see the beginning of this book, but by the time it finally arrives they may be able to read it.

TECHNOLOGY
IN THE
HOSPITAL

I

<center>~~~~~~</center>

PHYSICIANS, PATIENTS, AND
MEDICAL TECHNOLOGY

On Monday, April 23, 1900, a thirty-one-year-old single laborer living in Philadelphia, whom we shall call Mr. James Moran, injured his leg.[1] The injury appeared to be serious, so he was taken a few blocks to the Pennsylvania Hospital. There Mr. Moran was seen by a physician, who concluded, based solely on a history and physical examination, that both bones in Mr. Moran's lower leg had been broken. Mr. Moran was admitted to the hospital, perhaps because his broken leg made it difficult for him to move about and he had no one to look after him at home. Although the Pennsylvania Hospital had owned an x-ray machine for three years, no x-ray image of Mr. Moran's leg was taken; Mr. Moran's experience in this respect was like that of almost all of the other people with broken legs who were admitted in 1900. Someone looked at Mr. Moran's urine, once, on the day that he entered the hospital, but scant notice was taken of the results. No blood was drawn; no other laboratory tests of any type were done. This lack of interest in laboratory tests was a pervasive feature of hospital life. Fifty-one days after he came in, Mr. Moran left the Pennsylvania Hospital, pronounced "cured." Despite the length of his hospitalization, the entire hospital record consisted of only a single page.

About twenty-five years later, on Wednesday, November 11, 1925, a fifty-one-year-old widower, a cook whom we shall call Mr. Richard Scott, was also admitted to the Pennsylvania Hospital.[2] Mr. Scott, like Mr. Moran, was soon discovered to have broken his leg. In many respects, however, Mr. Scott's experience was very different from that of Mr. Moran. Like almost every other person admitted in 1925 with a broken leg, on the same day that he was admitted Mr. Scott had an x-ray image taken to confirm the diagnosis. His urine was examined, not just once but on four separate occasions. Although Mr. Scott stayed in the hospital only twenty-one days, his hospital record grew to eight full pages, including three forms and one graph. Thus, it was eight times as long as Mr. Moran's record had been, despite the fact Mr. Scott's stay was less than half the length of Mr. Moran's. Like Mr. Moran in 1900, Mr. Scott did well; he was noted to have "improved" during his hospital stay.

Why was Mr. Scott's experience so different from that of Mr. Moran? In this book I seek to understand why physicians in 1925 thought it important to confirm their clinical impression of a broken leg with a diagnostic test produced by a machine, the x-ray image. I wish to know why they decided that laboratory tests should be an important element of patient care. I want to know why physicians found it necessary, or desirable, to pepper the hospital chart with forms and graphs. In other words, I want to find out why medical care changed between 1900 and 1925 to a form dominated by machines and "science," a change that has persisted to the end of the twentieth century. I conclude that the fact of the invention of the machines, the creation of the physical artifacts, is not a sufficient explanation for the changes in clinical practice which took place between 1900 and 1925. Rather, to understand the clinical applications of technology we must look at the meaning of a medical technology, such as the x-ray machine, within a specific social and political context. In so doing, we may subvert the idea that scientific value (or truth) alone defines the clinical utility of a given medical technology and that scientific validity alone has determined how that technology is to be used or understood. Rather than simply attributing change to the march of science, it is far more interesting for the historian and valuable for the policymaker to examine when and how the appeal to science derived its current power.

Whenever possible, this book will address medical care at the level of individual, specific patients. The particular experiences of Messrs. Moran and Scott reflected widespread changes in how health care was provided in U.S. hospitals between 1900 and 1925. In 1900 few specialized tests were being done in the hospital. Few medical tests were being done at all. So it was for Mr. Moran. Although physicians chose to look once at his urine, the results of the urine examination did not influence either diagnosis or treatment. Physicians did no blood tests whatsoever, nor did they perform an x-ray examination of Mr. Moran's injured limb. Why should they? Someone looked at Mr. Moran's leg when he entered the hospital; it was obviously fractured. That was all there was to it. The clinical examination provided all of the diagnostic information needed to identify Mr. Moran's injury and to care for him; physicians saw no need to obtain any additional diagnostic information. This was the case for most patients, with most diseases. Physicians rarely used laboratory tests to guide their clinical decisions; patients rarely thought that science could be relevant for their day-to-day care.

By 1925 the hospital world that Mr. Scott entered had changed considerably. Blood tests played an important role in assigning a diagnosis to many patients' ailments. Ward laboratories near the patients' beds made it easier for house officers to do numerous tests on almost all patients; clinical laboratories, run by people who based their careers on administering laboratories, were active day and night. X-ray examinations had become routine for essentially all persons suspected of having broken bones as well as for patients with a variety of other conditions. Laboratory tests and x-ray images were thought to provide physicians with useful data about Mr. Scott, data they believed to be valuable, in large part, because that data was seen as objective and scientific. Patients, too, had come to share their physicians' faith in objective, scientific information.

Not just the laboratory tests—the entire hospital had become, by 1925, quite actively and self-consciously based on science. Moreover, the definitions of what constituted science were extremely broad. Just as was the case for U.S. society in general, within the hospital walls scientific ideals were perceived as having far-reaching importance, having value that extended beyond the immediate medical care of patients. The hospital's administrative structure had begun to be designed around something called the "efficiency movement," based on principles held to be scientific. Scientific ideas were also an essential part of a new financial and accounting structure, a structure that was as much a part of the new hospital as any modern medical theory, a structure that was based on new technology, albeit technology that we, at the end of the twentieth century, rarely think of as medical. By around 1925 the people who ran and financially supported the general hospital in the United States, as well as those who delivered health care within it, had come to see science as the essential tool for making the institution a central part of twentieth-century medicine.

Yet to look at the hospital only through the thoughts and experiences of physicians and administrators is to look at only half of the story, and, depending on one's perspective, perhaps not the most important half.[3] We also need to consider the question: What difference did the changes in hospital care, changes in how medicine and science existed within the hospital walls, make to people, patients, like Messrs. Scott and Moran? Some of the changes were invisible to patients. When confined to bed with a broken limb, patients had to urinate into some type of container, and it probably mattered little to them whether that urine was later examined in the laboratory or poured down the sewer. Similarly, it was unlikely to have any immediate impact on the patient whether the medical staff shared any new conceptions about the theoretical causes of disease. But in some obvious ways, Mr. Moran and Mr. Scott, and the others who joined them in the hospital in 1900 and 1925, had very different experiences during their hospitalization. Those who had blood tests probably noticed. Lying in bed while someone poked or prodded your arm with a needle was a new sensation for people in the early twentieth century, an unpleasant sensation, and one doubtless not easily overlooked, even by a lay observer. Having an x-ray image obtained was not an easy undertaking either. Mr. Scott was taken to a basement suite of rooms, where large, dirty, smelly equipment was used to produce an image of the inside of his body. Even if he did not see the actual "skiagram," also called a "skiagraph" (shadow picture)—it would later be called an x-ray image, or a roentgenogram—he was unlikely to forget the experience of having the picture taken.

On the other hand, having the latest medical devices may have helped the hospital entice different types of people into the hospital for care in 1925 than had been the case in 1900. Mr. Scott was joined in the hospital corridors by others of modest social standing, people who were not only laborers but also business owners and artisans. That this group of middle-class people was willing to enter the institution at all reflected changing ideas about the hospital's function. The decision to enter the hospital in the first place was, in

1925, a distinct shift for many patients from 1900, a shift that for some reflected a perception of the hospital as a scientific place in which to receive medical care.[4]

The new elements of the hospital which helped to define its new role in health care ultimately became part of a broader change in the relationship between physicians and patients, which involved health care at almost all levels and locations.[5] Much of that change was mediated by the use of shiny new machines, machines such as the radiologist's x-ray machine and the laboratory director's microscope, machines that reflected a growing desire on the part of both patients and physicians to see medicine as scientific. Today, in the late twentieth century, medical machines have become a part of routine medical care, accepted and expected by physicians and patients alike. Some of the technology that was new to people in 1925 seems by the 1990s to have disappeared. But not all of it has gone away. Rather, much of this technology has simply blended into the background of the usual. It has been observed that "the most profound technologies are those that disappear": "They weave themselves into the fabric of everyday life until they are indistinguishable from it."[6] By that standard most of the technologies I will discuss in this book are truly profound. Typewriters and adding machines are not seen today as new and exciting. Urine analyses, blood tests, even the "ordinary" x-ray, are no longer identified by most people and in most accounts as being remarkable medical technologies; they are simply part of routine medical care. Other machines have come to the fore; remarkable imaging devices now known widely by their initials, such as computed axial tomography (CAT) scanners, magnetic resonance imaging (MRI) scanners, and positron emission tomography (PET) scanners, produce the pictures that adorn newsstand magazines, pictures that are often given color specifically for popular consumption.[7]

Machines are not always depicted in positive terms. Late in the twentieth century medical machines have been assigned the blame for a wide range of evils, but perhaps two of these alleged failings are more important than others. First, technology has been blamed for the ever-increasing cost of medical care. The seemingly inexorable upward spiral of the amount of money that Americans spend on disease may impede the achievement of one of the most often talked about goals for health care reform, expanding insurance coverage for medical care to all Americans.[8] On the other hand, at the same time as technology is being blamed for costing too much money, technology is being credited with the relief of much human pain and suffering. Any attempt to impede the development of new technologies, such as by a meaningful attempt at cost containment, may simultaneously slow the development of newer and better treatments for diseases.

Second, technology has taken much of the blame for distancing physicians from their patients, both literally and metaphorically. As a result of this distancing, patients find that their personal, expressed accounts of their own illnesses are devalued, that information derived from machines is given a privileged position. Many people feel alienated from mainstream medical care. Some of this feeling may have been historically derived from a shift of care from home to hospital. When patients received care in their home, they (and their relatives) exerted considerable influence to define and shape what care they would experience, but once care moved into the hospital it became much more difficult for patients and relatives to have such input.[9] Although patients could still tell what hurt, and where, and could perhaps speculate about why, new, scientifically trained caregivers, often in hospitals, used machines to create "objective" data and used machines and science to write a new version of the patient's story.[10] An overuse of machinery may have made physicians better scientists but poorer healers.

How did we come to this state of affairs? The answer may lie in understanding how, why, and when physicians and the public came to see medical machines as useful devices for patient care, and when such machines started to be used routinely for patient care. In this book I will explore the relationship between technology and medical care in the United States between 1900 and 1925, focusing on what happened within the hospital but putting it in the context of general social ideas about science and machines. After considering how the hospital itself was shaped by medical technology, I will examine the use of three different types of clinical medical technology in the early twentieth century. One was a very old test, at least in name: the urine analysis. One was very new and very public: the x-ray machine. And one, blood counts, combined old ideas about blood with new ideas about the laboratory and became central to a debate over how to make the diagnosis of not only blood diseases but also diseases requiring surgical intervention, particularly appendicitis.

TECHNOLOGY: DEFINITIONS AND EXPLANATIONS

This book purports to be about "medical technology." We ought to consider just what has been meant by the term *medical technology*, what it meant within the institution of the hospital, and how its definition changed between Mr. Moran's hospital admission and Mr. Scott's. Around the turn of the twentieth century the structure of institutionalized medical care was much more integrated into the fabric of the larger society than has since come to be the case. Hospitals were designed along the same lines as orphanages and old-age homes and, like these facilities, were used primarily for the long-term care of dependent people.[11] The most important machines in these institutions were those that were essential to the daily operations of the facility. Thus, when asked what machines marked his hospital as modern and new, the proud, sanitation-minded hospital superintendent of the 1890s and 1900s would likely have pointed to the laundry room, the kitchen, or perhaps the telephone system.[12] Popular accounts of outstanding hospitals praised their sanitation, their cleanliness, and their facilities for the cold storage of food. Machines that were designed to be used primarily by physicians, such as x-ray machines, were not seen as particularly important means of defining a hospital's identity.[13]

New amenities were used to attract private patients into the hospital, people who could pay for some part of their care. These new funds presented hospital administrators with a new (though presumably desirable) problem: how to manage the money. Soon after the turn of the century some of the most important technology that started to find its way into the U.S. hospital existed to keep track of money. Although we would not now, in the late twentieth century, characterize adding machines as medical technology, they were important for many changes in the early twentieth-century hospital. Chapter 2 will explore the ways in which machines such as adding machines shaped the institution and affected the experiences of both patients and physicians.

Eventually, however, medical technology became conceptualized in terms of machines that were used directly on or around patients.[14]

A few decades into the twentieth century a new and modern hospital started to be defined, as it often is today, in terms of "fancy" medical equipment that was operated by physicians or, at least, directly supervised by them. How did this process take place? Was it the direct result of the invention of new places, such as the clinical laboratory, or devices, such as those used to take x-ray images? We shall see in chapter 4 that it would be a mistake to assume that the high-profile 1895 invention of the x-ray machine quickly resulted in a new perception of what it meant to practice modern medicine.[15] Rather, the technologies seen as being most directly important for medical care remained in the hands of non–medically trained people for at least a decade or so after the turn of the twentieth century.

While determining what technology is considered "medical" may seem somewhat problematic, the question of how to define "technology" has attracted even more critical attention.[16] Some leading historians of technology have questioned the need to give a single, cogent definition—we speak easily of "politics," for example, without seeking a precise meaning of the term—and are satisfied to let the meaning of the term be flexible, to point out that technology means different things to different people.[17] Using a narrow framework, many of those who have written about medical technology have taken *technology* to mean only the machine, the physical artifact itself. At the other extreme, some analysts have taken the definition of medical technology to be broad enough to include almost the entire health care system.[18]

Perhaps most useful are those historians who distinguish between three layers of meaning for the word *technology*.[19] First is the level of technology as physical artifact, as machine. The most obvious example relevant to medicine in the early years of the twentieth century is the x-ray machine. Second is technology as an activity, as a means of accomplishing some goal. Thus, one can speak of the various ways of doing a blood count as a technology, in addition to the physical apparatus necessary to accomplish the counts. Finally, what people know is another form of technology. Simply having the artifact and a description of the proper technique is not enough for a technology to have an impact. Users must also know how to apply the artifact and the techniques within a given sphere of activity.

I shall consider technology in this book using all three of these levels as valid meanings of the word *technology*. I shall consider the physical artifacts, such as the x-ray machines, but, in order to understand why people chose to use the machines as they did, I will also examine the organization within which the x-ray images were made. Such an analysis may help explain not only when people used (and did not use) the machines but also why they chose to assign certain meanings to the evidence produced by those machines. I shall examine the techniques used to do blood counts and will consider the social and professional reasons why some people saw the counts as useful while others disagreed. Those reasons may have had much to do with the ways in which technology, read broadly, informed the power relationships among those involved in caring for the patient.[20] I note the multiple ways in which medical technologies may be understood, without attempting to place each instance of technology use into a separate theoretical level. Throughout the book my ultimate goal will be to understand the clinical, medical uses of technology.

Having taken a broad view of medical technology, where should we seek explanations for how and why it has become part of the familiar fabric of medical care? How the question is framed will largely determine the answer that is obtained. Consider the case of the x-ray machine. Should we examine the development of better and better x-ray tubes, or should we look at how social relations shaped (and were shaped by) a new imaging device? Both matter. We cannot meaningfully understand the use of medical machines without taking account of both the scientific and the social.

A danger of writing for many audiences is that what is seen as radical by one may be seen as obvious by another. Hence, this direct assertion that machines are in part socially constructed will seem obvious to many readers, particularly those familiar with recent work in the social history of technology.[21] Yet the social history of technology has had a limited impact on the history of medical technology. Some writers have postulated models for technological change in medicine which deny, explicitly or implicitly, that social context is of much value for understanding the history of medical technology.

One standard model for understanding health care views the invention and dissemination of technology simply as a function of its efficacy in solving a particular problem. This approach tends to assume that technology is the same as the mechanical artifact, that

technical descriptions are the most important element for understanding the history of technology, and that the artifact itself primarily determines how it will be used.[22] Although widely criticized,
this approach still holds a great deal of sway. The reasons why this
model has been so pervasive for medical technology are not hard to
fathom. It is a useful myth for those who practice medicine and who
must daily make very real decisions about very real patients, hoping
always to make the best possible decisions. Moreover, it is a comforting story not only for medical caregivers but also for most people.
We are all future patients. We all wish to believe that when we fall ill
we will receive the very best health care possible. In the late twentieth century patients and physicians trust medical knowledge based
on machines, and many define the "very best" care as something
based on objective, scientific measurement. They wish deeply to
believe that, while culture and sociology may inform some aspects
of medical care, there remains a core, defined in part by medical
machines, which is transcultural—or acultural.[23]

The privileging of knowledge created by medical technology is
often not explicit. Rather than critically examining medical technology, some scholars simply ignore it. Social construction arguments
are commonly found in discussions of women's diseases, disorders
of sexuality, or psychiatric diseases, but not in diseases defined by
instrumental technology. Even when technology is examined in
light of gender differences, the questions that scholars ask tend to be
about how the technology can be equitably applied to women and
men, rather than about how gender has informed the creation of the
knowledge itself. To date, most social historians have implicitly
treated the medical knowledge produced by machines and by science
as more "real," more objective, than the knowledge produced by
theoretical arguments. We are only beginning to unpack the reasons
why technical knowledge was held to be better or more valid.

Technology was (and is) commonly found in hospitals. Hospitals
have now become temples for high-technology medical care, and
they have not escaped the attention of historians of medicine.[24] Yet
hospitals have received no more attention from urban historians
than medical technology has received from social historians. Some
of the best books to be written about the history of urbanization fail
even to mention the growth of hospitals.[25] Certainly, one need not
make hospitals central for an analysis of urbanization. But hospitals

clearly have come to dominate their local physical environment, and one might suspect that they would be at least occasionally the object of analysis in the same way as urban historians have studied factories, churches, schools, and housing, all of which have had a major impact on the areas where they are located. Perhaps the authors believe, or wish to believe, that decisions about medical care were, and are, based on "scientific facts" absent any social concerns.

Medical technology deserves the same level of critical analysis as does the definition of diseases or the growth of cities. To view the development of medical technology as simply the logical expression of scientific and clinical reality is unsatisfactory for several reasons. It will overemphasize the importance of the invention of a technology and underemphasize the process by which use of a technology becomes standard practice. Such an approach will also devalue any attempt to understand "failed" medical technologies, as the technology's failure can then be treated as simply the inevitable realization by a set of rational users that a given tool did not (i.e., could not) become clinically useful.[26] Perhaps most important, failing to engage critically with the process by which a medical technology becomes useful leads the historian away from listening to the voices of those who opposed a technology, even a technology that later become widely used, despite the fact that critical voices and the resistance they engaged may have made a great deal of sense at the time. Indeed, the reasons given for *not* using a particular technology, even one as ultimately successful as the x-ray machine, may provide insights into the process by which communities make decisions about how to practice medicine. Understanding that process may make it clear what choices were available to those who wished to use new technology without assuming that the choices that were made were somehow natural or inevitable. Moreover, such an analysis may give us a window onto how the larger community, of which patients and physicians were both a part, acted to define what the meaning of a new technology would be. Often discussions of medical technology focus on how technologies change the ways in which people view the world.[27] I shall attempt to attend as well to how the world changed the ways people viewed medical instruments.

THE OTHER END OF THE TUBE: MEDICAL TECHNOLOGY FROM THE PATIENT'S PERSPECTIVE

For some time social historians writing from a wide range of perspectives have been moving away from creating a litany of wars, treaties, political events, and biographies of great people and have started considering how the great mass of individuals lived their lives.[28] Birth and death are a fact of life for every person. In between these two major events few escape disease. So, it should come as no surprise that the social history of medicine has become increasingly relevant to social history in general. Rather than chronicling "great moments in medicine," social historians of medicine are treating history as a process rather than an event and are increasingly examining how medical care affected ordinary people.

Medical care has affected people in several different ways. One way is through innovations and changes in public health measures. Another way is through clinical care for individuals. In the 1960s the noted medical historian Erwin H. Ackerknecht called for increased attention to medical practice.[29] I shall heed his call in this book and focus primarily on the use of technology for patient care, paying relatively little attention to questions of invention and priority or of the relationship between science and technology and treating changes in medical theory as important primarily insofar as they relate to changes in medical practice.

One way of constructing the social history of medical technology might be to focus on the individual experience of sick persons. Can we understand what they felt and learn what they perceived to be the benefits (or lack thereof) of the new techniques? Rather than focusing exclusively upon the view from one end of the x-ray or the endoscopy tube—the view of the medical practitioner—we might consider what it was like to be at the other end of the tube.

As is always the case for history, this mode of analysis is ultimately constrained by the availability of sources. Historians have used letters, diaries, and memoirs to produce some extremely useful patient-centered studies of health and disease, often when examining the nature of mental illness.[30] But sources for understanding patients' perspectives on use of technology are limited. This is particularly true for hospital care around the turn of the twentieth century, when many patients were, at best, only marginally literate.

Available narrative sources tend to be highly selective: most patients left no diaries or memoirs; they either didn't write letters from the sickbed, or they were not so prominent that their personal letters were saved in an archival repository. If we wish to know how and when technology became part of the fabric of everyday care, we need to know something about the experiences of the persons who didn't leave an eloquent written account, a group that includes most of the people who were receiving medical care.

Published literature might be a useful source. Well-known literary works include descriptions of the new technology, such as Thomas Mann's 1924 novel *The Magic Mountain*. I will discuss further in chapter 5 how the images produced by the x-ray machine play an important role in Mann's novel. If this work gives us insight only into how Thomas Mann thought about the x-ray machine, we will not have gained much insight into the social history of medical technology. But, perhaps, people who read novels gained some of their ideas about the machine from fictional accounts. Thus, "elite" literature such as *The Magic Mountain* might have shaped, as well as reflected, ideas about the x-ray machine.

Short stories published in literary or popular magazines may offer a different kind of historical insight. Stories in popular magazines reached a wider audience than more sophisticated publications and had to resonate with the experiences of less sophisticated readers in ways that elite literature did not: if the general public had never heard of a new technology, that technology would have to be explained, or else the tale would make no sense. If the public could not understand the new devices or did not enjoy the way that the technology was integrated into the story, the magazine would not sell. Magazines and their stories were (and are) consumer commodities, which may be historically useful for recreating popular attitudes. Furthermore, much of what was published was genre fiction, made popular in large part through its very familiarity and predictability.[31] That the x-ray machine plays a central role in such material, as will also be discussed in chapter 5, tells us that people had heard of the new device and had at least some vague idea about its capabilities, possibly gleaned from speculative accounts in newspapers or other types of the popular press. Thus, popular writings that deal with medical technology can provide markers of social perceptions, or at least social awareness.

But stories need not accurately reflect either dominant medical opinion or standard clinical care of the time. Some literary critics around the turn of the twentieth century complained that authors too often used the "wrong" fictional diseases, choosing diseases that were thought not to exist, such as "brain fever," instead of "real" diseases, which would be better for dramatic effect, such as pneumonia.[32] Nor are stories necessarily accurate representations of typical experiences. Fiction engages readers in part through its originality, through its ability to create new worlds for the reader. Fiction of the early twentieth century incorporated such innovative visions as time travel and visits to the moon. Accounts of the x-ray machine may not accurately reflect the nonliterary experiences of typical people. Useful though they may be, these stories will not tell us when medical technologies became part of the routine experience of most people who broke a limb or required surgery. For such information we must turn to other sources, such as patient records.

Records created by physicians and others who were caring for patients may help us recreate the sick person's experience.[33] Obviously, patient case records are an indirect way of getting at people's experiences: they were created by the caregivers, not the patients. This presents a fundamental problem. The caregivers' records have enormous potential for distorting patients' experiences. On the other hand, these records may provide insights that we are unlikely to have through any other means. The historian Barbara Duden has recently used the casebooks of an eighteenth-century German practitioner to recreate the ideas of the patients whom he treated.[34] If, like Duden, we can learn to read *through* the elite accounts that health care professionals created, so as to use them but not to privilege them, we may be able to glean important insights from the case records.

Patient records may allow us to recreate some element of the patients' experiences if we are able to read the records in a patient-centered way and focus primarily not on knowledge claims but on what happened to hospitalized patients. From 1900 to 1925 the hospital world was changing in ways that must have been obvious both to patients and to other people who spent time within the walls of the institution. Case records, though they rarely relate the experience of a patient in his or her own words, can indicate when certain activities were done. These records can tell us when performing a procedure became routine. From that information we may be able to infer some aspects of a patient's experience. For example, in an era in which therapeutic bloodletting had fallen into decline, having blood taken to make a diagnosis was an unusual event. The magnitude of the procedure should not be underestimated: removal of blood was something usually done by physicians and was accompanied by emotion and pain. Therefore, knowing when blood tests became part of routine care tells us when that particular procedure became a common part of a hospitalized patient's experience.

Patient records document events that took place in newly created parts of the hospital, and, undoubtedly, those events were meaningful to the persons who experienced them. The late-nineteenth-century patient's room, or ward, or at least his or her bed, must have quickly become familiar territory, given the long periods of time that most patients stayed in the hospital. But patients in early twentieth-century hospitals were taken more and more often on trips away from the familiar ward to unfamiliar territory, to places like the x-ray laboratory, the "heart station" (or electrocardiogram room), and the cystoscopy suite.[35] There a patient faced a variety of bewildering experiences and a rather strange array of impressive-looking devices. The equipment in the x-ray room would give off sparks; in the heart station a patient would be required to immerse his or her limbs in buckets of saltwater.[36] In some cases a patient's body would be invaded, either by machines that could look completely through it or by equipment that would go directly within it. The visits to new places and experiences with new devices were meaningful events for patients who stayed in hospitals at the turn of the twentieth century. Patient case records are one way, perhaps the only way, to know when these visits started to become a regular part of a hospital admission.

These events took place within a changing hospital system, and that changing system was itself a new technology, one whose structure had a direct effect on each patient's experience. The hospital was becoming organizationally complex in ways that were apparent to both the caregivers and the patients that they served. Patients were having contact with a greater variety of people, people whose specific roles were being carefully delineated. The ophthalmologist was coming around to look into patients' eyes. The dietitian was deciding what patients could eat for breakfast. Medical students, new to many hospitals, were questioning patients, listening to their hearts, probing their abdomens, and trying out their new, scientific diagnostic and therapeutic techniques. Even the person who wheeled patients around to their various tests represented a new kind of worker in the hospital, and being wheeled around to various units was a new experience for the patient.

There are many advantages to shifting the frame of reference away from the technology and toward the patient, and toward his or her interaction with the health care system. This approach moves the gaze from the machine to the person, from abstract theory to individual encounter. In so doing, it moves us away from a sole focus on published clinical literature. We ought not to get too far from that literature; it is clearly valuable for understanding some of the reasons that physicians might wish to practice medicine in a particular way. But to focus exclusively on published accounts of medical practice will give a distorted image of how technology was used. It will look like the machine is central for health care in whatever period we choose to study, when, in fact, it may not have been. Whether or not we are ultimately successful in recreating a finely detailed, richly textured map of a person's experience, simply trying to make patients a primary object of study helps to put them back into the center of the analytic frame.

TECHNOLOGY IN THE HOSPITAL

Where should we examine the use of medical technology? When source material is available, looking at individual practitioners can be extremely revealing.[37] Using the patient records of individual practitioners in concert with other sources, one could track in some detail the life and training of a single practitioner. One could look at when and why that practitioner started to use a new machine and for which patients. He or she might have cared for some patients over a long period of time, thus enabling the historian to observe what happens to the physician-patient relationship as new tools and techniques are introduced. But the in-depth study of a single practitioner poses problems. Practitioners probably will be more likely to adopt new ideas and tools early in their professional lives, when they are most actively learning and training, than later in their lives. Any person will only be at one point in his or her career when a particular technology becomes available. More problematic, it is extremely difficult to locate complete case records of a given practitioner: most were thrown away. For the early-twentieth century there are occasional volumes to be found but very few series of records that document the complete practice patterns of a single individual. Even if such records could be found, one is left with comprehensive records of a single person, but in such a case it is often a fairly prominent practitioner, and there is little evidence that his or her style was in any way typical of other practitioners.

Considering technology use within hospitals solves some of these problems, while it introduces others. Hospitals tend to outlast practitioners. They have a life as an institution; they are ethically as well as legally required to save case records for some period of time. Thus, hospitals are more likely than practitioners to have preserved complete sets of patient care records, from which one can extract some type of meaningful sample.

Many hospitals served as training sites for medical (and other) students, particularly after the turn of the twentieth century, so that the ways that technology was used within each hospital were important in ways that transcended the care of each patient, helping to shape the practice patterns of that hospital's trainees and, thus, the care of the patients who came to see that practitioner. On the other hand, the presence of medical students, house officers, and attending physicians all caring for a single patient may at times make it difficult to identify precisely who made a specific decision.

Until fairly recently most histories of hospitals, often written to glorify the local hospital, were concerned with a single institution. However, along with an increased interest in the social history of medicine has come attention to the hospital as a signal U.S. institution that was invented around the turn of the twentieth century. The strong secondary literature that now exists on U.S. hospital history provides essential background within which to set the findings from reviews of case records. Between around 1890 and around 1925 the U.S. hospital underwent a dramatic transformation.[38] Initially nineteenth-century repositories for the dependent poor, by some time after the end of World War I hospitals had become self-consciously scientific institutions. The number of hospitals dramatically increased, an increase that far outpaced any rise in population. This growth was obvious to contemporary observers. Even allowing for the need for a self-congratulatory piece with which to start a new journal, the *Modern Hospital*, the breadth of the 1913 offering is remarkable: "Hospital Growth Marks Dawn of a New Era: Vast Increase in Numbers and Variety of Institutions Is Chief Factor in Reshaping Modern Society."[39] The author noted not only a remarkable increase in the number of hospitals but also an increase in the number of hospital beds available for patient care: the state of Illinois had more beds in 1913 than had existed in the entire United States only forty years before. These hospitals were marked by an increasing number of people who wished to enter them for medical care, people who were no longer dependent on charity but who might be able or willing to pay for that care. Hospitals were also marked by the increasing amounts of money being spent, money that the author felt would be wasted without proper systematization and standardization, two themes to which we shall return.

Hospitals became central for medical education.[40] Whereas a typical physician who practiced in the mid-nineteenth century might well spend his or her entire career without ever setting foot in a hospital—either as a student or a practitioner—by early in the twentieth century most medical schools either had a hospital affiliation or were seeking to obtain one. From that point on the clinical training necessary to be a physician took place largely in the wards of a hospital.[41]

Also in the early twentieth century medical care started to move out of people's homes and to become centralized, first in the physician's office and later, increasingly, in hospitals.[42] At the same time, technology became a prominent feature of medical care. At the end of the twentieth century U.S. hospitals have become havens for medical technology, so much so that technology is one of the defining characteristics of the institution.[43] Many devices, such as the x-ray machine, were (and are) difficult to carry about. Did the centralization of machines in hospitals help drive the increase in hospital care which occurred in the early twentieth century? Were those machines even used? In hopes of answering this question, chapter 4 explores the use of the x-ray machine in the hospital.

Hospitals were places in which people worked out new ideas that were later applied more widely. But hospitals are also important in their own right, as important case studies. If we are to come to grips with the ways in which new medical techniques are adopted by some community of practitioners, if we are to understand the relationships between theory and practice at the level of individual patients' care (and that is fundamentally the level at which care takes place), we must choose some venue in which to start. Looking inside a hospital, one can explore the ways in which specific institutional and organizational innovations were played out.

UNIVERSAL THEORIES, LOCAL PRACTICE

In order to understand the uses of medical technology, it is also important to examine geographic variation in medical practice, the ways in which theoretical ideas about medicine, including ideas about the appropriate use of medical technology, are put into clinical practice differently at different locations. The tension between universal theories and local practice has no doubt existed for some time, but it must have been particularly acute at the turn of the twentieth century. On the one hand, the growth of cities and hospitals meant that larger groups of people than ever before were working together, more medical schools were sending their students to train in hospitals, and more and more people were involved in the care of each individual patient. Thus, there was a greater opportunity for groups of people to develop their own specific standards and behaviors. They could do so within a theoretical framework that encouraged local theories of disease. American ideas about disease incorporated a strong belief in the importance of local conditions in understanding disease and in evaluating therapy, a belief that allowed American practitioners to incorporate a European theoretical framework about disease while at the same time maintaining the uniqueness of their North American environment.[44]

On the other hand, many physicians wanted to use the recently championed scientific basis of medical practice to produce universal guidelines for ideal clinical practice. Disease-causing organisms had only fairly recently been defined as the basis for important infectious diseases such as tuberculosis and cholera. If these organisms were the same everywhere, and if treatment was to be based on specific disease-causing agents, the process of optimum medical care could be systematically applied to all people in all areas of the country. This position was in part a reaction to the newfound power of the natural sciences in explaining the causes of human disease, a power most notably successful for microbial diseases. It was also an attempt to assert the primacy of scientific over personal knowledge, to assert the expertise of those physicians and scientists who were in a position to make use of the laboratory.

Machines well might have been used to support universal, rather than local, patterns of medical care. If the artifact defined its use, it could be picked up and moved about and applied equally, and well, in every site. But such was not the case. There was a continual tension between universal ideals and local practices, a tension that may be more apparent from day-to-day medical practice than from broader pronouncements. Thomas Misa, a historian of technology, has pointed out the critical difference in the answers one gets about the use of machines, depending on whether one looks at the level of the shop floor or at the level of the overall organization.[45] I wish to look both at the overall organization of U.S. medicine and at the shop floor—the care of individual patients—but to pay more attention to the shop floor than has heretofore been the case in most discussions of medical technology.

When we do that, we shall see considerable variation in the ways that new technologies were used for patient care. Medical practitioners with similar training, working in similar institutions, in the same area of the United States, used medical technology very differently between 1900 and 1925.[46] Were these differences due to differences among patients? Differences in the diseases? Differences in the organizational structures? The answers may not be clear, but the presence of variation is itself an important finding.

That ideal medical practice can be established by some authorities, and then uniformly applied, is an appealing idea. If true, it would have the potential to eliminate variations in medical practice caused by practitioners who do not know how best to apply the fruits of medical advances. Late in the twentieth century that idea has reemerged (or perhaps it never disappeared) in the form of practice pattern guidelines, routinized lists of what ought to be done for patients with certain characteristics and certain diseases.[47] Much of the contemporary debate over health policy concerns the "appropriate" use of technology. It presupposes that the existence of regional differences that cannot be explained by clinical characteristics means that the technology is either used "too much" in one group or "too little" in another. We have not reached a consensus about the validity of such an approach. This historical analysis obviously cannot decide whether we use (or used) technology too much or too little.

However, the continued existence of variation even in the late twentieth century justifies, in part, historical attention to its existence in the early twentieth century. One might logically wonder if the historical variation was simply a difference in the speed at which individual locales reached the same endpoint. The fact that we have not yet reached a homogeneous application of medical technology does not mean that we never will, but it implies that there still exist forces that lead to local practice variation and that such variation was more than merely a short-lived perturbation in response to the introduction of a new technology.

TWO CITIES, TWO HOSPITALS, TWENTY-FIVE YEARS

Much of this book is based on a detailed analysis of case records to identify when and how medical technology was used for patient care over a twenty-five-year period. Examining patient records to study technology use for specific patients is extremely time intensive. I have chosen to look at the New York Hospital, in New York City, and the Pennsylvania Hospital, in Philadelphia. The records are taken from patients admitted between 1900 and 1925. I selected the study years to bracket what appear to be the critical times in which medical technology became a part of routine medical care. In 1900 most hospitals retained a nineteenth-century flavor. The excitement of what was to be twentieth-century science was on the doorstep, but life within the institution as experienced by Mr. Moran and others was still not dramatically different than it had been for some time. By 1925 much of what we have come to recognize as the daily routine of hospital life was essentially in place, a routine that Mr. Scott and others came to know quite well.

Because the total number of patient records from each of these hospitals is too large to be usable, I have taken a sample of these records. The sample is designed to be statistically valid, meaning that every available record from the sample years had an equal and nonzero probability of being included in the sample. Record availability led to sampling from the New York Hospital in 1900, 1910, and 1920 and from the Pennsylvania Hospital for 1900, 1909 (which is compared with 1910 for the New York Hospital), 1920, and 1925. The sample for analysis includes 940 records from the New York Hospital and 1,622 from the Pennsylvania Hospital. (For details on the specific methodology used to construct and analyze the data set, see the appendix.) For each case record that was used, a detailed summary was prepared. That summary included detailed demographic information about the patient, such as their age, sex, marital status, race, occupation, nationality, and place of residence. Also included on the summary form was the diagnosis (initial and final, when both were given), along with operations and procedures and comments in the chart made by caregivers or others. The use of a wide range of technology was noted. In addition, characteristics of the chart were recorded, including its length, whether forms or graphs were used, and what kind of forms were included. All of this information was encoded for computer-aided analysis.

I selected these two hospitals for a number of reasons. First, they have each preserved large portions of their patient case records. Perhaps they did so because each retains a strong sense of its own historic importance. The Pennsylvania Hospital, founded in 1751, has long laid claim to being the oldest hospital in the United States.[48] The New York Hospital was the second to be founded in what became the United States, being granted a royal charter by King George III in 1771 and first receiving patients in 1791.[49] Well into the nineteenth century these two institutions were the only two private general hospitals in their towns.[50] The New York Hospital was distinguished for the achievements of its surgical staff, although by the end of the nineteenth century other hospitals in the area were beginning to deliver care of similar quality.[51]

The hospitals were similar in many respects. Both were urban hospitals on the eastern seaboard. Both were well respected and relatively stable institutions, but neither was an "elite" turn-of-the-century institution along the lines that one might characterize Johns Hopkins. Both were fairly large. In 1900 the Pennsylvania Hospital admitted 4,002 patients; the New York Hospital admitted 6,054 patients at the main institution (which will be the object of our attention in this book; another 2,386 were admitted to the House of Relief).[52] Both hospitals used their annual reports to note with some pride the total numbers of patients cared for during the institution's existence, albeit using somewhat different terms. The New York

PENNSYLVANIA HOSPITAL / NEW YORK HOSPITAL

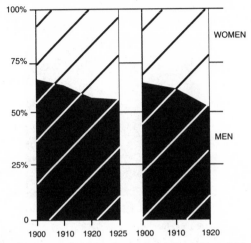

Figure 1.1   *Sex of patients admitted to Pennsylvania and New York hospitals, by year.*

Hospital noted in 1900 that it had cared for 966,847 people, both inpatient and outpatient, since January 3, 1791. Since its opening in 1751, the Pennsylvania Hospital had admitted 151,595 people. Whoever decided to include these figures in the annual reports was sending a clear message; these two institutions were large, and they had been caring for people for some time.

The annual reports for each hospital include many summary statistics, which agree closely with statistics derived from the sample of records used for this book. By using a computer-generated analysis instead of summaries from the annual reports, one can analyze the data in a wide variety of ways to obtain insight into technology use as well as the demographics of the institution. For now it may be useful to take a look at the characteristics of the patients who were admitted to the two hospitals as well as how those patients changed between 1900 and 1925. Figure 1.1 shows the sex of people who were admitted. Although there were more men than women admitted, the percentage of women being admitted to each hospital increased consistently after 1900; this was a statistically significant change.[53]

One might also wonder about the marital status of people who

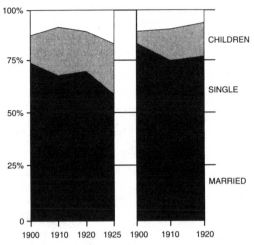

Figure 1.2 *Marital status of patients admitted to Pennsylvania and New York hospitals, by year.*

were being admitted. It has been suggested that one reason for the rise in the importance of hospitals in Boston was an increasing number of single men, perhaps such as Mr. Moran, moving to the city in search of jobs. When they became injured, these people had no one at home to care for them and entered the hospital for care.[54] At least for the New York and Pennsylvania hospitals, for these years that theory does not hold. As figure 1.2 shows, the percentage of married people admitted each year increased, along with a decrease in the percentage of single people. Although small, the change was statistically significant. The increase in the percentage of children (defined as people aged under fifteen years) admitted to each hospital reflects the increasing numbers of tonsillectomies and adenoidectomies being done, as will be discussed in the next chapter, and this change is the primary reason for a fall in the mean age of the patients admitted, from 31.7 to 27.9 at the Pennsylvania Hospital between 1900 and 1925 and from 32.4 to 29.1 at the New York Hospital from 1900 to 1920. The unlabeled section of the graph represents widows, widowers, and people for whom martial status was not indicated on the chart.

PENNSYLVANIA HOSPITAL / NEW YORK HOSPITAL

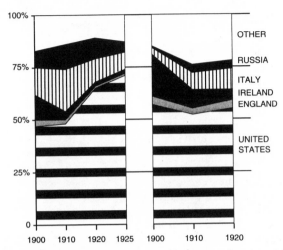

Figure 1.3 *Nationality of patients admitted to Pennsylvania and New York hospitals, by year.*

Figure 1.3 shows the nationality of people admitted to the two hospitals. Not surprisingly, because they were located on the eastern seaboard and, like most hospitals of the period, cared for a population largely unable to pay (much) for medical care, each hospital saw a fairly large proportion of patients who were from a country other than the United States. At the Pennsylvania Hospital the percentage of U.S. citizens increased from 47 percent in 1900 to 71 percent in 1925, an increase driven in part by the number of younger people being admitted, who were more likely to have been born in the United States. At the New York Hospital the percentage of U.S. citizens admitted stayed between 50 and 60 percent. The graph shows the changing patterns of hospital admissions; the block marked "other" includes people from a wide range of nationalities, primarily European, with Germans and Austrians making up an increasing proportion at the New York Hospital.

Table 1.1 displays the reasons that brought patients into these two hospitals, categorized according to a standard classification system used during the period. The overall pattern is not surprising. Infectious diseases were initially the most common reason for admission.

Table 1.1 *Discharge Diagnoses for Patients Admitted to Pennsylvania and New York Hospitals, by Year (as a Percentage of Total Discharges Each Year)*

Diagnosis	1900	1909	1920	1925
PENNSYLVANIA HOSPITAL				
Diseases of the tonsils	2.09	14.93	23.81	25.51
Infectious diseases	26.89	22.89	19.50	12.63
Injuries	12.53	10.20	6.12	8.59
Diseases of the nervous system	5.22	1.49	3.40	1.52
Diseases due to physical agents	4.18	0.75	0.45	1.52
Diseases of the circulatory system	4.18	3.98	2.27	4.04
Diseases of the kidney	3.92	1.99	2.72	1.77
Diseases of the intestines	3.66	9.20	6.35	6.06
Diseases of the bones	3.66	2.74	1.59	2.02
Diseases due to animal parasites	3.39	0.50	0.00	0.25
Diseases of the female generative organs	2.87	3.98	4.31	5.05
Diseases of the trachea and bronchi	2.87	2.24	2.95	0.51
Diseases of the rectum	2.35	1.49	3.17	0.25
Diseases and injuries of the eye and ear	2.35	2.24	2.95	2.53
Diseases of the male generative organs	2.09	3.23	0.91	0.51
Diseases of the stomach	2.09	1.49	0.91	0.00
Diseases of the abdomen	1.83	1.99	2.27	2.02
Diseases of the skin	1.31	1.49	0.23	0.00
Diseases of the lymphatic system	1.31	1.00	0.91	0.76
Tumors, benign and malignant	1.31	2.99	3.85	2.02
Poisonings and intoxications	1.04	1.49	1.36	1.52
Diseases of the liver	1.04	1.49	0.23	1.77
Diseases of the pleura	0.78	1.49	0.68	1.26
Puerperal state	0.78	1.99	1.13	2.02
Other	6.25	2.75	7.94	15.92

	1900	1910	1920	
NEW YORK HOSPITAL				
Diseases of the tonsils	0.52	2.50	19.02	
Infectious diseases	23.83	20.28	15.95	
Injuries	15.03	9.44	3.68	
Diseases of the nervous system	2.07	2.50	1.23	
Diseases due to physical agents	3.11	0.83	0.00	
Diseases of the circulatory system	4.66	4.72	4.91	
Diseases of the kidney	2.07	3.06	0.00	
Diseases of the intestines	8.81	13.06	23.31	
Diseases of the bones	0.52	1.94	1.84	
Diseases due to animal parasites	2.59	0.28	0.00	
Diseases of the female generative organs	8.29	9.72	5.52	
Diseases of the trachea and bronchi	1.55	1.39	0.61	
Diseases of the rectum	1.55	1.94	2.45	

Table 1.1   *Continued*

Diagnosis	1900	1910	1920
Diseases of the male generative organs	1.55	2.22	0.61
Diseases of the stomach	0.52	1.94	1.23
Diseases of the abdomen	2.59	5.83	7.98
Tumors, benign and malignant	4.15	4.17	2.45
Poisonings and intoxications	5.70	1.11	0.00
Diseases of the liver	1.55	1.67	2.45
Diseases of the pleura	0.00	2.50	0.00
Puerperal state	2.07	1.11	0.61
Diseases of the bladder	2.07	0.56	0.00
Diseases of the lung	1.55	0.00	0.00
Diseases of the urethra	1.04	0.83	0.00
Diseases of the breast	0.00	1.11	0.00
Other	2.59	5.29	6.14

Note: The coding in this table is based on a widely used diagnostic classification system from the period: *Classification of Diseases, as Adopted by the Massachusetts General Hospital, Boston City Hospital, Carney Hospital, Peter Bent Brigham Hospital, Massachusetts Homeopathic Hospital, and Others,* 7th ed. (Boston: Griffith-Stillings Press, 1926). The system listed forty-two different categories of disease. In order to make the table easier to use, of those forty-two different categories, only twenty-four are listed in the summary for the Pennsylvania Hospital. The remainder are subsumed under the category "other," which in this table includes disorders coded as diseases of the breast (male and female), blood and blood-forming organs, jaw, tongue, bladder, urethra (male and female), lung, nose and accessory sinuses, ductless glands (now generally termed endocrine diseases), or larynx; anaphylactic or metabolic diseases; congenital malformations; and diagnoses that were either omitted or illegible. All of these categories had at least one diagnosis coded in that group between 1900 and 1925. Some of what may appear to be surprising is a result of the diagnostic schemas used in this period. Asthma, for example, was included quite reasonably as a disease of the trachea and bronchi, rather than as a disease of the lung, where it might now be placed. In the interests of clarity, the diagnostic labels are somewhat abbreviated from the longer labels in the original description. The coding system included quite specific diagnoses, which are recorded in the data set. Investigators wishing to know about a specific diagnosis should consult the full coding system used. (See the appendix for details on the actual data set.)

For the New York Hospital the category "other" includes diseases of the lymphatic system, of the eye and ear, nose and accessory sinuses, jaw, esophagus, ductless glands, and of the blood and blood-forming organs; congenital malformations; metabolic diseases; diseases peculiar to infancy; and diagnoses that were either omitted or illegible. Because categories are only listed if they had at least one diagnosis coded in that group between 1900 and 1920, the summary for the New York Hospital lists different diagnoses than for the Pennsylvania Hospital. In addition, as the hospital records included many people admitted with injuries who did not spend the night in the hospital, this table includes only patients whose length of stay was greater than zero days.

PENNSYLVANIA HOSPITAL / NEW YORK HOSPITAL

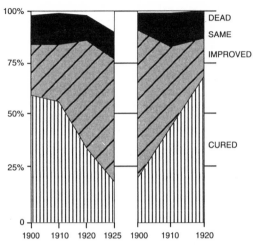

Figure 1.4   *Outcome for patients admitted to Pennsylvania and New York hospitals, by year.*

Injuries also ranked high on the list. Over the period of this study the percentage of patients who were admitted for diseases of the tonsils increased dramatically. The remainder of the patients suffered from a diverse range of conditions.

Some patients did well, some poorly. The condition of almost all patients was noted on discharge, although the meaning of the terminology can be unclear. For example, it is difficult to know the difference between those patients noted to be "cured" and those noted only to be "improved." As figure 1.4 shows, the percentage of people said to be cured fell at the Pennsylvania Hospital (along with a rise in those said to be improved), while the reverse is true at the New York Hospital. It may be that this change reflects primarily a change in the ways that house officers decided to fill out the paperwork. One measure, however, seems clear: death seems fairly straightforward as an undesirable outcome. Initially, people at the Pennsylvania Hospital seemed to die more often: over 10 percent of the admissions died in 1900. Yet by 1920 the two death rates fell to approximately the same level. As is the case today, one cannot make judgments about the quality of care without knowing more about how sick the patients were when they were admitted, an adjustment difficult to make in the 1990s and impossible for these patient records from the early years of the century. A small fraction of patients, who make up the unlabeled section at the top of the graph, did not have their condition recorded.

In this book patients at the New York and Pennsylvania hospitals will serve as windows into a changing world of health care. In chapter 2 I will explore the varying meaning of science in the early-twentieth-century U.S. hospital, paying particular attention to the importation of business methods into the hospital and to the implications of an active surgical service for that institution. Chapter 3 starts a shift to the level of individual patient care and looks at the urinalysis, a procedure ancient in its roots but modern in its implications for this period. Chapter 4 analyzes use of the most dramatic medical technology, the x-ray machine, and shows that, despite the drama attending its invention and the money expended to buy x-ray machines for hospitals, the structure of the hospital had to change before the x-ray machine could become a part of routine care. Chapter 5 looks at the x ray in terms of its implications for privacy, both in and out of the hospital, and considers how the machine might have been used differently for men and women. Chapters 6 and 7 explore use of the blood count, a diagnostic tool that played an important part in the debate on the effectiveness of laboratory tests versus the importance of a clinical examination.

In all of these chapters there is an attempt to capture a broad definition of what constituted medical technology for the period from 1900 to 1925. Also uncovered is the constant difference between theory and practice, between ideology and action, and the importance of local culture in determining how that tension was (and will be) played out. Attention is paid not only to national, published utterances in medical journals, but also to the ways that decisions were made in particular circumstances and involving specific people. Whenever possible, a patient's experience is taken into account, for all of medical technology ultimately has its impact on a specific person at a specific time and place. Before turning to the details of technology use for specific patients in these U.S. hospitals, it is helpful to consider the changing nature of the institution and how those changes reflected some broader-based social themes about science.

2

~~~~~

SCIENCE, SCIENTIFIC SYSTEMS, AND SURGERY

Technology and the U.S. Hospital

Toward the end of the nineteenth century Americans in all walks of life were becoming increasingly familiar with the idea of "science." The meaning of the word *science* has, of course, changed with time. But early in the twentieth century science seemed to be more than merely a body of knowledge, it was a "method and a spirit," one that was believed to be compatible with and beneficial for just about any aspect of society.[1] During that time science was perhaps most tightly bound up with a constellation of related ideas having to do with efficiency, which some called an "efficiency craze." As at least two generations of historians have described it, this was not a single, cohesive movement toward a clearly defined goal.[2] Those who advocated "efficiency" promoted a wide range of proposals, often contradictory. Nonetheless, the idea of efficiency became a national infatuation, thought to be applicable to any sphere of life.[3] One of the most important results was a joining together of people who worked in science with people who worked in business.

The most precise approach to efficiency was scientific management, the brainchild of the engineer Frederick W. Taylor. In 1895, the same year that the German physicist Wilhelm Röntgen first described x-ray images, Taylor published his first paper on scientific management. Taylor thought that one could apply the same principles of efficiency to human hands and muscles which others had applied to the gears and ratchets of machines. Using a stopwatch to analyze the movements of workers at the Midvale Steel Company, in Philadelphia, he claimed that he could determine the one best way for each of the workers to do his specific task. Thus, Taylor devised a system for supervisors to instruct workers in how to be more efficient.

In some ways the application of the idea of efficiency came in the form that Taylor had first envisioned, by detailing the movements of individual workers. But scientific management soon came to involve far more than merely an improved method of doing handiwork. It implied a complete "mental revolution" in the means of doing business. And that revolution—or so its proponents claimed—would result in a better world for all, a world without scarcity and constraint.[4] Proponents of the efficiency movement asserted that their ideas were not only rational but also universal, that the tenets of scientific efficiency not only could, but should, serve as a blueprint for reforming all types of social institutions engaged in all types of activities.[5]

Perhaps the most profound application of the efficiency movement came in the organizational restructuring of U.S. business. Starting with the railroad industry, U.S. entrepreneurs came to believe that the road to growth, success, and increased profits was paved by the precise application of scientific ideas to their business management. The links between railroads and medicine started early. Even before the efficiency movement railroads had been important for U.S. health care. They employed many people and produced far more than their share of traumatic injuries. These injuries required medical attention, often in hospitals. Some railroads set up their own hospitals, such as the Illinois Central Hospital in Chicago. Yet it was the railroad industry's experience in running the rails, far more than running its own hospitals, which was to have a major impact on U.S. health care. The efficiency movement's success for the railroad industry provided still more evidence for its broad value in all walks of life.

Health care was an obvious candidate for reform by the methods of scientific efficiency. Advances in scientific medicine and the reform of medical education attracted public attention. The changing structure of early twentieth-century health care delivery in the United States made it a field particularly susceptible to analysis and improvement, particularly as regards hospital care. Hospitals were expanding rapidly both in numbers and in size. They were increasingly seen as the proper setting in which middle- and upper-class people would receive medical care. Voluntary hospitals were supported financially by business owners, who insisted on the same efficiencies in the institutions that they supported as they did in the businesses that they ran. Within the hospital walls surgeons did more and more operations. The craft of surgery could be subjected to the same type of time-motion analysis as any other form of manual labor, while the increasing volume of surgical patients who passed through the operating rooms demanded new techniques for dealing with a new tempo and intensity to hospital care. In this chapter I shall consider how the ideas of science and efficiency became part of a changing world of medical practice and explore the ways in which new technology played a pivotal role.

SCIENCE, MANAGEMENT, AND PATIENT CARE

A central part of the new, scientific style of business management had to do with managing information.[6] As businesses became larger and developed a formal management system, they needed rationalized ways of moving information around the system. As hospitals also became larger and as they, too, developed a more formalized management system, they also were forced to deal with increasing amounts of information. Although some of that new information had to do with clinical medicine, a subject to which I shall return shortly, much of it had to do with money.

Money was increasingly important to hospitals for several reasons. Paying, middle-class patients entered the hospital more and more beginning around the turn of the twentieth century. Their arrival helped transform the fundamental nature of the institution from one in which money played little role to one in which money was a central part of its workings.[7] As more paying patients entered the hospital, physicians started to insist on being paid for their services, another reason that money management came to the fore. As the historian Morris Vogel has suggested, the "hospitalization of the middle classes changed the nature of the traditional institution as fundamentally as scientific medicine."[8]

In addition, as hospitals became larger, their scale made managing finances more difficult. A single person might be able easily to do the paperwork required to pay the bills for a fifty-bed hospital but not for one with five hundred beds. If the hospital wanted to buy new, expensive machines, the hospital needed funds to pay for those machines. And, perhaps most important, there was a widespread belief that careful, systematic, *scientific* attention to finances would enable the hospital to operate in a more efficient manner, to use its limited funds better in serving the needs of whatever community relied on it for health care.

The deployment of funds within the hospital depended on new technologies to manage that money, new technologies first used in factories but soon applied to hospitals. The new technology in this instance was more than merely a new machine. Rather, it was a new method of conceptualizing the relationship between the hospital's funds and activities, costs and charges. To manage money well within the hospital required a new means of accounting.

Accounting Technology

Scholars have recently demonstrated that the history of accounting, as the history of science, should not be taken as the ever more precise elucidation of basic principles. Accounting does not merely enable the performance of some established task; it actively shapes an organization, providing a tool by which certain groups of people may exercise their power and control in specific ways.[9] Any decisions by hospital managers to import from business new methods for keeping track of money had profound implications for the early twentieth-century hospital and also reflected their desire to reshape the nature of hospital management.

The most advanced accounting technique generally available in the 1880s was Italian double-entry bookkeeping, a technique that had changed little over five hundred years. Using that technique, most nineteenth-century business owners knew at the end of the day (or the month or the year) whether they had made or lost money, but they could not know which of their products had made or lost money.[10]

Railroads were the first major businesses to relate their financial status to each part of the overall enterprise. They did so in order to answer some very practical questions. After a manager decided to start a new railroad line or planned an extension of an old line, he or she wanted to know if that addition was profitable or not. The older methods of accounting would allow the manager easily to know if the business as a whole was making a greater profit, or taking a greater loss, but would not permit him or her to determine whether the change had resulted from the new line. To know which parts of a business were making a profit and which were taking a loss, the manager needed to be able to separate out the amounts spent and received by each unit. As a result, people who ran businesses were extremely interested in the development of cost accounting, a technique by which accountants could not only assign indirect as well as direct costs to each product but also could identify which parts of a business were making money and which were not. Managers who wished to apply the latest scientific tools began to demand cost accounting, and colleges and universities responded: in 1900, 12 institutions of higher learning taught accounting; by 1910, that number had risen to 52 and, by 1916, 116.[11] Cost accounting was rapidly adopted not only by railroads but also by all manner of organizations, including hospitals.

Hospital managers began to use cost accounting in an explicit attempt to emulate businesses, including not only railroads but also factories, the arena in which many Americans at the turn of the twentieth century saw science as having its most visible successes. In this period, to call the hospital "factory-like" was not to invoke the pejorative tone that one might use in making the same association late in the twentieth century. The hospital administrator was exhorted to apply "sound business principles" because "no superintendent who wants to keep up with the times will overlook the factory, store, or office which must apply modern methods to survive."[12] Numerous talks and presentations to hospital administrators admonished that the hospital should be established "on business principles." Those methods involved, basically, the need to "maintain an institution at the point of highest efficiency and lowest commensurate cost."[13] In order to do so, modern methods of accounting were thought to be a necessity.

The push toward cost accounting in hospitals came from without as well as within. Economic factors made issues of money management particularly acute. As the historian David Rosner points out, the financial crisis of the 1890s had made hospital deficits a major issue. Moreover, early in the twentieth century hospital boards developed a different character. They were increasingly made up of a new group of business owners, many of whom were leaders in the move toward industrialization. These people had succeeded by using the newer techniques of cost accounting. They shared less paternalistic emotion than their nineteenth-century predecessors, who had come largely from the older merchant families, and felt more of a sense of financial responsibility for the institution they were charged with overseeing.[14] The financial donors who sustained early twentieth-century voluntary hospitals were hard-nosed pragmatists who wanted to see the same efficiency within the charities they supported as that they insisted on in the businesses they ran. To document that efficiency these donors insisted on demonstrably accurate accounting methods: "Hospitals must not only know themselves what each item of service costs, but they must show the public that they know."[15] For hospitals supported by the state, such as the University of Michigan, the legislature at times provided the impetus to adopt modern methods of accounting, wishing to be assured that funds designated for patient care were not being spent on other tasks.[16]

One way to improve finances was to bring in more money, to attract private, paying patients. Toward that aim, hospitals often supplied such people with elaborately decorated rooms or a higher quality of food or nursing. These amenities cost money. Part of the rationale for keeping accurate financial records came from the desire to be able to compare the costs of the new group of private patients with the traditional group of charity patients, in order to see how much additional expense was going toward the increased costs of private patients. This was precisely the task that new methods of cost accounting were able to address. Often, the cost of caring for private patients was almost equal to the revenue they produced. But there were advantages to admitting private patients over and above the money spent on their rooms. If pleased with their care, private patients might decide to donate money to the hospital or perhaps endow a bed. Moreover, some thought that private patients were beneficial to the educational function of the institution and that, because of them, trainees would receive broader clinical training by being able to come into contact with different classes of patients.[17]

At times financial records were not up to the challenge of accurately establishing where funds were being spent. The lack of
uniform standards was a particular problem when one wished to
compare financial records among various hospitals.[18] In 1906 the
four major New York City hospitals, along with several others,
formed a unified system of accounts in an attempt to establish a
sound basis for accounting and in response to a perceived "agitation"
about the inability to compare accurately income and expenditures
among different institutions.[19] Philadelphia hospitals, on the other
hand, lacking a systematic system of medical or financial statistics,
were unable to compare either costs or the outcomes of care.[20]

In order to do cost accounting, either for industrial factories or for
hospitals, an institution had to be organized in a manner that would
permit such an analysis. Without a specific product, a specific railroad line, or, in the case of the hospital, a specific unit or department, such as social service or the X-ray Department, it was not
easy to identify what should be the object of analysis. As the early-
twentieth-century hospital became more organized, administrators
created various divisions for management and finances.

Financial reports became more detailed than before. Compare, for
example, the University of Michigan Hospital budgets for 1897–98
and 1919–20 in figure 2.1. Note how little the 1897–98 budget tells
us about the distribution of expenditures among the various departments. We are given no information about how much each unit
spent on payrolls or instruments. Such lack of detail was typical for
the budgets of other hospitals, even those with otherwise excellent
reputations.[21] The increased level of detail in the 1919–20 budget is
striking. Not only were more expenses kept track of, but those
expenses were specifically assigned to six divisions. Thus, one can
easily tell, for example, that, aside from general administration,
social service spent the most on traveling expenses, as would be
expected for a unit charged with visiting patients in their homes. Or
a reader of this report might conclude that the cost of equipment
repairs in housekeeping was surprisingly high.[22]

Previously, a hospital's superintendent had been the one to keep
track of financial records and to sign all checks for hospital expenses.
Figure 2.2, taken from the 1898 annual report of the University of
Michigan Hospital, shows the superintendent's office. Note the safe

EXPENSES FOR 1897-98.

Bread	$ 470.56	
Butter	597.08	
Canned Goods	177.03	
Eggs	328.13	
Fish	191.70	
Fruit	347.46	
Groceries	1015.33	
Milk	1173.07	
Meat	2020.45	
Poultry	190.51	
Vegetables	398.00—$	6,909 32
Dry-goods	215.35	
Furniture	773.14	
Freight, express, etc	77.63	
Hardware, shop work, etc	231.29	
Instruments	17.35	
Lumber	38.31	
Miscellaneous	277.25	
Medicines, dressings, and apparatus	2032.05	
Nurses' room rent	985.56	
Printing and stationery	177.75	
Pay-rolls	9323.59	
Telephone and telegraph	91.53—	14,240.80
Total		$21,150.12
Receipts from patients		$20,880.89
Other receipts		861.65
Total		$21,742.54

Figure 2.1   *Expenses, University of Michigan Hospital, 1897—98 and 1919—20. From* Annual Report of the University of Michigan Hospital for the Year Ending June 30, 1898 *(Ann Arbor), 8; and* Annual Report of the University of Michigan Hospital for the Year Ending June 30, 1920 *(Ann Arbor), 24—25.*

with a letterpress on top; the superintendent was himself keeping the forms and doing the paperwork to pay the bills.[23] This picture exemplifies the centralized functions of a late-nineteenth-century hospital superintendent, but a single superintendent could do only so much in the way of financial management. Part of the efficiency ideal involved the movement of direct responsibility for financial management from a single superintendent to a new group of administrators, many of whom would be well-trained accountants. New people were hired to keep track of the hospital's books, working daily to account for the flow of money.

Exhibit B

Disbursements from Hospital Funds, July 1, 1919, to June 30, 1920

	General Administration	Professional Care of Patients	Nursing	Housekeeping	Kitchen	Social Service	General House and Property Expense	Totals
Postage, telephone and telegraph	$ 912.36	$ 9.30	$	$ 7.96	$ .11	$ 5.21	$	$ 934.04
Stationery and office supplies	2,692.63	107.45	11.68	1.67	. . . .	38.47	. . . .	2,851.90
Publications and printing	13.18	1.17	1.60	12.60	.50	. . . .	. . . .	29.05
Traveling expenses . . .	193.45	. . . .	. . . .	. . . .	. . . .	75.00	. . . .	268.45
Freight, express, drayage	825.34	1.28	. . . .	13.58	28.61	. . . .	. . . . . .	868.81
Equipment repairs . . .	35.37	273.67	. . . .	53.95	28.85	7.75	. . . .	399.59
Supplies for instruction.	. . . .	. . . .	6.82	. . . .	. . . .	. . . .	. . . .	6.82
Material and General Supplies:								
Medical and surgical supplies	106.97	29,042.99	27.60	176.19	. . . .	. . . .	. . . .	29,353.75
Pharmacy supplies . .	. . . .	6,195.67	. . . .	. . . .	. . . .	. . . .	. . . .	6,195.67
Optical goods	. . . .	5,002.49	. . . .	. . . .	. . . .	. . . .	. . . .	5,002.49
Ice	. . . .	. . . .	. . . .	. . . .	. . . .	. . . .	5,896.33	5,896.33
Laundry	1,495.80	. . . .	. . . .	37,137.42	. . . .	. . . .	. . . .	38,633.22
Cleaning supplies . . .	. . . .	. . . .	. . . .	2,570.88	1.35	. . . .	. . . .	2,572.23
Linen, blankets and bedding	. . . .	. . . .	. . . .	15,266.80	. . . .	. . . .	. . . . . .	15,266.80
Not otherwise specified	2,783.94	661.55	1,125.74	6,347.78	1,234.43	6.92	. . . .	12,160.36
X-Rays	. . . .	5,473.00	. . . .	. . . .	. . . .	. . . .	. . . .	5,473.00
Food Supplies:								
Milk and cream	. . . .	. . . .	. . . .	. . . .	24,548.17	. . . .	. . . .	24,548.17
Groceries, baked goods	. . . .	. . . .	. . . .	. . . .	35,389.18	. . . .	. . . .	35,389.18
Butter and eggs	. . . .	. . . .	. . . .	. . . .	24,155.54	. . . .	. . . .	24,155.54
Fresh fruits, vegetables	. . . .	. . . .	. . . .	. . . .	18,158.67	. . . .	. . . .	18,158.67
Meat, poultry and fish.	. . . .	. . . .	. . . .	. . . .	33,758.24	. . . .	. . . .	33,758.24
Board of patients outside	. . . .	6,735.85	. . . .	. . . .	16.85	. . . .	. . . . . .	6,752.70
Heat, light and power. .	. . . .	. . . .	. . . . . .	. . . .	. . . .	. . . .	. . . .	. . . .
Water	. . . .	. . . .	. . . .	. . . .	. . . .	. . . .	. . . .	. . . .
Fuel	. . . .	. . . .	. . . .	. . . .	. . . .	. . . .	. . . .	. . . .
Rent:								
Nurses' homes	. . . .	. . . .	. . . .	. . . .	. . . .	. . . .	3,639.08	3,639.08
Rooms for employees.	. . . .	. . . .	. . . .	1,570.87	6.25	. . . .	. . . .	1,604.12
Rooms for patients . .	. . . .	3,305.00	. . . .	. . . .	. . . .	. . . .	. . . .	3,305.00
Repairs to buildings . .	. . . .	. . . .	. . . .	. . . .	. . . .	. . . .	. . . .	. . . .
Refunds	2,931.02	. . . .	. . . .	. . . .	. . . .	. . . .	. . . .	2,931.02
Pay Roll:								
Salaries of officers, superintendents, etc. . .	12,672.86	6,874.25	41,612.05	5,238.28	5,162.71	1,277.50	. . . .	73,137.65
Clerks, stenographers.	7,597.59	225.00	755.00	715.00	. . . .	3,301.13	. . . .	12,593.72
Labor and unclassified service	76.45	20.90	30.50	18,907.50	4,179.66	. . . .	758.45	23,973.46
Apparatus	56.91	4.07	3.37	. . . .	. . . .	. . . .	. . . .	64.35
Furniture and office equipment	472.05	630.77	79.49	4,714.50	251.21	171.62	1.00	6,320.64
Books	. . . .	. . . .	57.09	. . . .	. . . .	. . . .	. . . .	57.09
Machinery and tools . .	. . . .	. . . .	1.08	.95	1.96	. . . .	. . . .	3.99
Insurance	27.50	. . . .	. . . .	. . . .	. . . .	. . . .	. . . .	27.50
Hospital service	. . . .	363.28	. . . .	. . . .	. . . .	. . . .	. . . .	363.28
Totals	$32,893.42	$64,927.69	$43,712.02	$92,762.93	$147,222.29	$4,883.60	$10,294.86	$396,696.81

Figure 2.1 *Continued*

There was some resistance to the idea of hospitals becoming *too* much like a business or having hospital employees spend too much time and energy on the development of intricate systems of accounting. Some observers cautioned that the financial reports required by hospital superintendents simply did not need to be as detailed as those for other businesses and that the effort spent in tracking dol-

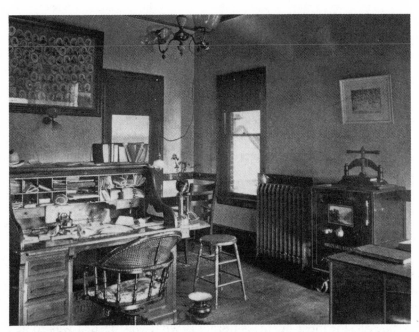

Figure 2.2 *Superintendent's office, University of Michigan Hospital,*
1898. From Annual Report of the University of Michigan for the Year
Ending June 30, 1899 *(Ann Arbor), facing p. 34.*

lars too carefully through the system would interfere with the ability of hospitals to serve the sick. Also, the inherent charitable mission of hospitals, it was pointed out, distinguished them from many
other organizations. Unlike most businesses, they needed to continue to operate even in the face of continuous deficits.[24] Nonetheless, there was nearly universal agreement that some level of cost
accounting was necessary, often coupled with the assertion that any
attempt to save money by *not* employing adequate bookkeepers
would in the end cost much more.[25]

New methods of financial accounting were associated with a new
set of relationships revolving around physicians and machines.
Physicians began to be reimbursed for services performed within the
hospital, often using hospital equipment. In chapter 4 I shall consider in more detail the impact of one of those decisions, the 1912
decision to return a percentage of fees from use of the x-ray machine
at the Pennsylvania Hospital to the radiologist. But before being

able to implement these types of decisions administratively, the hospital staff needed to be able to track accurately what funds were spent and received. For this they required not only new ideas about cost accounting but also new machines with which to do the calculations.

Calculating Technology

Hospital administrators were aided by dramatic improvements in adding machines in the 1880s. Mechanical devices had existed to do simple mathematical calculations since the seventeenth century, and by the 1870s there existed a thriving market in calculating devices.[26] But manufacturers of the time were aware that to be fast enough to be practical a machine had to use numbers that were entered by depressing individual keys. The only key-driven mechanical devices in existence prior to the mid-1880s were single-digit adding machines. These were adequate to do multiple calculations on a few numbers, as was needed for many scientific calculations. However, for most business purposes what was needed was to add long lists of numbers, and for this purpose the machines were so slow and unreliable that they could not compete with a good accountant doing the calculations by hand.

In 1885 the U.S. machinist Dorr E. Felt completed the first model of a new, key-driven machine capable of meeting business requirements, which he called a "comptometer." By the end of the decade business owners and hospital superintendents could purchase new adding machines, which would record the results as well as do complex calculations, including subtotals and totals. These tools were first used in banks starting in the late 1880s and the early 1890s. Adding machine manufacturers explicitly linked the mechanical advantages of their calculators with the efficient principles of cost accounting.[27]

Other devices were useful for analyzing information within businesses and hospitals. One important new technology for keeping track of information within the hospital was the punch card. Early versions were called the Hollerith card (see fig. 2.3), named for and patented by, in 1889, the engineer Herman Hollerith.[28] The card was a flat piece of stiff paper through which one could punch holes to indicate information. It resembles the punch card used by the

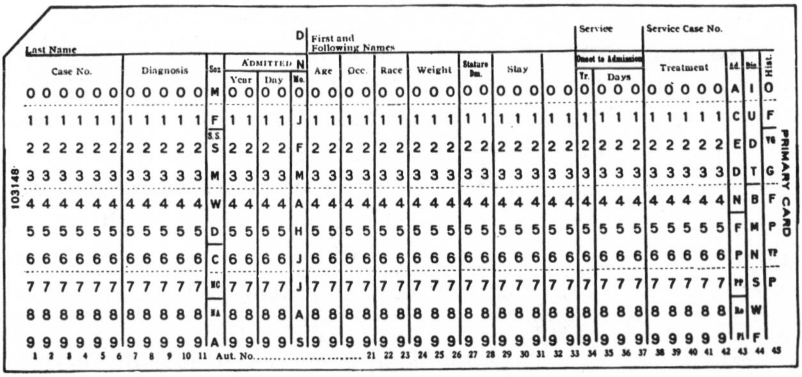

Figure 2.3 *Hollerith card. From Raymond Pearl, "Modern Methods in Handling Hospital Statistics," John Hopkins Hospital Bulletin 32 (1921): 184–94.*

International Business Machines Corporation (IBM) some decades later; indeed, Hollerith went on to become a founder of IBM. Information was recorded by punching holes in predetermined positions in the card. When the card was passed through a tabulating machine, an electrical contact could be made where a hole had been punched. Using the machine, workers could quickly summarize information stored on the cards.

Some of the earliest organizations to use the cards were health departments. Cards were useful for tabulating 1887 mortality rates in Baltimore and assembling vital statistics for the New York City Board of Health.[29] The Surgeon General's Office, in Washington, D.C., started using cards to keep track of diseased soldiers. The most dramatic early use of the punch card came with the 1890 census, which the Hollerith Electrical Tabulating Machine assisted to great effect. The average clerk was able to process almost eight thousand cards per day; some were able to do almost twenty thousand. By the 1900 census an automatic card feeder allowed up to eighty-four thousand cards to be processed by a machine in a single day. This was far faster than anyone could process information without the aid of mechanical devices. Cards and tabulating machines were quickly taken up by governments and organizations in a wide range of areas.

Hospital departments of statistics purchased similar card systems and tabulating machines. On each card they could record the patient's case history number, "ailment," sex, social status (single, married, widowed, or divorced), race, age, and many other items of information. Using the new technology, one could then, easily, select out all patients with a specific disease, of a specified age and social status. Tabulating machines could run at rates up to 250 cards per minute and in a few minutes could sort through a quantity of patient records that would previously have taken days, or weeks, by hand. These devices were used to advance the idea that medicine should be able to use analysis of case records to emulate the more advanced, more quantitative, more *accurate* sciences such as physics and chemistry.[30]

Cards were used to track financial as well as clinical information. Using a card sorter, hospital accountants could track expenditures by each of the hospital's units—such as the clinical departments, for example, or the nursing stations. Thus, a cost accounting system could be implemented using the punch card system.[31]

EFFICIENT RECORDS

Hospital workers thought that they could improve hospital care by creating efficient, scientific hospital records. These new hospital records, like the new methods of accounting and information analysis, were also explicitly modeled on business techniques. Some of the changes in record keeping reflected organizational developments that have already been mentioned, such as the invention of new departments. Some of the changes in record keeping reflected new ways of organizing information, such as forms, charts, and graphs. Although we now see such devices as natural, almost inevitable parts of the office landscape, their invention in the early years of the century was an active process, seen as an essential step in achieving a more scientific, efficient means of behavior. The new forms and charts did not grow out of contemporary theories of business communication, which lagged far behind practice. Instead, they were a practical response to scientific management, a managerial tool for controlling a growing business.[32] But their application to the care of human beings, particularly in hospitals, had clinical and medical implications that transcended the scientific and business intentions of their inventors.[33]

How were these records different? First, scientific hospital records of the early twentieth century became longer than those of the nine-

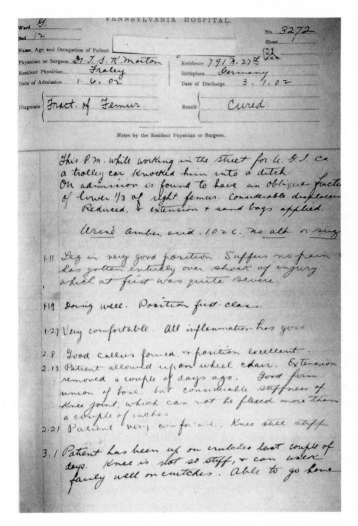

Figure 2.4 *Patient record, 1902. From* Pennsylvania Hospital Case Records *96 (1902): 3272.*

teenth century. They contained more forms and more information, created by more people. The single page shown in figure 2.4 is the complete record for a person admitted to Pennsylvania Hospital in 1902 with a broken leg, like Mr. Moran was in 1900. Although this person stayed in the hospital for almost three months, the entire record is only one page long. Such brevity was typical in 1900, when

PENNSYLVANIA HOSPITAL / NEW YORK HOSPITAL

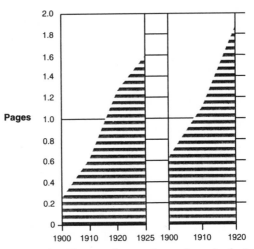

Figure 2.5 *Mean length of hospital record, per day of admission, Pennsylvania and New York hospitals, by year.*

the median length of a patient record at the Pennsylvania Hospital was only two pages. By 1925 the median length was six pages, a threefold increase. At the New York Hospital the median length of the patient record rose from five pages in 1900 to eleven pages in 1920. The raw length of the record is, however, only an approximation of the intensity of care. While the length of the record was increasing, the amount of time each person was spending in the hospital was decreasing. At the Pennsylvania Hospital, for example, the median length of stay fell, from fourteen days to six days.[34] Thus, a more meaningful indication of what was happening to the record may be provided by the length of the patient record produced *per day of admission*. This value increased more than fivefold over twenty-five years at the Pennsylvania Hospital and by over threefold at the New York Hospital, as shown in figure 2.5.[35] Also noteworthy is the fact that the increase continued over the twenty-five year span at the Pennsylvania Hospital: there was no sudden jump at a single point in time.

Patient records became longer in part because more and more people were becoming involved in patient care and leaving a written record of their presence. Medical education started to include clinical instruction, and medical students were found with increasing frequency on hospital wards. Many of them commented in the clinical chart. Some people reflected an increasingly specialized medical world. Consultants came by, saw the patient, and left notes—the eye specialist with the ophthalmoscope, the urologist with the cystoscope, the internist with the microscope. Some clinical tasks were handed over to allied health personnel. A newly professionalizing nursing corps was making more decisions about patient care, documenting those decisions on charts. They took temperatures more regularly. Some nurses even began measuring blood pressure and keeping track of the fluid intake and output of patients with metabolic diseases.

The increased length of patient records also reflected the creation of new administrative units.[36] Note that in figure 2.4 there is no hint of separate units within the hospital; few existed. As those units were created, each one—such as the Roentgenology Department or the Social Work Department—created its own, standardized forms. Each form in the chart served to reify yet another unit in an ever more balkanized hospital. Each form also served to isolate some aspect of the person lying in the hospital bed. The narrative of a single patient, the smooth flow of a story about a human being's travails, was starting to become fragmented, discontinuous.

Standardized forms did not arise spontaneously. Rather, their creation was taken quite seriously; their very existence reflected a larger set of ideas about record keeping. Again, many of the new ideas were exported from the business world to the medical world. Business people paid a great deal of attention to precisely how to design forms: what color they should be, what size, what shape. Those decisions, it was asserted, ought to be made with the same care as an engineer would use in designing a machine.[37] Properly designed forms made the day-to-day clerical work easier. They provided information that was easy to find, information that could then be used to make decisions. In some instances forms were themselves the means for carrying out decisions and policies; they facilitated administration and enabled those who defined the forms to exercise what the historian Jo Anne Yates has termed "Control through Communication."[38]

These same characteristics translated easily into the medical care arena. A properly designed system of forms made the delivery of patient care more efficient—a concept not taken lightly.[39] Medical reformers claimed that standardized records could speed the transmission of increasing amounts of information about each patient. Well-designed forms could also help hospitals manage the growing numbers of patients being admitted. For many of these patients, as we shall see, that care included surgery.[40] Forms enabled readers to locate information quickly, either for the care of the particular patient or for combining into summaries. Standardized forms also simplified the reporting of clinical information and facilitated comparisons between patients, a sine qua non of clinical research; they both defined and constrained the information that was to be provided by a given interaction between a patient and a hospital.

Starting around 1917, radiologists at the Pennsylvania Hospital used a standardized form, shown in figure 2.6, to report the results of gastrointestinal x-ray examinations. This procedure involved having the patient swallow a substance, often based on barium, through which the x rays could not pass. The radiologist observed the passage of a barium meal through the digestive system; the walls of the gastrointestinal tract would be outlined, and abnormalities, such as gastric ulcers or carcinoma, could be identified. Similar forms were introduced at many other hospitals, including the Mayo Clinic and the Massachusetts General Hospital.[41]

By deciding to issue reports using a form such as this one, an X-ray Department changed both the process of reading an x-ray image and the content of the report that was generated. First, the person reading the x ray did not need to consider what portion of the exam needed to be described or even the appropriate adjective to use in describing each part of the gastrointestinal tract through which the barium mixture passed; he or she needed only to check off the appropriate term. This made the process of generating a formal report much faster. The form also insured that the same set of terms would be consistently applied to each part of the gastrointestinal tract, no matter who was writing the report. This made it easier for the person reading reports that described the new x-ray images to learn how to understand them. Because the use of forms to report results of diagnostic tests standardized the information passed on to those who were caring for the patient, it made the transfer of information easier even for the experienced clinician. A physician reviewing a report would always read the same type of narrative description of the

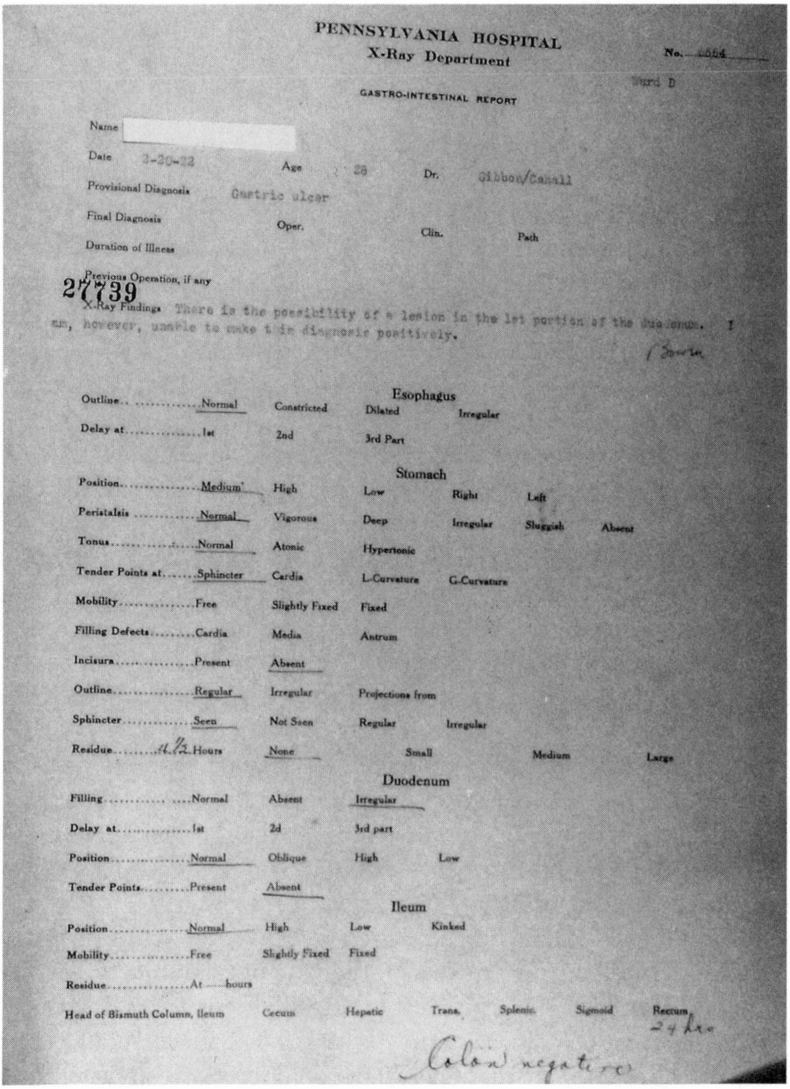

PENNSYLVANIA HOSPITAL
X-Ray Department
No. 6664
Ward D

GASTRO-INTESTINAL REPORT

Name

Date 3-20-22 Age 28 Dr. Gibbon/Cahall

Provisional Diagnosis Gastric ulcer

Final Diagnosis Oper. Clin. Path

Duration of Illness

Previous Operation, if any

27739

X-Ray Findings There is the possibility of a lesion in the 1st portion of the duodenum. I am, however, unable to make this diagnosis positively.

Esophagus

Outline.............Normal Constricted Dilated Irregular

Delay at.............1st 2nd 3rd Part

Stomach

Position.............Medium High Low Right Left

Peristalsis.............Normal Vigorous Deep Irregular Sluggish Absent

Tonus.............Normal Atonic Hypertonic

Tender Points at.......Sphincter Cardia L-Curvature G-Curvature

Mobility.............Free Slightly Fixed Fixed

Filling Defects.........Cardia Media Antrum

Incisura.............Present Absent

Outline.............Regular Irregular Projections from

Sphincter.............Seen Not Seen Regular Irregular

Residue........4 1/2 Hours None Small Medium Large

Duodenum

Filling.............Normal Absent Irregular

Delay at.............1st 2d 3rd part

Position.............Normal Oblique High Low

Tender Points.........Present Absent

Ileum

Position.............Normal High Low Kinked

Mobility.............Free Slightly Fixed Fixed

Residue.............At ..... hours

Head of Bismuth Column, Ileum Cecum Hepatic Trans. Splenic Sigmoid Rectum 24 hrs

Colon negative

Figure 2.6 *Standardized gastrointestinal x-ray form. From* Pennsylvania Hospital Case Records *746 (1922): 6664.*

roentgenological findings. Moreover, the precise organization of the form, the use of space, even the crisp typography, gave the form a very clean appearance, one that probably evoked the clear, manufactured, metallic lines of engineering science more than the fecal reality of what it was like to be a part of many gastrointestinal examinations.[42]

Standardized forms could encourage physicians (and others) to record essential information that might otherwise be overlooked. Such forms entered the hospital record in many areas other than x-ray reports. (Standardization of forms used to report urine analysis will be discussed in chap. 3 and the ways in which the use of the x ray was associated with the use of standardized depictions of the human body in chap. 4.) Most forms were designed to include spaces in which physicians could record comments in their own words, perhaps responding to critics who contended that standardized recording of information would constrain the ability of physicians to record accurately information about their patients which might not fit into the rigid format of the standardized form.[43]

Forms in the hospital were taken very seriously. They were designed to speed the flow of information about patient care as well as to shape the precise information that was to be recorded and transmitted. Rarely seen in the charts of 1900, forms had, by 1925, come to dominate the hospital record, as they continue to do as we approach the end of the century. Expressed in the quantitative terms of the period, one might note that people who worked in the early-twentieth-century hospital between 1900 and 1925 saw a 438-fold increase in the use of forms.[44]

As they paid increasing attention to accurate communication, hospital administrators borrowed other themes and machines from business. Figure 2.7 is particularly telling. The image is one from a group of pictures of an x-ray unit in the 1927 Pennsylvania Hospital annual report, a report that was distributed largely in an attempt to raise funds for the voluntary hospital. Because the picture is, in a sense, propaganda—as are all the pictures in every annual report—we can read it not as an impartial image of some arbitrary room but, instead, as a reflection of the values held by the people who took the picture or who selected the picture for publication. These people determined that a prominent part of the image, front and center, was to be the typewriter. Why?

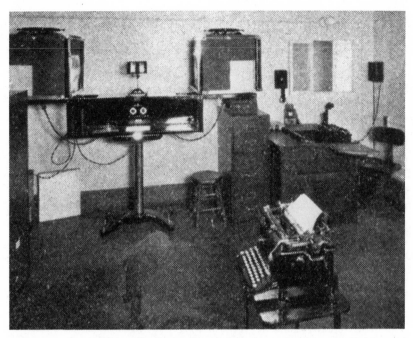

Figure 2.7   *Typewriter shown in illustration for annual report. From* Report of the Board of Managers of the Pennsylvania Hospital to the Contributors at Their Annual Meeting, Held May 4th, 1925 *(Philadelphia), facing p. 39.*

Although machines to aid in writing had been attempted since the 1700s, the typewriter was first patented in something like its modern form in 1868. In 1874 the first machines from the Remington factory started to reach the market. They could only type capital letters and cost from twenty-five to fifty dollars. In 1878 Remington started to sell a machine that could type lower-case letters as well. Typewriters were sold first to court reporters, lawyers, editors, and members of the clergy. By 1880 businesses started to use them. Very rapidly the typewriter became popular, and other manufacturers entered the market. From 1874 to 1878, 4,000 typewriters were sold; between 1881 and 1884, 18,000 were sold. By 1890 there were thirty factories in the United States making typewriters, and, by 1900, 144,873 had been sold.[45] Typewriters were easy to move about and inexpensive enough to be used by almost any institution.

The typewriter accomplished a number of goals. First, it vastly increased the speed at which a document could be created. Whereas with a pen a person could write 24 words per minute a person using a typewriter could write 75. With the development of touch typing in the 1880s, speeds increased to 120 words per minute, with an average of around 80—three times faster than handwriting.

The typewriter also signified a separation between the creation of the information in a document and the physical production of the document itself. The physician need no longer spend his or her time actually writing; someone else could do that. The image from the Pennsylvania Hospital annual report visually emphasizes that a person who operated the typewriter was assigned to work in the X-ray Department. This fact provided yet another marker of the importance of that unit for the hospital at the same time that it demonstrated the unit's ability to produce documents in the best possible way—with a typewriter.[46] Best in this instance clearly meant the most modern. Using a typewriter would, if you believed the advertising, "stamp your hospital records *modern* before all eyes that see them."[47]

Thus, we must look at the typewriter in this picture as a marker of something quite specific, as a new device that enabled the X-ray Department to accomplish goals it could not otherwise reach. The typewriter is in the picture for a reason. It did not need to be front and center; someone could have easily moved it out of the way before the picture was taken.[48] The fact that it was placed in such a prominent position should tell us that not only the x-ray images but also the x-ray reports—typed, standardized, efficient, scientific reports—were part of what was new and modern about the unit.

One reason for having an efficient reporting system was so hospitals could better follow up on the care they provided. Failure to convey information efficiently and promptly could result in the failure to use valuable information obtained by a new machine. For example, on October 21, 1925, a five-year-old girl was admitted to the University of Michigan Hospital with a provisional diagnosis of diabetes mellitus. Staff closely monitored her urine and blood sugar. On the fourth hospital day the patient's mother told the physician that she had once been told that her daughter might have tuberculosis. Examiners detected no clinical signs, but a chest x ray was ordered nonetheless. Two days later the patient was discharged because there was no evidence of diabetes. Meanwhile, the x-ray image was developed and evaluated. One week after the patient's discharge the chest x ray was reported as "suspicious for tuberculosis," and a letter was sent out that day. The patient did not, however, return for care. Thus, in this instance not being able to convey information rapidly was a problem. Partly as a result of this incident, hospital staff soon implemented procedures that resulted in a more rapid reporting of x-ray results.[49]

Patient records became longer between 1900 and 1925 in part because physicians wanted to include more information in the chart. Much of that information was selected specifically to be objective, and thus scientific. Sometimes that meant putting the information on a form in which words conveyed most of the message. But often that information was recorded in graphic form, a method of information transfer which was "fast becoming the international language of science."[50]

Like the public at large, the medical profession saw graphs as an important symbol of science, partly as a result of a new emphasis on laboratory instruction. During the late nineteenth and the early twentieth centuries medical education changed drastically, most notably by including science as a central topic for study.[51] Science made its way into medical schools not only in the lecture halls but also in the laboratories, in which instructors, some of whom had learned about science in German universities, taught students to use new instruments such as the kymograph, an instrument that recorded motion on a drum of smoked paper.[52] The motion might be a pulse wave or respiratory efforts. Sometimes students recorded these by tracing the motion in laboratory animals; often they used one another as experimental subjects. The recording was made in the form of a graph,[53] which was an important experience for two reasons: first, students became acquainted with the idea of using machines to acquire information, and they did so in a way that resembled what they would later do with patients; second, they became familiar with the idea of recording quantitative information in graphic form.[54]

Some graphs were produced not by directly recording a biological phenomenon but, instead, by charting observations made over time. When derived from patient data, graphs provided by medical technology made explicit the exact, quantitative, "objective" nature of such information. The first type of information to be placed routinely on a graph in the patient record was the temperature chart.[55] Producing this record was aided greatly in the late nineteenth century by the development of portable, registering thermometers as well as by the presence of a nursing staff who could take and record the measurements. Graphic recording of the temperature created a curve, and characteristically shaped waves could suggest the specific type of disease a person was suffering from. During the late nineteenth century hospital charts included graphs of the patient's temperature, but few others.

Graphs were by no means exclusively medical. They were central to new, scientific methods of business communication in the early twentieth century. Standardized forms and graphs enabled people to grasp quickly the essence of a mass of complex information and then use that information to make decisions. Manuals intended to help business people design graphic methods sometimes included medical examples.[56]

Between 1900 and 1920 hospital charts started to be filled with graphs for all manner of information. Some graphic reports recorded routine observations of the patient, such as his or her temperature and weight. Rubber stamps helped produce nice, neat, standardized dots on the graphic charts and reduced the time needed to make the graphs by one-half.[57] Some forms were more specialized. The pulse and blood pressure were recorded graphically on an anesthesia form. To look for the presence of gastric disease the amount of stomach acid produced was recorded as a graph on a separate form. The electrocardiogram was laid directly into the patient's hospital chart, itself a diagnostic, graphic form. The number of graphs per patient, per day, increased ten-fold at the Pennsylvania Hospital between 1900 and 1925.[58]

The graph in figure 2.8 dramatically (and beautifully) charts the fluid intake and output of a seventeen-year old-schoolboy with acute nephritis, a type of kidney disease. Clearly, producing this graph required a great deal of work. In return for the effort required to produce it, the person who created this graph made a very individualized depiction of a patient, one that allowed the viewer to obtain a great deal of information at once, to see the day-to-day variations in the fluid intake and urine output far more clearly than would have been the case using a numerical table. Like the other graphs that were filling up patient records, it not only conveyed vital informa-

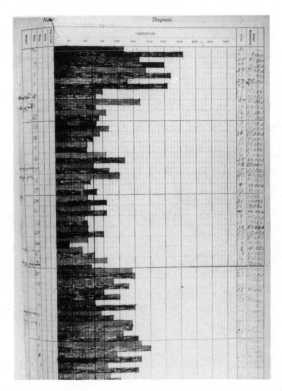

Figure 2.8 *Graph of urine output. From* Pennsylvania Hospital Case Records *1036 (1927): 4253.*

tion; it exemplified a specific, new, graphic method of conveying such information.

It is also interesting to note that there was a transitional phase for some of these charts as they changed from being handmade and specific to a patient to being a standardized, stamped document. The diet chart for diabetics, for example, was once laid out by hand, as shown in figure 2.9. This was an effective way of charting the diet because it allowed for variation among patients; one could omit a column or two, depending on a patient's specific condition. This method required that someone redraw the chart each time it was used, although with modest effort an attending physician could arrange to have charts made specifically for his or her service.[59]

When the chart became a printed, standardized form, like the one

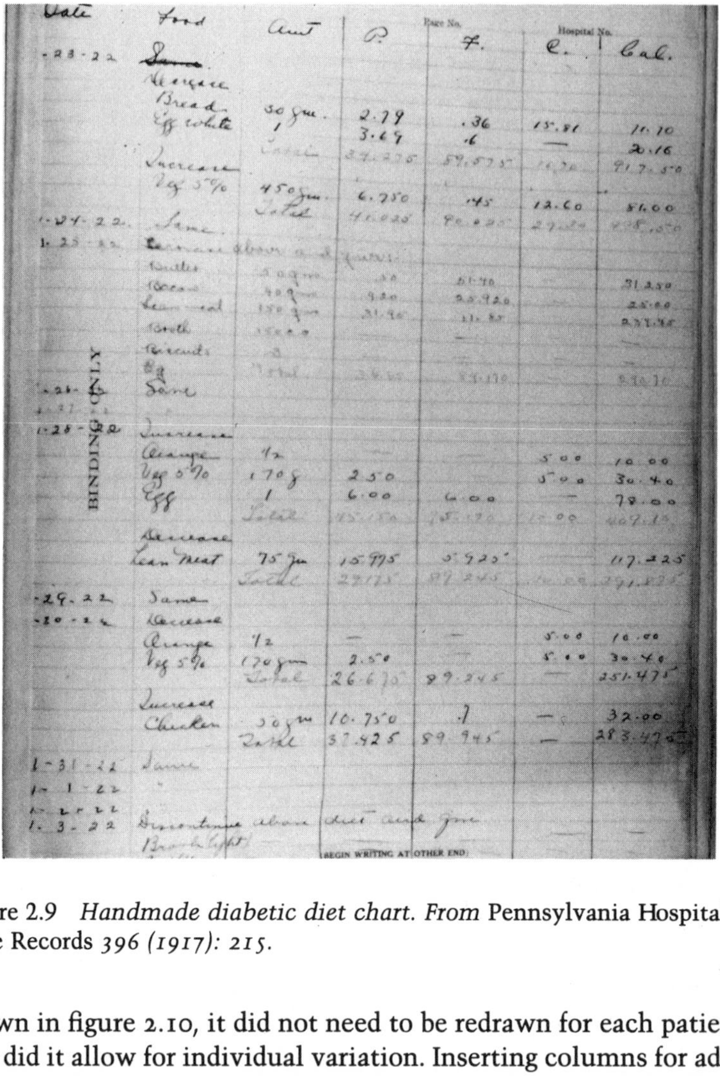

Figure 2.9 *Handmade diabetic diet chart. From* Pennsylvania Hospital Case Records *396 (1917): 215.*

shown in figure 2.10, it did not need to be redrawn for each patient. Nor did it allow for individual variation. Inserting columns for additional information would be difficult, and it was obvious when any of the requested information was omitted. Similarly, the bold, colorful, hand-drawn graph of kidney intake and output was soon superseded by a series of standard graphic pages—again, a transition from a more to less individualistic depiction of information.

By the 1920s hospitals had adopted many aspects of the business world. Some of the change with regards to the management of

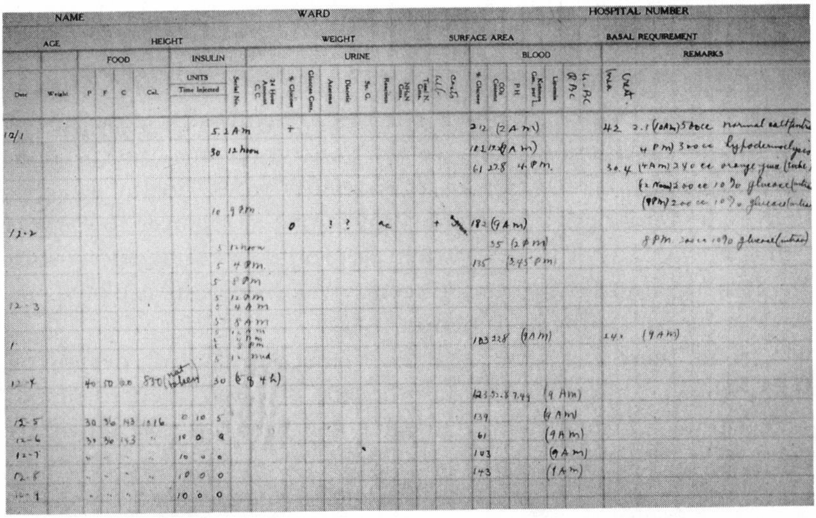

Figure 2.10   *Standardized diabetic diet chart.* From Pennsylvania Hospital Case Records *1026 (1927): 5675.*

money will be taken up in chapter 4 for a specific technology, the x-ray machine. In some ways, the factory-like nature of the hospital was most central for the surgeons and for the operation of the operating rooms, a topic I shall explore shortly. But let us for a moment consider the kinds of changes we have seen in the overall appearance of patient records. There is a distinct, consistent transition from about 1900 to about 1925, one that may help us understand some of the changing ideas about patient care which I will examine in later chapters.[60]

First, there is a change from a more to a less individualistic type of record keeping. Earlier charts, with their dramatic handwriting and graphological nature, allowed those creating the charts to explore a considerable range of expression in how they chose to indicate results. Compare the big, bold word CURED in figure 2.4 with a single punch on the Hollerith card in figure 2.3. Both convey the same information, but they do so in very different ways. The bold CURED appears to give voice to excitement and emotion; the punch on the card appears to reflect scientific objectivity.[61] The written CURED seems to reflect a state of being, one in which the patient's feelings and attitudes would play a part; the punch on the card seems to bespeak the finality of a diagnostic test, a precise laboratory finding. Similarly, compare the description of the fracture setting as "first-class," a narrative description found in occasional patient records, with the dichotomous choices presented in figure 2.6 for describing the x-ray findings of the gastrointestinal tract. Again, both methods for reporting an x-ray result "work" in the sense of conveying information, but one allows for the reporter to express some individuality, even excitement; the other does not. Along with the loss of narrative descriptions comes the increasing use of visual devices for conveying information.[62]

Second, there is a fundamental difference in control, depending upon who gets to decide how information is to be presented. Handmade forms can reflect the initiative and needs of the individual drawer; the standard forms allow whoever designs the forms to determine precisely how information is to be presented. Standardized forms can be used to control the communication of information and thus to define how procedures are to be done, as in the case of reporting the results of urinalysis, as will be discussed. The fact, however, that the patient records first contain handmade versions of some forms, which are then followed by a printed version of that form, suggests that more is going on here than merely the imposition of order from above, although that may be the end result. The assumption that it is good to present information in a systematic, standardized format was shared by both those people writing in the charts (who created the handmade forms) and those running the hospital (who purchased the standardized forms). The pressure of increasing caseloads and the presence of increasing amounts of information made it useful to be able to summarize large quantities of information and make them accessible at a glance.

These changes were important parts of how the ideology of the efficiency movement was operationalized in the hospital setting. Ideas and ideologies must have their effects through specific mediators, and an important one of these had to do with the ways in which information was created, recorded, and used in the changing hospital system.

SURGERY

The most dramatic medical changes in the United States in the late nineteenth and early twentieth centuries were based on surgery. In England, as well as other European countries, surgeons had been relegated to a more subservient role on account of the craft nature of their trade. But in the United States the heroic nature of surgery was particularly appealing. Surgery, though perhaps a craft, was a practical one, and it yielded measurable results. This resulted, by the mid-nineteenth century, in surgery having become a reasonably high-status field of clinical medical practice.[63] By the turn of the twentieth century surgeons were regarded as having surpassed their more dignified and traditional physician-colleagues in other medical fields and found themselves at the center of a rapidly changing world of medical practice.[64] They reigned supreme in the new medical universe but no longer only on account of their skill and courage. Surgeons were central for a changing medical world in part due to new medical ideas, in part due to new operations, and in part due to a new hospital structure within which they could work, a structure that was centered on Taylorism and the efficiency movement and the search for one true answer. As the medical historian Christopher Lawrence has put it: "In surgery, the fiction that medicine had nothing to do with politics reached its fullest expression. Surgical intervention could be represented as the inevitable, scientific solution to disease."[65]

Hospitals were increasingly becoming the center of both medical education and medical care. They provided surgeons with a workplace, a new location in which to operate on their patients. Certainly, surgeons were not the only medical practitioners to benefit from the hospital. Physicians—internists—might also derive many advantages from a hospital setting. Their patients could be cared for by a trained nursing staff; the diseases they treated most often could be more quickly diagnosed because laboratory facilities were nearby and easy to use. Almost all of what internists did, however, *could* have been done in the traditional setting for medical care, the patient's own home. One could argue that this was also true for surgeons. After all, operations were performed in patient's houses, on kitchen tables, sometimes by candlelight, and could have continued to be done there.[66]

The hospital was, however, more central for the surgeon than for the physician for at least two sets of reasons. First was the physical setting of the operating room. Although operations could, and had, been performed with illumination provided by sunlight alone, electric lights dedicated to operating room use offered a far more reliable and constant source of light, one that could be made available on cloudy days as well as sunny, on late-winter afternoons as well as late-summer days, one that could be manipulated to shine on the precise part of the body under scrutiny. Some houses had electric lighting even before hospitals, but major hospitals were wired for electricity before most private homes. Even when a home had electric power, it lacked the complicated equipment that allowed visualization of deep parts of the body as well as the marble walls that were believed to promote aseptic conditions.

Both the New York and Pennsylvania hospitals went to great lengths to supply their surgeons with the very finest facilities for doing operations. Near the end of the nineteenth century the Pennsylvania Hospital opened the Walter Garrett Memorial Building, complete with a 45-by-46-foot operating theater. This theater had provisions for lighting which looked forward to the electrified twentieth century while simultaneously retaining nineteenth-century roots. It had a large glass dome for lighting during the day, as would most nineteenth-century facilities, but electric lights for use on cloudy days or at night, in keeping with the new technology.[67] The new operating theater of the New York Hospital, which opened a decade later, in May 1907, exemplifies what was thought to constitute a new facility of the very highest quality. Unlike in 1877, when the New York Hospital boasted that the new hospital building would make surgery there as safe as if it were being done in the "most luxurious home,"[68] this new setting was far better than any private home could provide. The new suite was designed throughout with cleanliness and sterility in mind, complete with details such as the copper screens on the surgeons' lockers having wires one inch apart, to allow for air circulation, or the placement of a shelf to prevent a careless member of the audience from dropping items into the surgical field. The heating and ventilation system, the paint, the sterilizing room, and the Vermont marble that lined the students' galleries, were all described in detail in the celebratory volume that announced the new facility. The light fixture, called an "illuminator," was precisely designed so as to avoid problems with either shadows or adverse effects on the surgeon's eyes from the intrinsic brilliance and glare of the lights.[69] One aspect of the technology which made surgery a leading part of the early-twentieth-century hospital was that related to lighting and equipment.[70]

Another part of the operating room was the increasing availability of new instruments that could be used for aseptic techniques, which were becoming widely adopted. Traditionally designed instruments could not withstand the high heat necessary to destroy bacteria. After around 1890 a new breed of machined tools made the old artisanal instrument manufacturer less and less important, even in the face of the increasing status of the surgeon.[71] Certainly, a surgeon could own his or her own set of operating equipment, and many did. But others—more junior or less busy, or both—found it convenient to be able to use a hospital's equipment as well as its sterilizing facilities.

Yet a second element that made the hospital particularly important for surgeons, at least as important as the operating room itself, was the hospital's system, the organizational framework within which the surgeon could operate. This, too, can be considered a form of technology.[72] Moving the act of surgery off the wards and into a special place was one way of differentiating the procedure from normal ward activities. As the pace of procedures increased, patients needed to be moved rapidly in and out of the operating room. More and more people became involved in the course of each operation. As a result, surgeons needed a place in which the rapid flow of bodies could be coordinated.

That flow dramatically increased in the first few decades of the twentieth century. Consider surgery at the Pennsylvania Hospital. In 1895 the most frequently performed operation was excision of cervical adenitis, usually tuberculous, which was done only 25 times. Three decades later, in 1925, surgeons performed 1,356 tonsillectomies and/or adenoidectomies, 234 appendectomies, 98 inguinal hernia repairs, and 39 thyroidectomies.[73] We can look at this change in at least two different ways. First, we can note a change in the *types* of operations performed. Excision of tuberculous glands in 1895 might have been encouraged by the recent microbiological revolution, although such excisions had been commonly done even before the mycobacterium specific for tuberculosis had been discovered.

The most common operations in 1925 were also consistent with what physicians and public perceived as modern, scientific ideas.[74]

By far the most frequent reason for patients to enter the operating room in 1925 was to have a surgeon remove their tonsils, their adenoids, or both. Tonsillectomies and adenoidectomies were consonant with the popular theory of focal infection, the idea that microbes, newly discovered and assigned specific roles in disease causation in the microbiological revolution, could, when hidden in pockets such as those found around the tonsils and adenoids, cause diseases ranging from arthritis to nephritis:[75] "The lacunae of the tonsils, ... offer nides for the reception and culture of micrococci that may give rise to more serious trouble. These depressions are sometimes very deep ... and form an ideal nest for the development of microorganisms. There are warmth, moisture, decomposing secretions, and a harbor from the currents of air or friction of fluids and food that might otherwise dislodge them."[76] Diseases of the tonsil received increasing attention in the medical literature. The first series of the *Surgeon General's Index Catalog*, in 1893, includes barely three pages of references on surgery of the tonsils.[77] When the references were updated for the 1913 second series, they included eighteen pages on surgery of the tonsils alone, now listed as "excision of the tonsils," and thirty-two pages in all.

The indications for removal of the tonsils became so broad as to be practically coextensive with the presence of the organ itself. As one leading physician recalled in the 1930s; "The operation of tonsillectomy, complete excision of the tonsil, had [at the end of the nineteenth century] recently become recognized as one of the most important in surgery. Almost all children had diseased tonsils that were a menace to life and health."[78] The indications for operation were of two types: physiological and pathological. Physiological indications included impairment of some type that could be attributed to the tonsil, such as an unpleasant quality to the voice, impaired hearing, or "certain failures of the body metabolism, leading to a lack of resistance or to a general indefinite *below-par-ness.*" Pathological indications included evidence of infection elsewhere or simply prophylaxis—because the tonsils were there.[79] In other words, based on the latest scientific evidence, one could justify removing the tonsils in almost any person.

Despite the active operating rooms, many more people, primarily schoolchildren, needed the operation than were having it done. A 1920 survey of children in New York City revealed that between 10 and 20 percent of them had either enlarged tonsils or defective breathing; both findings were indications that an operation was needed. Operating facilities needed to increase their output. Because more tonsils needed to be removed, some medical leaders considered allowing less-experienced practitioners to extract the offending organs. An early, draft version of the survey report was even willing to suggest that pediatrics interns do some of the operations, but, perhaps because the operation was felt to be too difficult for such inexperienced trainees, that advice was later omitted.[80]

The operation was held to be one of the most important weapons in the surgeon's armamentarium. It was asserted that "no operation in surgery yielded (and it is the same today) a higher percentage of satisfactory results." Of course, it was also the case that the operation produced a high percentage of satisfactory results in terms of benefit to the physician's bank account, making up a "major portion of the . . . income" for some practitioners.[81] With so many indications for removing tonsils, many people could benefit from the operation. The dual goals—of improved health (for patients) and improved wealth (for physicians)—could only be met by an efficient system for moving patients in a machine-like fashion in and out of the operating room.

The other operations frequently done in 1925 were thought to be just as scientific. Appendectomies carried the search for bacterial infection further and called upon surgeons to dive boldly into the abdominal cavity to drain and destroy pockets of pus. (Appendectomies are discussed in detail in chapter 7, particularly with respect to the role of a new diagnostic laboratory test, the blood count.) Hernia repair was an important, though often overlooked, example of what reformers considered the wedge of modern, progressive surgery. Inguinal hernias were the battleground between modern surgeons and the self-styled mechano-therapeutists, the latter with tried-and-true trusses, the former with what was called the "radical cure" for hernia.[82] Thyroidectomy was linked to an exciting new idea—that substances produced by a gland in one location could act at a distance, throughout the body.

Thus, the types of operations performed reflected a new scientific ethos. They helped surgeons to see themselves, and to be seen by others, as far more than merely highly skilled technicians. Rather, they were bold, progressive, scientific reformers. In comparison with surgery, medicine was seen as far less exciting. Students were advised to start their clinical studies with medicine, because after surgery it would seem dull. As the noted British *physician* (not surgeon) Sir John Burdon-Sanderson remarked in 1899: "If a comparison be made of the two great branches of medical practice—surgical and medical— . . . one of the most striking points of difference is that the influence of scientific discovery has been much greater in surgery than in medicine." He went on to say, "The surgeon has during the last two or three decades acquired new powers for the preservation of life and relief of suffering."[83]

Yet it was not only the *types* of operations at the Pennsylvania Hospital which changed from 1895 to 1925; there was a dramatic increase as well in the total *number* of operations performed. In 1900 the total number of operations was 870. In 1925 the number was 4,180, of which 3,606 were done in the hospital, the remainder being done in the outpatient department. The almost fivefold increase in the number of operations performed far exceeds the increase in the number of patients seen in the hospital. The total number of patients treated in the wards in 1900 was 4,345. The total number of patients treated in 1925 (for the wards and private rooms) was 6,668, an increase of only about 50 percent.

Another way to examine the increasing importance of surgery within the hospital is to look at the percentage of patients who had an operation (see fig. 2.11). (One cannot merely divide the number of admissions by the number of operations, because some patients had more than one operation performed during their stay in the hospital.)[84] In 1900, 20 percent of the patients admitted to the Pennsylvania Hospital had an operation performed. That percentage increased to 40 percent in 1909, 45 percent in 1920, and 52 percent in 1925. In other words, whereas in 1920 only about one person in five would have an operation, by 1925 over half did. Similarly, at the New York Hospital the percentage of patients admitted who underwent an operation increased from 18 percent in 1900 to 40 percent in 1910 to 69 percent in 1920.[85] All of these numbers serve to confirm a central idea, that the number of operations being done went up dramatically

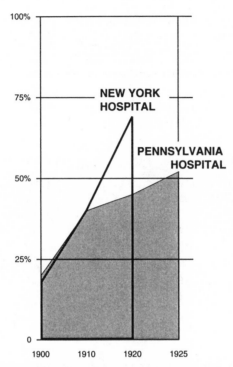

Figure 2.11 *Proportion of patients having operations, Pennsylvanina and New York hospitals, 1900–1925.*

and that more and more patients who entered the hospital walls found themselves being operated on at some point during their stay.

These people tended to be younger than those who did not have an operation. This is not a surprising finding on purely clinical grounds. It seems reasonable to assume that, like those of the late twentieth century, the early-twentieth-century surgeon disliked seeing the death of patients he (or, rarely, she) had operated on. Thus, those people who were sicker tended to be less likely to have an operation, and those people who were older tended to be sicker. This tendency was true at the Pennsylvania Hospital, even excluding people (mostly children) who were admitted for reasons other than tonsil disease, as shown in table 2.1. Interestingly, at the New York Hospital, after removing those people admitted for diseases of the tonsils, there was not a consistent trend toward a lower age for people who had an operation. The people who were being operated on also

Table 2.1 *Ages of People Undergoing an Operation*

	1900	1910 (1909)	1920	1925
Mean Age of Patients, with and without an Operation				
Pennsylvania				
with	30.8	21.6	22.3	22.0
without	31.9	30.1	30.1	34.2
New York				
with	32.9	27.7	28.5	—
without	32.2	30.9	30.5	—
Mean Age, with and without an Operation, for Patients not Admitted for Disease of the Tonsils				
Pennsylvania				
with	31.3	28.0	30.6	28.4
without	32.2	30.3	34.3	35.5
New York				
with	32.9	28.7	33.8	—
without	32.3	30.9	32.3	—

tended to be somewhat better off financially than the typical nine-teenth-century patient. As the historian Rosemary Stevens has pointed out, the clean, sterile, efficient hospital helped to attract people who could pay for medical care into the hospital who might otherwise have been operated on at home.[86]

Why the increase in the numbers of operations on hospitalized patients? The cause for the increase cannot be the two reasons often positivistically invoked: anesthesia or antisepsis.[87] Anesthesia had been an important element in increasing the respectability of surgeons, who no longer needed to operate amid the suffering cries of their patients. This not only improved the aesthetic environment of the operating theater; it also enabled surgeons to concentrate more intensively on the technical aspects of their work. Yet anesthesia had been described over half a century earlier.[88] By 1900 it was widely accepted in the United States, and *all* of the patients who had an operation at both the Pennsylvania Hospital and the New York Hospital were given anesthesia.[89] Thus, the advent of anesthesia cannot be used to explain the increase in the number of operations during the early twentieth century.

Nor can the introduction of antiseptic surgery be used as an explanation. In 1867 the English surgeon Joseph Lister described a technique to reduce infections based on a carbolic spray, which he called "antisepsis."[90] Shortly thereafter surgeons modified the procedure, changing to an "aseptic" technique in which sterile procedure, rather than Lister's original carbolic acid, was used to eliminate potential sources of infection. The initial description of the technique did not result in a significant increase in the number of operations being done.[91] What was defined as the proper use of these techniques remained quite controversial through the 1880s.[92] Yet some elite hospitals, such as the Massachusetts General Hospital, boasted of having quickly adopted the technique.[93] Although, by comparison with the use of anesthesia, we cannot create such clean statistics to measure the impact of the theory of antiseptic or aseptic technique, some form of the technique appears to have been widely used by around the turn of the century.[94] Thus, neither anesthesia nor aseptic technique can provide a plausible explanation for the early-twentieth-century explosion of surgery.[95]

For whatever reason, early in the twentieth century there was an astonishing increase in the number of operations performed in hospitals. The most commonly performed operation at the Pennsylvania Hospital in 1895 was done 25 times; the most commonly performed operation in 1925 was done 1,356 times. The total number of operations went from 870 in 1900 to 4,180 in 1925. These raw figures start to suggest the overall transformation that took place in the hospital. The impact of this new activity was felt at every level: housekeeping, nursing, cooking, accounting. The volume forced house staff to work at a frantic pace just to keep up with the paperwork necessary to shuffle people into and out of the system. One occasionally finds humorous asides amidst the ceaseless, monotonous lines describing patients admitted for a tonsillectomy or adenoidectomy. One house officer must have become bored during a long series of repetitious admission workups of children admitted for these procedures. For almost all of his workups he noted that the heart and lung of each child were "normal," though he slipped in, for humorous relief, that one heart and set of lungs were "present."

The increased use of operating rooms required an efficient system for managing everything from supplies to soap, from patients to patient records. The increase in scale forced the hospital to start to resemble a factory. Part of what this meant came from a direct importation of methods and tools from the world of U.S. business, methods and tools most prominent as part of scientific management and the efficiency movement. Hospital reorganization was necessary for this change in hospital affairs. It was not sufficient—but it was necessary. Anesthesia, antisepsis, and all of the other new ideas typically subsumed under the heading of the new, scientific surgery were certainly also necessary, but they, too, were not sufficient. Forms and charts were in the hospital, as in business, the tangible evidence of the work going on in a fluid and ever-changing institution. Those who used them well could share with physicians a new-found certainty in knowing what was happening in their domain. As the author of a book on forms pointed out, "An executive watching the flow of work through his office is like a doctor with his finger on the pulse of a patient."[96] More than simply documenting activities, the new systems enabled and shaped activities. The increased attention to organization had a direct impact on clinical medicine: forms, charts, and a new institutional structure allowed and encouraged the rise of surgery.

The technical aspects of surgery did not escape the attention of proponents of the efficiency movement. Ernest Amory Codman, an iconoclastic Boston surgeon, argued vehemently for what he termed an "end-result system," a systematic accounting of the outcome of each patient who underwent an operation. He felt this would enable people to compare the results of various surgeons as well as improve medical practice.[97]

Although they were implemented at individual institutions, there was a national base for the move toward standardized records led by the American College of Surgeons.[98] Meeting for the first time in 1913, the group soon decided to ask prospective fellows to submit case records of their operations for analysis. The inadequacy of the documents that were submitted provided dramatic evidence of the sad state of record keeping. When the American College of Surgeons examined hospitals with more than one hundred beds, they found that most could not meet its standards.[99] The college then embarked on a mission to upgrade and standardize not only clinical records but also surgical training in general, to make U.S. hospitals more efficient. Just as an efficient factory would be known by the quality of its work as reflected in its products, so, too, the quality of the care provided in a hospital would be reflected in its case records.[100]

Others tried to apply Taylorism directly to surgical practice. Most prominent among them were the Brooklyn gynecologist Robert Latou Dickinson and the engineer Frank Gilbreth.[101] Gilbreth claimed to have at one time considered a career in surgery. Later, when he first visited an operating room as an engineer, he hoped that he could learn from surgeons about how to make business more efficient. Instead, he found that "surgeons could learn more . . . from the industries than the industries could learn from the hospitals." Part of the problem was that much of the literature applied to the shop and not to medicine.[102] To help remedy that situation Gilbreth observed surgery in several countries and, as consultant engineer to the New York Hospital, took moving pictures of operations. Gilbreth concluded that between 10 and 30 percent of the time spent under anesthesia could be saved with proper training in Tayloristic methods. Dickinson outlined the preliminary results of what he hoped would be a systematic improvement in the efficiency of operative procedures, ranging from the proper lighting to how to place surgical instruments on a table to how best to suture an abdominal incision.[103] There were too many types of surgical instruments, he felt, and this impeded the optimum performance of operators. But much of his message went far beyond operative technique: overall, surgeons needed to pay far more attention to management science than they did. As leaders in society, they had an obligation to be aware of new tools and techniques that could aid their practice. As Dickinson put it, for those who did not pay adequate attention to modern techniques of management, there was "an excuse for a man of the industries who has not had the advantage of a general or a special education," but there was "absolutely no excuse for the surgeon."[104]

To what extent did surgery lead hospitals to adopt a new style of record keeping, and to what extent did a new style of record keeping allow surgeons to practice as they did? Obviously, both were important. The reformers of hospital management looked to industry for their models and to efficiency for their ideology. Some even admitted that "the term hospital efficiency has grown to be a fetish for many."[105] On the other hand, as surgery gained in power and prestige, surgeons acquired the power and authority they needed to play a key role in reshaping the hospital. The new hospital organization was itself an important new type of technology.

In addition, much of the other medical technology that was introduced in the early twentieth century could not have existed as it did without the new shape of the hospital. There is no reason to believe that the invention of the x ray, or certainly the electrocardiogram, drove hospital reorganization in the same way as did surgery or a desire to emulate industry. But, as we shall see, hospital reorganization was essential for using the new machines. It was most important for those that were large and bulky, such as the x-ray machine, and for systems that required the interaction of many people, such as surgery. The ideas and ideology of science were, however, part of a larger culture, both medical and nonmedical, and those who preached the utility of science may have found an easier means of introducing scientific practice in the form of the familiar urine analysis.

3

THE CHANGING MEANING OF
URINALYSIS
"Old Wine in New Bottles"

Let us now move our gaze from administrative offices to clinical wards, from operating rooms to diagnostic laboratories, in order to consider how new ideas about science and medicine were applied by those who cared for individuals admitted to the early-twentieth-century hospital. Just as the idea of science permeated the business community in different ways, it also came to have an impact on many different aspects of medical practice. By the latter part of the twentieth century many people *define* excellent clinical practice in terms of scientific medicine and scientific testing. How did we come to see science as the touchstone of modern medicine? The first intimations of change to a scientific model for making medical diagnoses might have been the use of scientific instrumentation or the institutionalization of new chemical or microbiological tests, but, instead, one of the earliest systematic scientific changes in clinical practice took place in a very familiar form of diagnostic testing: examining a patient's urine.

Urinalysis was not new. Medical practitioners had looked at urine for centuries, searching for evidence of disease, attempting to differentiate one ailment from another.[1] Artists from at least the fifteenth century have depicted the practice of uroscopy, examining the urine, as a central feature of medical life.[2] Urine analysis was mentioned in at least two of the works of William Shakespeare. In *Henry IV,* part 2, a physician tells Falstaff that "the water [urine] itself was a good healthy water, but for the party that owned it, he might have more diseases than he knew for." Here the urine analysis is used to poke fun at the idea that the urine might be healthy but the patient (Falstaff) might still be sick. In *Twelfth Night* the urine is treated as a fluid that can be used to establish a person's mental health; the test is used in an attempt to prove that Malvolio is mad, which he is not.[3] Urinalysis was clearly a familiar topic to audiences of the day, commonplace enough to be made fun of in a pair of popular plays.

One feature of urine is its very ubiquity. A person did not, and does not, need expert training to perceive changes in the color, odor, or quantity of urine. Urine is part of the constant cycle of bodily intake and outgo, its features obvious to everyone. Thus, in a nineteenth-century world in which observing the character of the body's excretions provided one of the most important manifestations of the body's functioning, observing the urine made a great deal of sense to physicians and the public alike.[4]

By the 1850s, at the handful of U.S. hospitals that had been established, urine analyses were not just done on patients suspected of having a specific disease but were said to be "nearly routine" for all.[5] Toward the end of the century some of these hospitals created specific areas for doing laboratory tests. Although historians studying clinical care have spent a good deal of time examining the shift of medical care from the home to the hospital, the dominance of the laboratory, both a century ago and today, in the creation and application of medical knowledge has received somewhat less attention.[6] This despite the fact that, when chemists, physicists, and physicians asked a wide range of questions about the natural world and about the nature of the human body in health and disease, they increasingly turned for their answers to the laboratory.

Not surprisingly, given the central (and obvious) role of urine in the functioning of the human body, many laboratory scientists turned their attention to that fluid. The general idea that practicing physicians ought to attend to their patients' urine had long been a familiar concept. Urinalysis was routinely accepted into the physician's diagnostic armamentarium without a great deal of debate or justification. Throughout the latter part of the nineteenth century and the first part of the twentieth century, people writing in the medical and scientific literature described many new physical, chemical, and microscopical tests for the examination of urine.

And what was the urinalysis? How ought the historian to approach new attempts to examine urine? The introduction of various new tests as parts of urinalysis might be taken, at first glance, to be a relatively straightforward process. Perhaps these tests simply reflected the increasingly scientific nature of medicine, as manifest in the rise of laboratory-based medicine. Perhaps as each new test was shown to be useful, it was simply incorporated into the existing diagnostic routine. Perhaps the urinalysis, having been long ago accepted into routine medical practice, was simply having its parameters refined. Indeed, one might wonder about the historical value of paying any attention at all to the urinalysis in a discussion of the changing practices of typical physicians at the turn of the twentieth century, particularly in light of the more dramatic changes of the period, such as the introduction of aseptic surgery or the invention of the x-ray machine. Yet, as we shall see, the fact that the label of "urinalysis" remained the same during the first few decades of the twentieth century should not obscure the fact that the fundamental idea of the test for hospitalized patients underwent a dramatic transformation. The change was, to some extent, a change in the types of tests that were applied to the urine. But this was true to a lesser extent than one might anticipate from the amount of discussion in the scientific and medical literature about the new ways of analyzing urine. The "old" urine analysis largely disappeared between 1900 and 1925, and urine soon became the center for a "new" test, new both in terms of the ways that the test was applied (when, to whom, and how often) and also in terms of the meaning of the test itself (what it meant to "do a urinalysis").

In this chapter I will first describe how often the urinalysis was done for a systematic sample of patients admitted to the New York and Pennsylvania hospitals between 1900 and 1925. I will then describe changes in how often some selected components of the analysis were done. Finally, I will consider how best to explain these changes and their consequences and will suggest that the urinalysis changed from an admission ritual into one of the first examples of a scientific monitor of a patient's clinical status: by 1925 the urine had become "old wine in new bottles" in ways that allowed it to serve as the prototype for a whole range of new scientific laboratory tests.

WHEN TO DO A URINALYSIS

Published primary sources include increasing discussion of laboratory tests for patient care during the late nineteenth and the early twentieth centuries.[7] Let us examine how often a urinalysis was recorded on patients entering the Pennsylvania Hospital and the New York Hospital during the first few decades of the twentieth century. Figures 3.1 and 3.2 show both the overall percentage of patients who had any urinalyses done and the number of urine analyses done on each patient at the two hospitals. The figures indicate the overall percentage of patients admitted, for each year, who had a urinalysis done (at least the indicated number of times). First, consider how commonly even one urinalysis was done for hospitalized patients. In 1900, 82 percent of the patients admitted to the Pennsylvania Hospital had at least one urinalysis of some type done. In other words, more than four out of five of all the people who were admitted to the hospital had a urine specimen collected, examined, and

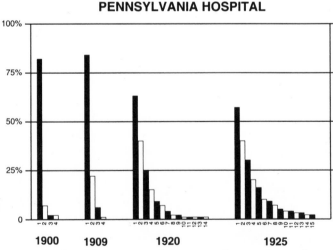

Figure 3.1 *Number of times urinalyses were done at Pennsylvania Hospital, 1900–1925 (as a percentage of total admissions).*

the results recorded in the chart.[8] What were physicians doing with all that urine?

One might wish to explain the ubiquitous nature of urinalyses in 1900 by suggesting that the test was being used to make clinical decisions, such as to establish diagnoses, to change diagnoses, or to guide therapies. Yet this appears to have been unlikely. There is almost never any suggestion within the written record that the urinalysis was taken into account in making clinical decisions. Rather, the test was done, the results were recorded, and the subject was never again mentioned. Certainly, the absence of explicit discussion in the chart does not mean that no one paid attention to the results. Perhaps the value of the urinalysis for guiding the clinical care of all patients was implicit, understood by all, and needed no mention within the written record. One could suggest that the urinalysis served to "rule out" diagnoses that were very real concerns for the physicians caring for the patient, diagnoses that were no less real for having been eliminated by the results of the urinalysis, although never, perhaps, committed to pen and paper. Perhaps. This might have been the case for the thirty-four-year-old laborer admitted with edema on Wednesday, January 17, 1900, for whom the differential

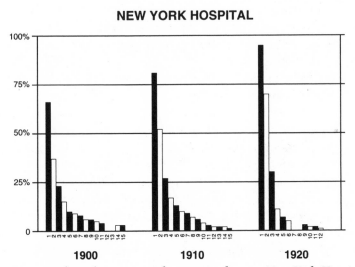

NEW YORK HOSPITAL

Figure 3.2 *Number of times urinalyses were done at New York Hospital, 1900–1920 (as a percentage of total admissions).*

Table 3.1   *Urinalysis, by Disease, at Pennsylvania Hospital*

Disease	1900	1909	1920	1925
Kidney disease	87	100	100	86
Infectious diseases	82	86	86	84
Injuries	81	76	70	50
Diseases of the trachea	91	67	100	100
Nervous diseases	75	50	87	67
Diseases of the tonsils	87	82	8	9

Note: This table shows the percentage of patients who had at least one urinalysis done as part of the diagnosis of one of six diseases, in 1900, 1909, 1920, and 1925. The diagnostic classifications were taken, as described in the section on methodology in the appendix, from a standard classification scheme of the time. For the sake of clarity and brevity only selected diagnostic groups are shown.

diagnosis for physicians of the day included diseases of both the heart and the kidneys. A normal urine might direct physicians' attention to the heart; an abnormal urine to the kidneys. But the suggestion that the results of the urinalysis guided patient care is harder to sustain for tests done on the twenty-one-year-old clerk admitted on Tuesday, February 13, 1900, for surgical repair of his hammer toes (done the next day), or for the fifty-three-year-old woman admitted Thursday, June 21, 1900, for constipation and sent home two days later, cured.[9] Try as one might, it is difficult, if not impossible, to hypothesize a likely rationale for the clinical value of urinalyses in these cases.

A systematic tabulation of selected, common diagnoses, shown in table 3.1, confirms that urinalyses at the Pennsylvania Hospital were done not only for patients for whom the urine might have provided clinically useful information but also for those with a wide variety of diagnoses; a similar picture holds for the New York Hospital. Table 3.1 evokes an obvious question. Why were physicians doing all those urinalyses in 1900? One can easily imagine why physicians did the test for most of the patients with kidney disease. By 1900 the kidney was believed to make urine, and examination of urine was thought to be valuable in the diagnosis of kidney disease. Similarly, the attention to urine in patients with infectious diseases is not hard to fathom. Such diseases—at the time the major cause of admission to a hospital—were thought to affect the entire body and could easily produce characteristic changes in the urine. But what about the number of urinalyses done on patients with injuries (81 percent of all patients classified in this diagnostic group)? What about those patients with diseases of the trachea (91 percent) or those patients with nervous diseases (75 percent)?[10] Recall that the overall percentage of patients, with all diagnoses, who had a urinalysis done was 82 percent. Neither clinical notes nor published medical literature supports the idea that examining the urine would be of any specific benefit in caring for most of the patients who were admitted.

Other possible explanations for the prevalence of urinalysis seem unlikely. The examination would have been of little value in promoting the hospital to the general public because the test was old and already used widely. Moreover, unlike blood tests, a urine examination was done without any ceremony surrounding the acquisition of the specimen, and, unlike the x-ray machine, it produced an output that was not particularly impressive to the lay viewer. There is no indication that the urinalysis was advertised to draw patients into the hospital, nor is there any notation to show that in 1900 the hospital charged patients an additional fee to have one done.

Another way of learning whether the urinalysis was done in response to specific clinical needs might be to consider when in a given patient's hospital stay the analysis was performed. Was it done as soon as a person entered the hospital? Or, was it done further into that person's hospital stay, perhaps in response to a specific clinical situation? For these two hospitals the test was almost always done immediately on admission. In 1900, for both the New York Hospital and the Pennsylvania Hospital, the median number of days between admission and first doing a urinalysis (for those cases in which a urinalysis was done) was never greater than one day. In fact, the 75th percentile was less than one day[11]: in other words, more than three-fourths of all patients who had a urinalysis done had their original test done within twenty-four hours of admission. This pattern of use suggests that people decided to do the initial urinalysis not on the basis of a considered decision or discussion among the people providing health care nor on the patient's diagnosis and unique characteristics. Rather, the test was part of a routine history and physical examination. It was part and parcel of the admission process, an admission ritual, a ceremony that was repeated without question for (practically) each and every patient who passed through the doors of the hospital.[12]

But did the meaning of the urinalysis change between 1900 and 1925? Any change is not to be found, at least not in any dramatic fashion, in the decision merely to look at urine. The overall fraction of patients who received a urinalysis at the Pennsylvania Hospital did fall from 0.82 to 0.57, yet that decline is less important than it may appear at first glance. One must take into account the increasing number of persons admitted for tonsillectomy and adenoidectomy in 1920 and 1925. Patients admitted for these surgeries were seen as falling into a separate category. Because they typically were admitted for a very short period of time—only a day or two—they were not subject to all of the standard rituals.[13] As table 3.1 shows, most of them did not have a urinalysis done. If one omits those patients admitted for tonsillectomy and adenoidectomy, the percentage of the remaining patients who had a urinalysis done in 1920 was 83 percent; in 1925, 76 percent. Thus, there was little change in the overall percentage. And the initial examination continued to be done immediately—more than three-fourths within one day, from 1900 to 1925.

THE BIRTH OF MULTIPLE TESTING

Thus far, we have considered only whether or not physicians examined the urine of each patient admitted to the hospital, that is, whether the test was used at all. Yet one might also ask how often a urinalysis was done on each patient. Here one sees a dramatic change in practice between 1900 and 1925. As is shown in figure 3.1, in 1900, of all of those patients who had a urinalysis done, over 90 percent had it done only once. Only one person in the sample of patients from the Pennsylvania Hospital had it done as many as five times. Consider this observation in light of the clinical course of patients after they were admitted to the hospital. Some improved and went home; some worsened. Some of those who worsened later improved; others died. Some patients had a diagnosis that was obvious on admission; some had a more obscure picture that later became clarified. Some who were thought to have a clear diagnosis had their diagnosis become more confusing to physicians over the course of their hospital stay. Sometimes medical therapies appeared to work, and sometimes they did not. Some patients had an operation; others did not. In other words, the clinical course of those who were admitted to the hospital varied a great deal. Still, in 1900, after the initial examination, very few patients ever had their urinalysis repeated. The urinalysis was a test to be done on admission to the hospital, a ritual to be recorded once and not to be done again. For most patients their hospital stay began, and their laboratory investigation ended, with an examination of their urine.

This was true for all patients, even those who had a disease for which the urinalysis might be perceived as particularly relevant. Consider patients thought to be suffering from kidney disease. In 1900, of the patients with kidney disease in the sample who had a urinalysis performed, 54 percent had it done only once.[14] Patients with kidney disease were seen, not surprisingly, as needing multiple urinalyses more often than most other patients. Still, for more than half of those patients thought to have diseased kidneys, the test was done only once, as was the case for the vast majority of patients admitted to the hospital.

But that pattern of use changed. By 1925 it had become typical for physicians to do urinalyses many times on a single patient. For those patients at the Pennsylvania Hospital who had an examination of their urine, by 1909, 73 percent had only one done; by 1920 that percentage had fallen to 37 percent, and by 1925 to 30 percent. Figure 3.1 illustrates the trend toward the increasing frequency of urinalysis in a different way. It charts the number of urinalyses noted for each of the patients, for each year of the study, and shows that there is an increasing trend toward more and more urinalyses being done for each patient. The bars indicate the percentage of patients who had a urinalysis done once, twice, up to—by 1925—fifteen times. For example, while, in 1900, 82 percent of patients had at least one and 7 percent had at least two urinalyses, almost no patient had as many as five urinalyses done. By 1925, although the number who had it done at least once had fallen to 57 percent, 40 percent of patients had their urine examined at least twice, and almost 20 percent of the patients had five or more of the tests performed; an appreciable number had between ten and fifteen tests done.

Restricting the analysis again to patients with kidney disease, we see a pattern similar to that among the general population. The number of patients are not sufficient to support a fine-grained statistical analysis, but there is a clear trend toward more attention to urine, as one would expect. In 1900, 54 percent of those patients with kidney disease had only one urinalysis done; by 1925 that percentage had fallen to 17 percent.[15]

Changes in the pattern of using a urinalysis are even more striking when looked at in the context of other changes taking place in the hospital. For, at the same time that patients were having more urinalyses done, the length of time that they were staying in the hospital was decreasing. Thus, the intensity of use of the urinalysis—how often someone examined the urine of each patient—increased even more than the numbers of urinalyses per patient would indicate. One can calculate the number of these tests administered per patient, per day, by dividing the total number of urinalyses done for each patient by the number of days he or she was in the hospital, the length of stay (LOS). At the Pennsylvania Hospital, for those patients who had a urinalysis done, the mean number per day was 0.12 in 1900, and the value steadily increased to 0.26 in 1925. Similarly, at the New York Hospital the mean number rose from 0.15 in 1900 to 0.31 in 1920.[16] In other words, at the Pennsylvania Hospital, for those patients who had a urinalysis done, it was done about every fourth day; at the New York Hospital it was every third day.

This changing pattern marks a change in the meaning of the test. By doing multiple urinalyses on the same patient, physicians were using the test in a new way, one that presaged a whole new attitude and approach to the use of laboratory tests in general. By 1925 the urine waiting to be examined was like "old wine in new bottles": more than merely a different kind of technical approach to the same old urinalysis, this was, instead, a new urinalysis.

I shall consider later in this chapter some of the clinical implications of doing a urinalysis multiple times on a patient. But before considering why the use of the urinalysis changed, we should delve a little more deeply into the test itself, to look at precisely what physicians were doing with the patient's urine.

URINALYSIS: METHODS AND RESULTS

People have for centuries tried to discover whether someone was sick or healthy from their urine's color, its froth, its smell, and even its taste, characteristics that can easily be appreciated without any special training or equipment.[17] Early attempts at instrumental aids for urinary diagnosis may now appear somewhat fanciful. They included flasks to hold the urine which resembled the bladder and complicated distillation devices in which the site of the urinary residue was thought to provide evidence about the site of disease.[18]

Starting around the eighteenth century, people started to analyze the urine in ways that would now seem somewhat more familiar. One attribute that could easily be measured was the specific gravity of urine, its weight compared with the weight of the same quantity of water. Another attribute was the presence of solid matter sometimes found in the urine. After heating urine in a spoon over a candle, people noted that, once the urine had evaporated, a coagulated substance remained behind.[19] The white material was called albumin. In a magisterial series of mid-nineteenth-century clinical studies, Richard Bright, working at Guy's Hospital in London, associated the presence of albumin in the urine with characteristic pathological changes in the kidneys.[20] In so doing, he defined the kidneys, for the first time, as the location of an important disease.[21] Others working with him analyzed the urine and blood of patients with kidney disease for the presence and the amount of albumin and urea. These methods were usually applied to patients with profound alterations of bodily function called at one time dropsy and later Bright's disease.

During the nineteenth century physicians and scientists, including several German physiologists, used new techniques in clinical chemistry to describe additional ways of examining urine, hoping to discern physiological processes going on within human bodies.[22] Additional techniques were invented within an American world of analytic and experimental sciences. The chemical analysis of body fluids, such as urine, was one place in which clinicians and biological scientists could interact, and many did so within the changing institutional context of the new discipline known as "biochemistry."[23] At Harvard University, in 1905, Otto Folin applied procedures he had observed in German breweries to describe new methods for analyzing urine for urea, ammonia, creatine, and uric acid. His series of papers attracted widespread attention from some chemists but also some skepticism from physicians, who wondered about the relevance of biochemical investigations carried on by a nonclinician.[24] Stanley R. Benedict, in the Department of Physiological

Table 3.2 *Books Cataloged in the National Library of Medicine by the Word* Urine

Decade	No. of Books	No. of Books per 100 Cataloged
1881–90	21	.194
1891–1900	33	.252
1901–10	27	.174
1911–20	14	.095

Note: Data taken from the NLM CATLINE database on September 11, 1992. This does not include the many laboratory manuals and clinical guides that included sections on urinalysis but not the word *urine* in their titles. Nonetheless, it includes most of those books in English for which urine was the primary focus.

Chemistry at Cornell, also contributed to the available techniques for estimating sugar in urine. Around the turn of the twentieth century, within the community of German research scientists, and to some extent within the community of those U.S. physicians who also carried on research and paid attention to the new tests and techniques, a new form of careful, scientific analysis of urine was becoming seen as a matter of some importance. Their new methods were used by investigators to excellent effect.[25]

Scholars wrote a significant number of books about how to examine urine. Descriptions ranged from slender guides on diagnostic methods to massive compilations of complex chemical diagnostic procedures. Some of the works were by U.S. authors, and many were translations of foreign-language texts, a good number of them written by German authors. There was sufficient interest that one German work appeared twice in the United States, in two different editions, with two different translators and two different publishers.[26] Obviously, someone thought that there was an active market for works on how to examine urine.

Table 3.2 shows both the raw number of books in the National Library of Medicine which include the word *urine* in their title and that number corrected for the total number of books added to the library during each decade. This is a crude measure, to be sure, but it provides one way of establishing a broad base of interest in urine. Both the absolute number and the fraction of the books cataloged show a rise to the decade 1891–1900, with a decline thereafter.

Drawing from both these books and the published literature, at the turn of the twentieth century U.S. physicians could choose from a wide range of tests to study urine. Which ones did they use? How did that pattern of use change? While the scientific changes of the late nineteenth and the early twentieth centuries certainly gave physicians new tests to use, many of the changes in the ways that physicians chose to do a urinalysis reflected the increasing standardization of laboratory test results and had very little to do with new medical technology, at least not in the traditional sense of laboratory equipment and apparatus.

In this chapter I focus on four specific tests of urine: color, specific gravity, sugar, and urea. These tests cover a range of parameters that might have made a difference to clinicians trying to decide what test to do with their patients' urine: whether the test required sophisticated laboratory methods, whether it involved new concepts, and whether it was perceived as having clear and obvious linkages to treatment of disease.

Color and Specific Gravity

The first step in examining urine is to look at it. To the eyes of an early-twentieth-century physician any change in the normal pale-straw tint of the urine could indicate a morbid condition. Darker colors suggested disease in general; bile gave an olive-green tint; blood gave a smoky or frankly reddish appearance; pus could lead to a milky coloration. Even as other chemical aspects of the urine became more central to academic discussions, the color still was held to provide important clues about the urinary constituents. Guides to designing modern clinical laboratories of the early twentieth century did so with the importance of color measurement in mind, pointing out the need for adequate natural light with which to look at urine.[27]

Another old test, perhaps the oldest one that required some type of apparatus, was measuring urinary specific gravity. The specific gravity was defined as the weight of some fluid as compared to the weight of an equal quantity of water. It was easily measured by an instrument called a hydrometer (or, if the instrument was specifically designed for use with urine, a urinometer). The urine was placed within the vessel and a urinometer inserted; the specific

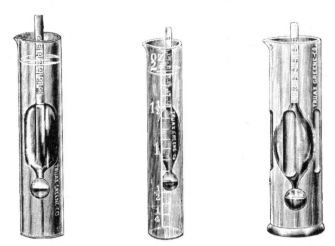

Figure 3.3 *Urinometers. Left, ordinary urinometer; center, urinometer
with graduated test glass; right, Squibb's pattern urinometer. From
Charles Traux,* The Mechanics of Surgery *(Chicago: Hammond Press,
1899), 76.*

gravity could be read from a scale on the side of the instrument
according to the height at which the urinometer settled. Figure 3.3
shows three different types of urinometers, ranging from the sim-
plest to the most sophisticated (which was not very). The specific
gravity varied according to the amount of solids and liquids present
in the urine and was thus a general index of the metabolic processes
taking place within the body.[28] It tended to be high in inflammatory
conditions, including acute nephritis, and low in chronic Bright's
disease.[29] Because it was so easy to obtain, the value was often used
without other chemical or physical determinations as a quick index
of health and disease.[30] Even in the mid-nineteenth century the
urinometer was at times considered important enough to be carried
along on home visits.[31]

Authorities claimed that these two tests, color and specific gravity, along with the twenty-four-hour quantity, were the most important tests to be done on urine.[32] How consistently were the color and
specific gravity recorded for those instances at the Pennsylvania
Hospital and the New York Hospital when there was a urinalysis
performed? Figures 3.4 and 3.5 show how often these attributes, as
well as two others, were recorded for patients in these two hospitals.

PENNSYLVANIA HOSPITAL

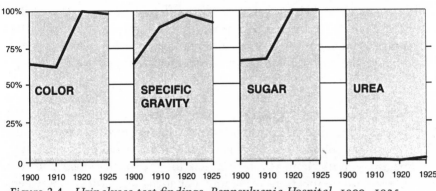

Figure 3.4   *Urinalyses test findings, Pennsylvania Hospital, 1900–1925.*

NEW YORK HOSPITAL

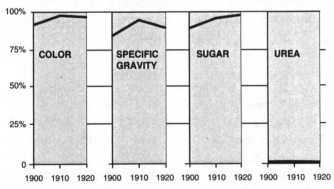

Figure 3.5   *Urinalyses test findings, New York Hospital, 1900–1920.*

At the Pennsylvania Hospital, in 1900, color and specific gravity were recorded about two out of every three times that a urinalysis was done. Over the next twenty-five years there was a striking increase in the consistency with which the tests results were recorded. After considering two more types of urine tests I shall explore why the color and specific gravity were described with increasing regularity. For now it should simply be noted that the shift cannot be due to any change in the technology associated with doing the test. Color is ascertained simply by looking at the urine, and the method of measuring specific gravity did not significantly change between 1900 and 1925.[33]

At the New York Hospital we see a different pattern. Most of the time that the urine was examined in 1900 the color and specific gravity were recorded, and this finding shows far less variation over the period of the study than for the Pennsylvania Hospital.

Sugar

Measuring urinary sugar provides a contrasting example to measuring urinary color and specific gravity. Unlike the case for color and specific gravity, both the techniques for measuring sugar and the therapeutic implications of finding it changed dramatically between 1900 and 1925. Sugar was long recognized as an abnormal substance in the urine, perhaps most characteristic of patients with diabetes. During much of the nineteenth century several methods for measuring sugar were available to the practitioner, each method having its own advantages and disadvantages, the accuracy of each a subject of debate.[34] Perhaps because of these methods' impracticalities, experienced clinicians might not actually measure urinary sugar at all, even if they were prone to testing the urine for other substances.[35] Despite the lack of standard methods, most guides to urinalysis recommended measuring sugar, because knowing if sugar in the urine was elevated, and approximately how much, was thought to be important for patient care.[36] The precise methodological details of so much concern to chemists were thought to be of doubtful clinical relevance, in part because medical practitioners could accept a lower standard of accuracy than was necessary for scientific investigators.[37]

As illustrated in figures 3.4 and 3.5, urinary sugar was measured often in 1900. Between 1900 and 1925, the medical literature described several new tests for measuring urinary and blood sugar. These new methods may have increased physicians' desire and ability to do the tests. A more important reason for paying attention to the importance of sugar in many bodily fluids, however, was an increased interest in diabetes, an interest that intensified after the discovery of insulin.[38]

Even before insulin, diabetes was one of the diseases for which monitoring of the urine was held to be most important. Consider, for example, a sixty-three-year-old nurse who was admitted to the Pennsylvania Hospital with diabetes on March 22, 1920.[39] Over the following two and a half weeks her urine was examined almost every single day, a total of fourteen times. She was not receiving insulin (it had not yet been described), so the tests were not being used to monitor the dosage of that new drug. Nonetheless, her caregivers were attempting as best they could to treat her diabetes, to lower her blood sugar. Most treatment efforts for diabetes before the advent of insulin therapy involved some aspect of dietary manipulation.[40] The success of the treatment regime was defined as the elimination of any trace of sugar from her urine. The urine test (certainly after the first one) was being used not for diagnosis but, rather, as a monitoring device, to track the status of her disease.

The discovery of insulin made measuring urinary sugar even more important than before. By 1925 insulin was routinely used to treat diabetic patients at major U.S. hospitals. Physicians were still trying to figure out how best to use insulin: too little insulin would not bring the blood sugar down low enough, and the patient would be at risk for dehydration and infection; too much insulin would cause a too severe lowering of the blood sugar, and the patient would be at risk for seizures, coma, or death.[41] Changes in diet or exercise would lead to changes in the blood sugar, which were difficult to predict. Moreover, the insulin preparations themselves were not well standardized, so that even for a single patient the response to a given dose of insulin was inconsistent. Blood sugar would be the ideal parameter to follow, but measurements of blood sugar were difficult. Urinary sugar could provide a useful proxy for blood sugar and could help physicians decide on a daily, patient-by-patient basis, how to treat persons with diabetes. In 1925 many patients with diabetes were having their urine tested daily for sugar.[42] Perhaps as a result of increased attention to diabetes, perhaps as a result of the efficiency movement, probably as a consequence of both, physicians measured sugar in the urine with increasing consistency. As was the case for color and specific gravity, the consistency with which blood sugar was reported increased between 1900 and 1925 at the Pennsylvania Hospital, when 100 percent of all urinalyses recorded the presence or absence of sugar; in 1920 at the New York Hospital 98 percent did.

Urea

But the history of urine tests is more than merely the gradual, seemingly inevitable inclusion of scientific tests in clinical practice. The textbooks and laboratory handbooks of the period are replete with literally hundreds of recommended tests—tests that, despite their basis in the very finest in scientific theory and research, seem rarely to be done in practice. One example of the split between science and practice is measurement of urinary urea. Urea was known to be a normal product of tissue metabolism. Some key nineteenth-century studies of the kidney and of the urine had focused on the measurement of urea in the urine and in the blood of patients thought to be suffering from kidney disease.[43] By around the turn of the twentieth century urinary urea was thought to be characteristically elevated in some conditions, such as most febrile conditions (but not in yellow fever), and diminished in other conditions, such as cholera and many kidney diseases, in which case the measurement of urea was thought useful for both diagnosis and prognosis.[44] Summary tables of urinalyses in general medical journals, which might include only five characteristics of the urine, sometimes included a column for recording the measurement of urea, suggesting that the authors (or editors) thought that urinary urea was important.[45] Methods for measuring urea are found in almost all guides to examining urine from the latter third of the nineteenth century. As was the case with sugar, manuals often gave the practitioner a choice between several different tests, some pointing out that, whereas the practitioner usually sought out the "more rapid and easy method," a more exact (and more difficult) method would give more reliable conclusions.[46] In 1912 measurement of urinary urea was held to be "one of the three most important tests to be performed" (the other two were albumin and sugar).[47] Thus, the test was widely discussed. But how often was it actually done?

Despite authors' exhortations, and a physiological rationale, essentially nobody was measuring urea in urine. Only 0.6 percent of the patients had their urea measured at the Pennsylvania Hospital and at the New York Hospital (a total of 16 out of the 2,562 patients in the sample). In one instance, a twenty-seven-year-old male laborer with acute creosote poisoning had urea measured; we might surmise that his physicians were concerned about metabolic damage to his kidneys.[48] Another patient was admitted for what was thought to be a malignant bladder tumor, although the physicians eventually concluded that it was not. Here, perhaps the urea was thought to provide general diagnostic information about the urinary tract. On the other hand, what are we to make of the two patients admitted for inguinal hernia repair who had their urea measured? Or the fifteen-year-old boy admitted with bronchitis?[49] For most of the patients, as with these, the medical rationale for measuring urea is not obvious and cannot easily be inferred.

Perhaps some physicians were simply partial to measuring urea, as a personal idiosyncrasy. Of the fifteen patients at the Pennsylvania Hospital who had urinary urea measured, four had the same attending physician, Dr. Charles Mitchell; although this data is suggestive that he was more interested in examining urea than his colleagues, Dr. Mitchell accounted for a very high fraction of the patients admitted to the hospital; 13 percent of 1920 admissions and 15 percent of those in 1925.[50] With such a small number of patients having their urinary urea measured, one cannot tell if, in fact, he was any more likely than his colleagues to ask about the urinary urea.

Perhaps the physicians at these two hospitals simply did not believe that urea was important. Perhaps the techniques were too difficult, although there was far more agreement about how to measure urinary urea than there was about how to measure urinary sugar. In any event, measuring urinary urea was not a test of any significance at the Pennsylvania Hospital or the New York Hospital in the first two and a half decades of the twentieth century.

It is certainly possible that urea was, in fact, more often measured at institutions other than the two I have chosen to study in detail. In some settings urinary urea was said to be frequently tested for, although it was generally useless.[51] Studies of medical practice at other hospitals and in other practices could help us ascertain to what extent physicians anywhere routinely measured urinary urea. If some physicians did so, it will be important to understand the reasons for the differences. In the meantime the example of urinary urea should remind us, once again, that published descriptions of test procedures may not be associated with actual application of those procedures—of the differences between science as symbol and science as method, between theory and practice.

More Tools, More Tests

Many other tests to examine urine were proposed. Some were based on the direct examination of urine under the microscope. For these tests a new machine, the centrifuge, proved extremely useful. Because the centrifuge was not only used to aid in examining urine but was also central for many other laboratory tests, it will briefly be described here, along with the rationale for its use in examining urine.

Most normal urine appears clear. Nonetheless, the fluid contains solid particles, visible under a microscope, but there are so few particles for the amount of urine that to examine those particles some method for concentrating the substances of interest is needed. During most of the nineteenth century, physicians who wished to examine the urinary particles did so by letting the urine stand in a tube for a period of time, often twenty-four hours. The solids gradually fell to the bottom of the tube, the urine was decanted, and the material that remained in the bottom of the tube was referred to as the urinary sediment. Under a microscope one could see in the sediment crystals, blood cells, microorganisms, and collections of material called "casts."

This technique for concentrating the urinary solids presented a problem that was well-known at the turn of the twentieth century. Much of the solid matter found in urine will dissolve long before twenty-four hours have passed. Preservatives could be added to the urine, but the physician still had to wait a full day before an examination could be made. The centrifuge, a device that spun the fluid in order to concentrate solid material, allowed physicians to examine urinary sediment immediately after the specimen was obtained. The centrifuge quickly came to be seen as an important device for scientific medical practice; after the microscope it was said to be the next item that physicians would wish to acquire for their laboratory. It would increase the physician's "efficiency," a term that, as we have seen in chapter 2, carried with it a good deal of implicit meaning.[52] Some centrifuges were operated by hand, such as the rather basic, low-speed device shown in figure 3.6. These were satisfactory if they were to be used only for urinalysis but would not be sufficient for other tests, such as blood tests. Better, if possible, to obtain one that could run on electricity (often designed to run on both AC and

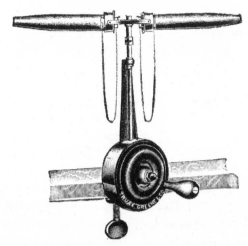

Figure 3.6   *Urinary centrifuge. From Charles Traux*, The Mechanics of Surgery *(Chicago: Hammond, Press, 1899), 39.*

DC current) and could be used for blood and sputum in addition to urine.[53] If the physician could not purchase a centrifuge, he or she might be able to make one from scrap, perhaps using a discarded electric fan motor.[54] Using the centrifuge, it was far easier to detect small amounts of solid constituents in the urine than it had been with earlier techniques. (We shall consider this widely used laboratory device for assessing the red cell content of blood in chap. 6.)

UNDERSTANDING THE CHANGING URINALYSIS

The urinalysis appears to be the first "laboratory" test to be applied many times to the same patient. Why did practitioners begin to use the urinalysis this way? I shall consider several possible explanations. Between 1900 and 1925 the test may have started to be seen as a more sensitive diagnostic device, perhaps as new ways of testing urine were described. Physicians had access to new treatment methods which might have made looking at urine more relevant. The way that most U.S. physicians were trained also changed. The modern hospital was invented as a new place for patient care, a place in which a new technology of hospital charts and systems was introduced. Finally, the urinalysis, when done many times, was used as a device to monitor the patient's clinical status. Each of these changes played a role in a more general transformation, not only of the urinalysis but of many other laboratory tests as well.

An Improved Diagnostic Device: New Methods of Care

Doing many urinalyses on a single patient could help physicians make more accurate diagnoses or arrive at difficult diagnoses by at least two mechanisms.[55] First, improved techniques could have enabled clinicians to detect abnormal substances in minute concentrations: if those substances were characteristic of a particular disease, then their presence would establish a diagnosis; if the substance were difficult to detect, the chances of finding it might be increased by doing the examination several times.[56] But, as the example of urea demonstrates, one cannot predict changing patterns of use based solely on the scientific rationale for a test's application.

Another reason to do multiple tests for improved diagnostic accuracy is that urine is a primary means by which the body excretes metabolic substances and that "the variations in nutrition and waste are accurately recorded in the urine hour by hour."[57] Thus, findings from just one examination might not be representative of the patient's condition. Only by looking at changes over time could the physician use urine to make an accurate diagnosis. Rather than doing multiple tests, some experts advised another way of summarizing the urine over a long period of time, by taking aliquots from a sample of the urine produced by a patient over twenty-four hours.[58] Both of these rationales for improving the diagnostic usefulness of urinalysis would imply that, once a diagnosis was made, the role of the urinalysis was over. The physician would know the proper treatment, and the urine need not be looked at again as a diagnostic device. This does not appear to have been the case for the urinalyses at the Pennsylvania Hospital and the New York Hospital after about 1920. In most instances the diagnosis was arrived at early in the patient's hospital stay, and the urine examinations did not abate.

The new use of the urinalysis might have been necessary as a result of having new methods of treatment available. The prototypical example of such a disease would be diabetes. Yet although diabetes may have been an important exemplar for the measurement of urinary or blood sugar, especially after the discovery of insulin, it cannot be used to explain much of the increase in urinalysis: the trend toward consistent and frequent measurement of urinary sugar existed well before 1925, and patients with diabetes made up a very small proportion of patients admitted to the hospital.[59]

Physician Training: A New Site for Care

Although both the New York Hospital and the Pennsylvania Hospital had long employed trainees to help care for patients, by the late nineteenth century these physicians had been educated in a new medical world, one in which the laboratory had become familiar territory. During the early twentieth century allopathic medical schools in the United States were coming to dominate the scene, and these places were coming to emphasize science as a means of knowing and of teaching.[60] Medical colleges started routinely to build teaching laboratories and to employ people to work in them. Rather than simply reading and listening in the lecture hall, by soon after the turn of the twentieth century most medical students received active training at the laboratory bench in how to examine urine. Perhaps they received too much training in the subject; the noted Boston physician Richard Cabot claimed that some Harvard graduates "always knew how to examine urine, even when they knew little else."[61] Nonetheless, British observers praised the practical instruction that U.S. medical students received in laboratory analysis and attempted to emulate the practice in their own country.[62]

Although part of the rationale for building laboratories had to do with allowing some students to join their mentors in doing original research, as was the case in Europe, part of the mission also had to do with a desire to teach laboratory techniques to all students. As the historian Robert E. Kohler points out, U.S. laboratories were, in fact, something quite different from those across the Atlantic. Whereas the European laboratories were intended for a select few, the U.S. version was intended for all students.[63] These new laboratories were meant to have an impact on all medical practitioners. Increasing numbers of young trainees, both medical students and house officers, arrived at the bedside already quite comfortable with the concepts and procedures of the laboratory.

Trainees and patients found themselves meeting more and more frequently in the hospital. This, too, had an enormous impact on the practicality with which laboratory tests could be done, particularly

the possibility of examining a patient's urine many times. True, practitioners could do some tests in the patient's home, such as observe
the urine's color. Even more complicated tests could be done in the
home using a portable centrifuge or microscope, although this made
the issue more difficult. But for tests requiring complicated laboratory equipment, patients seen at home who required a laboratory
test, or their specimens, had to travel to a medical facility. Issues of
transportation—still a problem even in the late twentieth century—
were even more of a concern in the early twentieth century. Without
an automobile patients had to travel on foot, horseback, or some
form of public transportation. None of these were especially easy
ways of reaching a medical office in order to have a test done multiple times. The hospital, however, was a place in which physicians
could do multiple urinalyses within a short period of time, and many
more patients than ever before were being admitted to the hospital.

Moreover, that urine could often be examined only a few yards
from the patient's bedside. Clinical laboratories gradually became a
routine feature of hospital design, placed on the wards so that clinicians could move easily from the patient's bedside to the laboratory
bench. Staff was available to assist in doing the work. Nurses could
collect samples at any hour of the day or night. House officers
and (later) nurses could do the tests. Interns were expected to be able
to do basic laboratory tests, including those on urine.[64] The two
hospitals selected for this study were near the forefront of the new,
laboratory-based approach to medicine and had clinical laboratories
before other, less well-established hospitals did.

Who was to claim expertise in the laboratory? Ward laboratories
allowed physicians to preserve diagnostic tests within the work domain of the clinically active physician.[65] Practicing physicians took
great pains to point out that laboratory findings could not be properly interpreted absent the perspectives of those clinicians who were
actually caring for the patient. For example, urine that was reported
from the laboratory as typical of chronic kidney disease might, in
fact, simply be urine from a patient known to have typhoid fever
who was drinking large quantities of water.[66] The criticisms went
both ways: clinicians' tales of misinterpretation were matched by
those of laboratory experts, who related the difficulties when poorly
trained practitioners attempted to do their own diagnostic procedures in the laboratory.[67]

Eventually, improved communication using the automobile, train, telegraph, and telephone could bridge ever larger distances and thus allow rural practitioners to enjoy the benefits of a fully equipped urban clinical laboratory.[68] At least at the start, however, hospital laboratories were the easiest places to learn how best to examine urine or do multiple analyses.

A Monitoring Device

The urinalysis may have started as a diagnostic test, but between 1900 and 1925 it also became a way of documenting and understanding a person's changing clinical course. In one sense this kind of monitoring was quite old: frequently, both temperature and pulse were measured many times on the same patient, and these two parameters had been represented graphically for some time.[69] Yet the urinalysis was a different type of examination. It was the first fairly common test that involved taking a part of the living patient away, going into the laboratory, and studying that specimen with microscopes and test tubes. Moreover, the urinalysis was multidimensional: it provided a variety of results, including those related to color, appearance, and albumin, among others. The results were of several different types: some were qualitative, such as color; some were dichotomous (i.e., a substance was either present or absent), such as casts; and some were quantitative, such as levels of sugar.[70]

The urinalysis was becoming part of a new, scientific program, a program drawn from the newly asserted relevance of laboratory science for clinical medicine. Previously, a physician had assessed a patient's condition by talking to him or her, by listening to the patient's story, and, perhaps, by examining the patient. The urinalysis served as a part of an early wedge of a whole new systematic approach to assessing a patient's status. No longer would the patient's own assessment of his or her condition be most important. Instead, the laboratory would come to dominate the criteria by which a patient would be evaluated. Soon urinalyses were followed by blood counts, later by a whole host of chemical tests on blood and urine.

The urinalysis was not the first technology-based tool to provide information about patients. But it appears to have been the first to be used in a systematic attempt to follow patients over time. When a physician does a urinalysis on admission as a matter of routine, he or she is doing a ritual that provides information about a patient at a single moment. When a physician does multiple urinalyses throughout the course of a hospital stay, he or she is using the laboratory test as a means of monitoring a patient, as a means of obtaining information over a prolonged period of time. This is, in one sense, a way of improving diagnostic accuracy. But it represents more than that; it also reflects the use of laboratory tests as a means of assessing the changing nature of a patient, even when the diagnosis is already certain. For example, a fourteen-year-old schoolboy with acute nephritis was admitted to the Pennsylvania Hospital on September 2, 1920. His urine was examined no less than fifteen times within the first three weeks of his admission.[71] That physicians examined the urine of a patient with kidney disease is not surprising or new. The first urinalysis probably made the diagnosis. What is new is the intensity of the testing and the use of the testing not only as a ritual of admission or a diagnostic test, but as a monitoring device.

One might wonder if the analysis was done more often simply because the requirements to do the test were more available—because there were clinical laboratories close at hand as well as trainees who had learned how to do the test. Were that the only rationale, one might expect to see a general increase in the use of urinalysis for most patients, but such was not the case. The urinalysis was used more often on patients who were clinically most active, whose health was less stable. Whereas in 1900 urinalysis was done on almost every patient regardless of the severity of illness, by 1920 the tests were done on fewer patients. Yet the fall was not a random, across-the-board decrease. Not only did the number of urinalyses performed on each patient who had one increase; the urinalysis was more likely to be done on patients who were sickest.[72] An increase in the availability of laboratories or the numbers of medical students and other trainees cannot fully account for the increasing numbers of urine tests. They were done more times on patients who had a number of clinical problems.

STANDARDIZATION AND SPECIALIZATION

Physicians did urine tests within not only a changing world of scientific ideas and clinical treatments, but also within a changing world of medical systems for recording and transmitting information. Standardization and systematization within the increasingly factory-like hospital had an impact that reached from the level of adding machines and accounting methods to choices about what to do with a patient's urine. Hospital administrators tried to use the best possible way to record and communicate information within the hospital (as discussed in chap. 2). Using standardized forms for recording the results of many types of information became part of the daily routine. Those forms helped shape and define what kind of tests were to be done when someone examined the patient's urine.

Among the many possibilities, what should be measured? For some time nurses had occasionally recorded the daily amount of urine excreted by a given patient.[73] As we have seen, by the end of the nineteenth century there existed a long list of possible tests that *could* be included in a urinalysis but little guidance about the specific items that *ought* to be included in one.[74] The turn-of-the-century record reproduced in figure 2.4 shows the way that the urinalysis was usually recorded. The house officer simply wrote down whatever he or she chose to measure, and depending upon the setting and the individual doing the test, that could be a great deal or very little.

Forms could diminish that variation, guaranteeing (or at least strongly encouraging) both consistency and the accessibility of information.[75] The use of standardized forms for urinalysis provided one way of both increasing hospital efficiency—by insuring that information was recorded in the same place, the same way—and simultaneously defining precisely what constituted a proper urinalysis. Near the end of the nineteenth century a few books started to include forms on which to record urine examinations, and some began to list those elements of a complete urine analysis that ought to be done in every instance.[76] By 1920 almost all urinalyses done at both the New York Hospital and the Pennsylvania Hospital were being recorded on standardized forms, which guided the person performing them to conduct certain specific tests. At the Pennsylvania Hospital the use of forms went from none in 1909 to all but 1 of the 279 urinalyses in 1920 (99.6 percent) being recorded on a printed, standardized form that listed specific tests to be done. At the New York Hospital the increase was more gradual, from 40 percent in 1910 to 99 percent in 1920. The forms at the New York Hospital were printed and indicated specific items to be done, but, unlike those of the

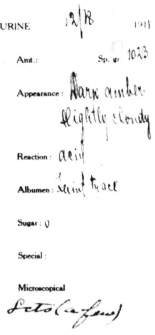

Figure 3.7 *Urinalysis form. From* Pennsylvania Hospital Case Records *196 (1912): 3165.*

Pennsylvania Hospital, they were not part of a general laboratory form.

The forms guided the physician to choose certain tests. At the Pennsylvania Hospital around 1911 the initial form (fig. 3.7) was introduced for urine alone. It was pasted into the patient record: one side listed the patient's name and the physician's name; the other side, shown here, prompted the person who did the test to note the date, amount, appearance, specific gravity, and reaction of the urine as well as the presence of albumin and sugar, anything "special," and whether a microscopic exam was done. On the form reproduced as figure 3.7, as on many others, not every blank was filled in. Later a summary sheet (fig. 3.8) again asked the physician to note the color, reaction, and specific gravity of the urine as well as the albumin and sugar. The microscopic examination now referred specifically to casts, blood cells, pus cells, urates, and phosphates. (The microscopic identification of urate crystals should not be confused with

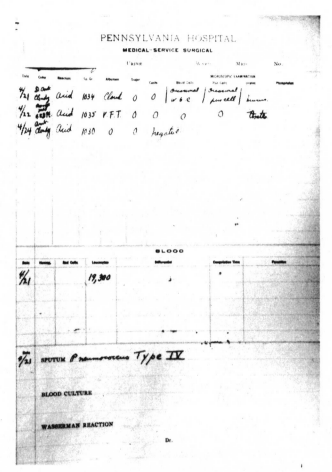

Figure 3.8   *General lab form. From* Pennsylvania Hospital Case Records *396 (1917): 3198.*

the chemical determination of urinary urea, which was described earlier.) Other lab tests were also recorded on the same form, gathering the process of pathological examination under the common heading of a single diagnostic laboratory.

What role did technology play in changing ideas about the urinalysis? Color, of course, is the ultimate in low-technology urinalysis. Forms, however, are an important technology, one that may have played an important role in defining the test. At the Pennsylvania Hospital once a form started to be used consistently—a form that indicated the color of the urine as an element to be noted—color was recorded with a great deal more regularity than before.

Specific gravity required technology in the form of an instrument, but one that was well-known by the turn of the twentieth century and one that did not change appreciably over the period of this study. The rate at which the specific gravity was measured went up markedly between 1900 and 1909, even when a specific form was generally not used to record the test results. But in 1920 and 1925 both color and specific gravity were recorded, essentially, each time the urine was examined. Thus, part of the change in clinical practice can be attributed to changes in the way that information was recorded; in these two instances change was not caused by the invention of any new type of laboratory equipment.

If forms were important determinants of practice, it would be useful to know more about how people made decisions about which tests to include on the forms. Some forms were described in nationally circulated journals; for example, those used at Bellevue Hospital in New York City were published in a 1900 volume of the *Journal of the American Medical Association (JAMA)*, including forms for reporting examinations of urine.[77] The forms list, among other items, color, specific gravity, and sugar (by several methods), but not urea. The forms used at the New York and Pennsylvania hospitals appear to have been specifically designed for use in those institutions, although they may have been patterned on nationally circulated models. Obviously, if forms routinely used elsewhere were different—that is, if they listed measurement of urea or the results of other tests that appeared to have been done rarely at these two hospitals—knowing whether physicians in these other settings actually did such tests would help us understand better the determinants of what constituted urinalysis.

The practice of doing urinalysis was clearly different at the New York and Pennsylvania hospitals. At the New York Hospital color, specific gravity, and sugar—three items routinely measured—were indicated in essentially all of the urinalyses from 1900 to 1920. The use of forms to record the test appears to have made little difference. At the Pennsylvania Hospital physicians behaved quite a bit differently. We are hard-pressed to come up with explanations for this difference in terms of diseases or in terms of the types of knowledge or equipment that were available to hospital practitioners in these two East Coast towns. The most likely reason for the difference, one that we will see again when we consider blood counts, is that the local environment, the local culture, was different in the two hospitals.

The fact that urea was not listed on the standard forms undoubtedly had something to do with the lack of attention to its measurement. But this cannot be the complete explanation, for urea was measured far less frequently than many other substances, such as sugar, even in 1900 and 1910, before standardized forms became commonplace.

CONCLUSION

By the third decade of the twentieth century there was growing concern that the value of urinalyses had become overrated. Some of the concern was based on questions about the ability of urinalysis to detect kidney disease. Output from the kidneys varies from hour to hour. Thus, some authors asserted, it made no sense to measure the urinary constituents quantitatively unless one was doing so on a complete, twenty-four-hour specimen.[78] Others pointed out further difficulties inherent in drawing inferences about kidney disease from urine, such as the fact that the urine is (usually) made by two kidneys and that abnormalities in one kidney (or in parts of one or both kidneys) may produce an abnormal urine that is not detected because the abnormal urine is mixed with the normal urine from the other kidney.[79] Other concerns were based on questions about the ability of urinalysis to detect specific diseases, diseases for which blood tests—which by the 1920s were becoming easier to use—may have given a better index of a patient's condition. The urinalysis began to be relegated by many physicians to the sidelines as a simple test whose results were rather uninteresting.

So, how are we to understand historically the humble urinalysis? In one of the more thoughtful works of medical history to appear in the recent past, Robert E. Kohler, working from the perspective of the clinical chemists, stated that by 1900 the "remarkable innovations" in microbiology "overshadowed the old craft of urinalysis."[80] In one sense they certainly did. It would have been hard for the urinalysis to compete with microbiology, a new science that had recently identified the specific agents responsible for much human death and disease. The same could be said of other breakthroughs. The newer, more self-consciously scientific and more dramatic innovations that I will consider in the following chapters, such as the blood count and, particularly, the x-ray machine, were seen at the beginning (as well as at the end) of the twentieth century as far more important, more meaningful elements in the way that medicine was practiced.

On the other hand, in one sense the "old craft of urine analysis" went away, and clinicians used the urinalysis in new and different ways from 1900 to 1925. One can explain some of the changing attention to urinalysis by the addition of new tests. Yet this explanation is not totally compelling, for several reasons. First, although some of the tests were new, or could be done with new methods, many were not; in fact, some of the most common features described in the urine, the color and the specific gravity, were quite old. Moreover, the tests required no equipment, in the case of color, or minimal and easily obtainable equipment, in the case of specific gravity.

Analyzing urine might have been linked to the scientific study of the human body. Although they were a prominent part of the mission to understand the meaning of human metabolism, some of the new tests that were being described appear to have had little application to clinical care. The authors of books about these new tests may not have concerned themselves with the clinical application of their techniques. For example, a 1900 text, which stated that it was written for general medical practitioners, included 167 densely packed pages on how to measure urine chemistry. It assured the clinician that "in ordinary clinical work the barometric pressure, as well as the tension of the aqueous vapor may be ignored."[81] There follows in this text a series of tables designed to correct for temperature. This would have been meaningless to most general practitioners and could actually be implemented only in the best-equipped laboratories. The section reads throughout like a difficult organic chemistry text and, in 1900, was unlikely to have been of much use (or interest) to most practitioners. Similar approaches can be found in many other books and articles.

That does not mean that descriptions in books and articles are unimportant. They obviously were important, to somebody, or else why would people have gone to such lengths to publish them? But patient records from the New York and the Pennsylvania hospitals suggest that those descriptions had little to do with the daily care of patients. Rather than asking why nobody was doing most of the tests, one could turn the question around and ask why there were so many books available and what difference they made. The answer may have something to do with a desire by the authors to appear scientific.[82]

A declining interest in writing about urine after 1900 may have been a response to increasing interest in other, newer, perhaps more scientific types of laboratory tests on other bodily fluids. Clinical investigators may have seen the urinalysis as part of a new scientific program, one that would move eventually from colorimetry and gasometry to a wide range of devices to investigate the acid-base status of blood or to study the electrolytes. What role did the urinalysis play in this transformation? It has been eclipsed as a marker of scientific, laboratory medicine. In the late twentieth century, despite the fact that the urinalysis is the second most common medical test, done on almost forty million people per year in the United States, it hardly stands as a marker of medical progress.[83] Yet it is interesting to note the extent to which the urinalysis was used for a time as a symbol of scientific progress early in the twentieth century. When the blood count (which I shall discuss in chap. 6) was first being promoted for clinical practice, the urinalysis was presented as an explicit model of its importance.[84] Time and time again, when people were asked to talk about the role of laboratory medicine or pathology, before moving on to other forms of tests they referred to the importance and usefulness of the urine analysis.[85]

Why did people pay such attention to urine? In part, because by the 1910s and 1920s there was an ever-increasing list of tests and examinations that could be done on body substances, including urine. But that does not explain why they paid attention to urine, when many of the same tests were being applied to blood, sputum, and other fluids, even to solid pathological specimens. Moreover, many of these people who continued to refer to urine were laboratory directors, for whom the relative inconvenience (for the physician) and pain (for the patient) of a venipuncture or other invasive procedure would matter little, once the specimen was ready for analysis at the laboratory bench. Instead, they continued to refer to the analysis of urine as "the first step in the way leading to a medical laboratory."[86] Clearly, for a time the idea of the humble urinalysis, both ancient and modern, resonated to early twentieth-century commentators, even if it was soon to be eclipsed by other ideas and tests.

Still, the urinalysis had changed, even if practitioners ignored most of the published material about it. The story of urinalysis shows that one can have a new medical technology—in this case, a new urinalysis—without many (or any) new techniques or machines. Changes in the patterns of how the urinalyses were applied in hospitals presaged some of the more important changes in medical practice. Specifically, urinalysis served as a model for the continuous monitoring of patients and as a substrate for the application of routinized, standardized procedures to medical examinations. From 1900 to 1925 this very old test helped physicians become familiar with the idea of doing multiple, systematic, standardized tests on their patients. As the meaning of the urinalysis changed, patients probably did not notice much difference; their experience with the medical world was little affected by either the theory or the practice of urinalysis. But that was not the case for the next diagnostic technology I will consider, the x-ray machine.

4

CLINICAL USE OF THE
X-RAY MACHINE
The Newest Technology at the
Oldest Hospitals

Late in the winter of 1895 a German professor of physics, Wilhelm Conrad Röntgen, decided to report on some interesting findings. He had discovered that by passing an electrical current through a partially evacuated cathode-ray tube he could produce a new form of radiation. This new radiation could penetrate solid objects, and it could be used to make a photographic image.[1] Röntgen called the new rays "x rays" because he did not know what they were made of and sent in a paper describing his findings to the Physico-Medical Society of Würzburg on December 28, 1895.[2] On New Year's Day, 1896, Röntgen mailed a picture of his wife's hand taken with the new rays to a number of his colleagues—further dramatic evidence that he had devised a means of seeing within the human body.[3] Röntgen's findings shocked and amazed the world. His pictures, as well as others taken with these new rays, soon appeared in both popular and technical magazines and newspapers. To be able to see within the human body had a profound impact on both the medical and lay communities, on medical thought, and on fundamental ideas about the human body. It is difficult to overestimate the profound impact the invention of the x ray had on the broadest possible scope of humankind.

In chapter 5 I shall discuss public reaction to images created by the new x-ray machine; here I shall explore the use of this new technology within the hospital walls and shall briefly compare its uptake with that of another new technology, the electrocardiogram (ECG) machine.[4] I shall explore how the clinical application of the x-ray machine was related to the people who made the images and to their positions within the hospital organization. To do so I will consider both the published medical literature and evidence provided by patient records from the Pennsylvania Hospital and the New York Hospital.[5]

Soon after Röntgen's description, x-ray machines appeared throughout the United States. The apparatus needed to produce the amazing new images was inexpensive, initially costing fifty dollars or less.[6] Because cathode-ray tubes were often found in scientific laboratories, and photographic plates were a common commodity, it was reasonably easy to assemble the equipment needed to produce pictures using the new technique.[7] Not even two full years after the initial invention of the machine, the Pennsylvania Hospital, like many other U.S. hospitals, purchased an x-ray machine, the symbol of advanced scientific medicine.[8] The New York Hospital also purchased an x-ray machine soon after its invention.[9] What is somewhat surprising, given the widespread public attention paid to this amazing new tool, is that for at least a decade following its purchase the machine played little or no role in patient care. In brief, although the x ray had an immediate and widespread impact on medical ideas, its incorporation into medical practice was far slower than the medical literature would suggest. Moreover, routine use of the x ray depended on the creation of a new hospital structure, the origins of which were sketched in chapter 2.

On one level the x-ray machine would appear to have been quickly accepted by medical practitioners. The x ray was widely described in the medical literature as being a useful aid for diagnosis, particularly for identifying foreign bodies and detecting abnormal conditions of bones. It was, by the end of 1896, the subject of over 1,044 articles and 49 books.[10] People claimed that no hospital could provide adequate care without one of the new machines.[11] Not only was the use of x rays written about in books and journals; it was also a common topic for presentation at local medical meetings and a subject about which hospitals boasted at world's fair exhibits.[12] Around the turn of the twentieth century one could not go far in the description of medical care at any level without coming across some comment on the amazing new x-ray machine.

FRACTURES

Despite all the public attention, how much was the x-ray machine actually used? To answer this question it may be best to examine not only the total use of the x ray but also its use for a specific diagnosis. Among specific clinical conditions broken bones—fractures—offer a particularly useful choice for two reasons (see fig. 4.1)[13] First, they

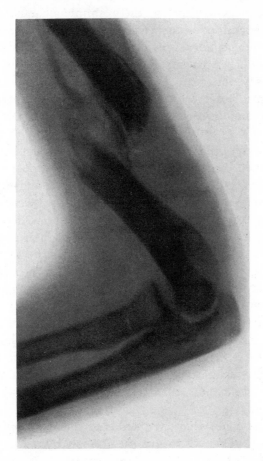

Figure 4.1   *Broken bone. From Lewis A. Stimson. A Practical Treatise on Fractures and Dislocations, 3d ed. (New York: Lea Brothers, 1900), facing p. 36.*

were a common problem; thus, both clinical examples and discussion in the published literature are easy to locate. Second, deciding whether to use an x ray for diagnosis of a possible broken bone was important not only for the physician but also for the patient.[14] Prior to the invention of the x ray, fractures were usually diagnosed by manual manipulation. Signs held to be pathognomonic of a fracture (i.e., to definitively establish the diagnosis) included deformity and abnormal mobility—that is, the movement of pieces of bone that would otherwise be solid. Another helpful diagnostic sign was crepitus, assessed by, literally, moving the bone so that the "crackling and grating of multiple fragments" of broken pieces of bone could be appreciated, either by the examiner's hands, or, occasionally, by the examiner's ears.[15] Scraping together the damaged fragments of bone was not without risk. By moving the broken pieces about, one could further damage an already injured limb.[16] Moreover, needless to say, this type of examination was quite uncomfortable for the patient. Observers saw the x-ray plate as a means of sparing a person the unnecessary "pain and agony" that usually accompanied the diagnosis of a fracture by standard methods of examination.[17] The x ray could also help patients by establishing that a bone was not broken. Because it detected "even the most minute fracture," it could exclude the possibility of a fracture and prevent people from spending unnecessary time in bed. The tool worked well: any problems that might appear were the fault of unskilled operators.

Wartime persuaded early users of x rays of their medical value. Conflicts in 1896 and 1897 convinced European military forces that an x-ray examination could help make the diagnosis of fractures and foreign bodies, both of which were found with some regularity upon the battlefield.[18] The U.S. Army also found x rays useful during the war with Spain in 1898.[19]

X rays were soon used not only in military conflicts but also in the civilian conflicts that took place in courtrooms. In what may have been the first such case, a court in Montreal allowed use of x-ray evidence in April 1896. Other courts soon followed suit, one allowing x-ray evidence to be introduced in December 1896 to show the conditions of bones that are "entirely hidden from the eye of the surgeon."[20] Demonstrations of how an x-ray machine works were presented to the jury, and a large crowd of onlookers gathered to see the x-ray photographs.

Wars and courts both reflected and created a general belief in the value of the x-ray image—the idea, stated as early as 1896, that x rays provided a means of "definite and exact diagnosis" of conditions such as fractures.[21] Less than two full years since Röntgen's original description, in October of 1897, a surgeon claimed to have seen five thousand pictures taken by the new machine.[22] By 1899 authors could claim that "it is probably unnecessary at this late date to assert, that the Röntgen-rays have proved to be of inestimable value in the diagnosis and treatment of fractures."[23] By 1900 the use of x rays to diagnose fractures was well described in many standard medical works.[24] One of the first major texts specifically devoted to fractures was dedicated in 1900 to "William Conrad Röntgen, without whose discovery much of this book could not have been written."[25] By 1905 one could claim that for a surgeon to fail to use the x ray "either shows his ignorance of a valuable modern method or his willful neglect of his patient's interests."[26] Radiologists outside of the most prominent teaching hospitals spoke easily of x rays as an "absolute necessity" for fracture work and stated that one might "almost as soon do without splints as without a Röntgenogram."[27] Even in country hospital settings people wanted to have a rudimentary x-ray apparatus available.[28]

But was uptake of the x ray really that rapid? True, the x ray was eventually seen as essential for the diagnosis of broken bones. This has perhaps led some historians to overlook the process by which the x ray came to be widely used.[29] Instead, most historians have focused on written evidence in the published literature and so speak of the unprecedented "rapid acceptance" of the new technology; others have concluded that "the use of X-rays in the study of fractures . . . led to an abrupt change in the method[s] of treating these injuries."[30]

After 1895, however, there were voices that remained skeptical for some time about the value of the x ray for patient care. Some medical experts were enthusiastic about its possibilities, particularly for localizing foreign bodies, such as needles and bullets. Yet when President McKinley was shot in the fall of 1901 his surgeons elected not to use an x-ray machine to locate the bullet and were widely praised for their restraint.[31] Other clinicians tried to temper the enthusiasm for the x ray by claiming that it rarely added information of practical importance which could not be obtained by other means.[32] Their skepticism was greatest for diagnosing fractures.

After all, the surgeon's techniques were well established, based on "methods of diagnosis and reduction [which had] evolved through centuries of observation and investigation."[33] Physicians had for some time been trained in a "*tactus eruditus* [that] is certainly a delicate and reliable sense in investigating fractures."[34] With adequate knowledge of the relevant anatomy, even fractures of joints that were difficult to examine, such as the elbow, could be diagnosed without the x ray.[35]

Even among those who advocated widespread use of the x ray for the diagnosis of fractures, there was still a sense of the value of physical examination and a clearly expressed reluctance to declare that an instrumental examination would always be superior to the best-trained clinician. Having claimed that it was unnecessary to assert the value of roentgen rays, as this was already obvious to all, the authors of one paper go on to claim that "no one will for a moment suppose that the vacuum-tube and induction-coil [which produced the x rays] will, or ever can, displace the sense of touch guided by a well-balanced and experienced mind." The outstanding physical examination is not just based on a superior sense of touch; it is an examination guided by superior judgment and intellect. But the mind can be fooled, for, of course, "there are many cases of comparatively slight or obscure injuries that may easily be overlooked." This would seem to be arguing for universal use of the x-ray examination, but the final sentence reveals that the truly exceptional clinician need not rely on the rays, because these slight or obscure injuries would not be overlooked by "a man of very extensive experience or exceptional abilities."[36] In the final analysis bedside diagnostic acumen reigned supreme over the x ray.[37]

Even if useful, an x-ray apparatus was not always available. Waiting for an x-ray image to be taken would subject the patient to unnecessary delay and discomfort.[38] If the machine was not close at hand—a likely proposition—traveling to a site where an x-ray machine was located would require transportation via either automobile or rail or, more likely, on foot or on horseback. The first U.S. census to reveal more than 50 percent of the population living in urban areas was that of 1920, and for purposes of that census the definition of *urban* encompassed all people who lived in towns of more than two thousand people. It is unlikely that many communities of fewer than two thousand people had an x-ray machine or even that many two or three times that size were able to support the use of such a machine. Thus, for the first few decades of the century most Americans who were unfortunate enough to suffer a broken limb probably did not do so within easy reach of an x-ray machine. For them the trip to have an x-ray image taken would lead to more pain and, potentially, more disability.

An American Surgical Association Committee charged with examining the medicolegal relations of x rays concluded in 1900 that x rays need not be taken in every instance of a fracture.[39] This conclusion must, of course, be read within the professional context of an association report. Had the American Surgical Association come to any other conclusion, it might have obliged each of its members to obtain access to an x-ray machine. This could have been difficult for members who did not live in a major urban area. In its report the committee noted concern over the seeming plethora of lawsuits based solely or primarily on radiological evidence.

As late as 1916, again in relation to the law, a surgical journal asserted that x rays were not needed in all cases of fractures.[40] The argument had to do, in part, with the professional expertise of medical practitioners and the fact that a competent physician, particularly a rural practitioner, did not need to call in a "special consultant," such as an x-ray specialist, for all difficult cases. Two other arguments in this article presage late twentieth-century concerns about the effects of medical malpractice suits. First, it was claimed that many x rays were taken not from medical necessity but, rather, out of fear of lawsuits. This type of argument has been recreated near the end of the century in concerns about the ordering of expensive, unnecessary tests, so-called defensive medicine. Second, the article concludes with a not-very-well-veiled threat that, if the x ray is held by the courts to be essential for care of fractures, "the prospect of litigation will prevent those most competent from undertaking the care and treatment of cases of this character." Again, this concern is being recreated in the 1990s, as some obstetricians, viewing increasingly expensive malpractice insurance premiums, are electing not to deliver babies.

THE NEWEST TECHNOLOGY AT THE
OLDEST U.S. HOSPITALS

By 1900 most major urban hospitals in the United States owned an
x-ray machine.[41] There patients had, at least, the potential for having the machine used for diagnosis. Moreover, those patients might
be a group of people for whom the x ray would be particularly useful.
Although some hospitals had by 1900 started to see an influx of
paying, middle-class patients, most patients admitted to large, urban
hospitals were similar to those who had traditionally sought care
there throughout the nineteenth century:[42] they were, some people
said, "somewhat below the average of intelligence," and such patients tended to wait for a long period of time before seeking appropriate medical care.[43] This belief could produce a self-fulfilling
prophecy. If physicians believed that their patients were unable to
provide a reliable history of their injuries and symptoms, those
physicians would probably not devote as much time and effort
toward obtaining a history from their patients. The x-ray image
might be particularly useful if it could provide diagnostic information without requiring active patient participation. The x ray could
tell the truth, even when the patient could (or would) not. Even
when a patient might be unable to recall an injury, the x ray could
reveal, for example, fragments of lead which would reveal that the
person had been shot.[44]

How much was the x ray used for hospitalized patients? If we wish
to know how and when the x ray became a routine part of medical
care in hospitals, we may find it useful to once again turn to case
records from the Pennsylvania Hospital, near the docks in Philadelphia. There, at the turn of the twentieth century, it was common for
people, usually men, to be brought in with trauma, often suffering
from encounters with tools and traffic of the newly industrializing
city.[45] Despite the fact that the hospital owned an x-ray machine and
that trauma accounted for four of the five most common surgical
diagnoses, in a sample of six hundred records taken from Pennsylvania Hospital case histories of 1897, I found no mention of x-ray use.[46]
A more systematic analysis of records in 1900 from both the Pennsylvania and the New York hospitals confirms the initial impression,
that the x ray was at first used very infrequently.

Table 4.1 *X-ray Use at Pennsylvania and New York Hospitals*
(as a Percentage of Patients Having an X Ray Taken)

	All patients	Excluding Patients Admitted with Diseases of the Tonsils	Patients with Fractures only
	PENNSYLVANIA HOSPITAL		
1900	1.31	1.33	8.7
	(.426–3.02)	(.434–3.08)	(1.01–28.0)
1909	6.97	8.19	50
	(4.68–9.91)	(5.51–11.6)	(26.0–74.0)
1920	16.78	22.02	100
	(13.4–20.6)	(17.7–26.8)	(76.8–1.00)
1925	25.25	32.54	85.7
	(21.0–29.8)	(27.2–38.2)	(57.1–98.2)
	NEW YORK HOSPITAL		
1900	0.52	0.52	4.35
	(.063–1.87)	(.063–1.88)	(.110–21.9)
1910	8.18	8.38	24
	(5.6–11.3)	(5.8–11.6)	(9.35–45.1)
1920	19.39	23.88	83.33
	(13.6–26.2)	(16.9–32.0)	(35.9–99.6)

Note: 95 percent confidence intervals are given in parentheses

Table 4.1 shows the percentage of people who had an x-ray examination done at the New York and the Pennsylvania hospitals, with 95 percent confidence intervals given in parentheses. The percentage is shown in three different ways. The first column gives the percentage of the entire patient population in each hospital which had an x-ray image taken. This number reflects the likelihood that a patient admitted to the hospital would have had an x-ray image taken. As discussed in chapter 2, however, by 1920 a major portion of the patients admitted to hospitals were admitted solely for procedures upon their tonsils or adenoids. These people were typically admitted for only a day or two, and very few of them had an x ray taken. The likelihood of patients admitted to the hospital for reasons other than disease of their tonsils and adenoids (and this includes most adults) having an x-ray image taken is therefore given in the second column.

The effect of this correction is to raise the overall percentage of patients who had x rays in 1920 and 1925.[47]

The patterns for these two groups of people are remarkably similar at the two hospitals. In 1900, when the equipment was still quite new, very few people had an x-ray image taken. About a decade later having an x ray taken was still a rather unusual event for the general patient population. Fewer than one out of every ten patients admitted had any experience with the machine, and those images that were made were often done out of curiosity, not for patient care. In one instance, an unfortunate, malnourished, blind, and "mentally deficient" nine-year-old boy with cyanotic congenital heart disease had x rays taken of his enlarged heart and of his deformed, "spatula-like" fingers.[48] The examination was performed to see if the finger deformity was bone (it was not) and to see how the heart appeared with the new instrument (it was enlarged). The x-ray image had no impact on the patient's therapy or prognosis, nor was the x ray taken as part of any clinical research. Rather, the machine was used to answer a simple structural question: What was the nature of the deformed fingers? It was used, in other words, not for patient care but out of medical curiosity.

By 1920 a significant number of people were having an x-ray examination done during their hospital stay. Excluding patients who were admitted for a simple procedure upon their tonsils, at both the Pennsylvania Hospital and the New York Hospital more than one out of every five patients had an x-ray image taken. By 1925, at the Pennsylvania Hospital, that number had risen to almost one in three. Clearly, by 1925 the x ray had become a familiar part of the hospital scene, in ways that it had not been in years past.

There could be many reasons for this increase in the numbers of patients having x-ray examinations done. An important factor might have been a change in the types of patients admitted to the hospital. We have already partially corrected for this variable by eliminating from the discussion a special case: patients admitted for diseases of the tonsils and adenoids. Let us now focus on use of the x ray for a diagnosis that was among the most widely cited early uses of the x-ray image, broken bones. By restricting our gaze to patients with a specific condition, one that had attracted widespread attention as being susceptible to x-ray diagnosis, we may sharpen our understanding of why and when the x ray became a part of routine patient care.

Of those patients diagnosed as having a fractured bone at the Pennsylvania Hospital in 1900, only 8.7 percent had an x-ray image taken. A similar percentage, 4.35 percent, is seen at the New York Hospital.[49] Although fewer than 10 percent had an x ray taken, not surprisingly, patients with broken bones had x rays done far more often than patients with other conditions. Still, in 1900, despite the fact that both of these well-respected hospitals owned an x-ray machine, and despite the fact that the medical literature was replete with descriptions of the machine's value for diagnosing broken bones, the vast majority of patients with broken limbs were not examined with the new ray. The slightly lower percentage of patients with fractures having an x-ray examination at the New York Hospital, as compared with the Pennsylvania Hospital, does not reach statistical significance, but one might speculate about possible differences. The New York Hospital had a reputation for particular skill in the treatment of fractures. Practitioners there might have held a higher estimation of their clinical diagnostic skills and, thus, would feel less need (or desire) to employ a new diagnostic instrument.[50]

About a decade later x-ray examination was still quite an unusual event for the general hospitalized patient, yet at both the Pennsylvania Hospital and the New York Hospital x rays were being used to diagnose fractures more often than they had been in 1900. About a quarter of those patients with broken bones at the New York Hospital and half of those at the Pennsylvania Hospital had an x ray taken to make or confirm a diagnosis. Nonetheless, the use of the x-ray image was not universally seen as a necessary test for patients with broken bones, including those with severe enough injuries to require surgical repair in the operating room.[51]

The issue of the appropriateness of x-ray examination for fractures made its way to the hospital's governing body. In 1914 the Pennsylvania Hospital Board of Managers considered the outpatient care of accident victims who had been seen without charge. They concluded that, "in justice to patients and also as the result of recent decisions, surgeons generally feel that all cases of fracture or suspected fracture should be examined by X-ray."[52]

Perhaps this type of discussion had an impact. World War I also influenced attitudes toward the use of x rays. By 1920 physicians at both hospitals seem to have decided that x-ray examination should be routine for diagnosing people with broken bones. In the sample of patients used for this book, of the only two people not to receive x rays for broken bones at the Pennsylvania Hospital in 1925, one was a sixty-five-year-old man with a fractured skull, a condition thought then (and now, at the end of the century) to be difficult to diagnose with x rays, and the other was an infant who was brought in after suffering trauma, including a broken leg, and who soon died, probably before an x-ray examination could be arranged. But the general practice in 1925, as at the end of the century, was routinely to obtain an x-ray examination for people with suspected broken bones.

CHANGING TIMES, CHANGING PRACTICES

Thus, between 1900 and 1925 there was an important change in the pattern of x-ray use, one that has persisted for at least seventy years. To explain this change we need to try to avoid thinking in terms of a "failure to recognize" something important, such as the value of an x-ray image for diagnosing fractures, simply because we now see such use as meaningful and obvious. Rather than attempting to explain why in 1900 physicians did not ask for an x-ray examination—and fall prey to the difficult task of trying to explain someone's lack of action—it may be more useful to consider why in 1910 and 1920 physicians decided that they did want to obtain an x ray. To do so, it may be useful to consider who was creating these images.[53]

At the Pennsylvania Hospital, from 1897 to 1909, the chief resident operated the x-ray machine, one of his many duties, which also included running the operating room, sterilizing room, and photography room and being responsible for the maintenance and care of "all apparatus and instruments." The position of chief resident had only been created and defined in 1897.[54] Clearly, the Board of Managers did not anticipate that dealing with medical instrumentation would occupy a large part of his day. X-ray equipment was stored in one corner of the new surgical building, in a room devoted also to microscopic and photographic work.[55]

X-ray instrumentation eventually assumed more of the chief resident's time, and in both 1910 and 1911 the former chief resident stayed on for an extra year specifically to run the x-ray machine. The first, Walter Estell Lee, promptly declared the old equipment obsolete and insisted on the purchase of $940 worth of new x-ray machinery. Lee went on to a successful career as professor of surgery at the University of Pennsylvania, where he put his familiarity with x rays to good use in some studies of pulmonary atelectasis. His successor, Charles Montgomery, with some difficulty, negotiated a pay raise from twenty-five to fifty dollars per month.[56]

The year 1912 marked a critical turning point in the operation of the x-ray machine, for in that year the responsibility for running the machine was shifted from a series of chief residents to a single physician, who devoted his career to roentgenology. That person was David Bowen, radiographer in charge to the Pennsylvania Hospital.[57] Bowen, an 1894 graduate of Jefferson Medical College in Philadelphia, had started his career as a country general practitioner. In 1906 he came across some discarded x-ray equipment in Rome, New York, which he was able to repair and use. The following year he studied roentgenology with Sydney Lange for two weeks, in Cincinnati, and attended the annual meeting of the new American Roentgen Ray Society. From 1907 onward he tried to limit his practice to the taking and interpreting of radiographs. He received additional training as an assistant to Willis Manges, in the Jefferson Hospital Radiology Department, from 1911 to 1920.[58] Whereas the earlier appointments at the Pennsylvania Hospital had lasted for only one year, Bowen remained in his position into the 1930s. In 1913 his title was changed to the slightly more formal "Roentgenologist," in honor of the x ray's inventor, and perhaps prompted by Bowen's election as secretary of the Philadelphia Roentgen Ray Society. In 1919 Bowen was elected president of the American Roentgen Ray Society, thus holding an official position in two early specialty groups. During his career Bowen published several articles and was an editor of the *American Journal of Roentgenology and Radium Therapy*. From 1907 he was, as we would now define the term, a specialist and an active member of the group of early radiologists who practiced and taught in Philadelphia.[59]

The terms of Bowen's employment differed significantly from those of his predecessors, marking a qualitative change in the relationship between the physician, the machine, and the hospital. In return for devoting 50 percent of his time to the X-ray Department, Bowen received a salary of fifteen hundred dollars per year. In addition, his income was to include 75 percent of all fees generated by taking x rays of paying patients; the hospital retained 25 percent. This agreement reflected the growing number of patients who paid for some part of their hospital care.[60] Also in 1911, the same time as Bowen's appointment, contributions from an anonymous donor allowed the hospital to purchase sixty-five hundred dollars' worth of new x-ray equipment, allowing a sharp increase in the capital investment in diagnostic machinery. The fact that this donor was willing to give such a large sum of money to purchase x-ray equipment is also an indication of the growing interest in the use of x rays among the general public.

Like the administrators of most voluntary hospitals of this period, the Board of Managers of the Pennsylvania Hospital became increasingly concerned with financial matters. Because the x ray symbolized the exact, scientific nature of medicine, it was seen as a way to attract more paying patients. X rays were ever more conspicuous in the annual reports of this period, which were sent not only to potential contributors but also to potential patients. Indeed, the number of patients examined by the x ray rose steadily, and in 1916 a nurse was assigned part-time to the X-ray Department. Physicians also requested x-ray examinations more frequently.

The situation at the New York Hospital was similar to the experience at the Pennsylvania Hospital. James H. Kenyon did most of the x-ray work from 1900 to 1903, first as a member of the house staff, then on "special assignment" from the New York Hospital Visiting Committee.[61] He eventually resigned the position because the work was dirty and bad for his hands and fingernails and because photographic work in a darkroom was "quite unhygienic." He also did so, and this reason is perhaps the most telling, because he felt that the work was of no value for other fields, either medical or surgical, and he wished to become a general surgeon.[62] Thus, skill in the taking of x-ray images in 1903 was not seen, at least to Dr. Kenyon, as an essential skill for becoming a general surgeon. Or, perhaps, he had just had enough of taking x rays and did not wish to become a radiologist.

Kenyon was replaced by Archibald Henry Busby. Three years after taking the job, Busby found it necessary to renegotiate his position with the New York Hospital.[63] He claimed that his work was a great help to surgeons, particularly for the diagnosis of fractures and foreign bodies.[64] Not only valuable, the work was difficult as well. It was essential that the hospital employ a skilled operator, as a few mistakes could easily cost the hospital "from $25 to $200 in one minute" or, worse, cause severe burns to the patient. Aside from performing excellent technical service, Busby had worked to make the department more clinically responsive, placing an x-ray image in every case record in which one was taken—and claiming that the New York Hospital was the first hospital to do this. Busby had worked hard, but he could no longer do so for only six hundred dollars per year; he would need twelve hundred dollars. After canvassing the city of New York to see what policies other institutions had in place, the administrators of the hospital agreed in 1907 to allow Busby to use the X-ray Department for his private patients.[65]

In striking similarity to the experience at the Pennsylvania Hospital, the director of the x-ray unit at the New York Hospital in 1912 asked to have his title changed from "actinographer," a title about which he had received many adverse opinions, to "physician in charge of the Roentgenological (or the Roentgen Ray) Department." This name change emphasized the fact that the person who held the position was a physician as well as honoring the inventor of the new technology. The department expanded, and more personnel were added.[66] A desire for more personnel, more equipment, and more space seems to have been a consistent feature of x-ray departments.

WORLD WAR I AND POSTWAR EXPANSION

In 1917 the United States formally entered World War I. This conflict encouraged x-ray use in three ways. First, medical personnel gained experience in using the new diagnostic technique. Of those patients admitted to U.S. Army hospitals over half were examined by x ray.[67] Several U.S. hospitals established units overseas, and dozens of nurses and physicians from the New York Hospital and from the Pennsylvania Hospital, staffed base hospitals numbers 9 and 10. While caring for an unprecedented flow of casualties, these nurses and physicians witnessed daily the x ray's value for diagnosing fractures and foreign bodies.[68] When there was only limited access to a machine, people sometimes traveled up to eighteen miles—a considerable distance, given the available transportation—in order to have an image obtained.[69]

Second, World War I stimulated technical advances in x-ray techniques. X-ray pictures were originally taken on glass plates imported from Belgium, but after 1914 the plates could no longer be imported. Thus, they became difficult to obtain and more expensive when they could be found. The New York Hospital had spent $289 on x-ray plates in the first six months of 1910. It spent $5,218 for the first six months of 1915, which was an unacceptable increase. More control was needed. The Executive Committee, like governing bodies up to the 1990s, decided that house staff would be more likely to order a test, without regard for its cost, than would the attending staff. Thus, they decided that house staff alone could no longer sign for an examination, that the attending physician would have to do so.[70]

As a result of the difficulty and expense in obtaining glass plates, manufacturers were forced to start making film for x-ray pictures, and they soon had an incentive for improving the film that they were selling. Portable x-ray units were often used near the battlefield; some of these units were carried about in specially equipped automobiles.[71] Such x-ray machines were less powerful than the stationary ones and required faster film to take high-quality pictures. To improve the machines new x-ray tubes were developed for use in portable units at the front.[72] Thus, World War I led to both improved portable units and the use of faster film,[73] and these advances were rapidly incorporated into civilian use.

Finally, the war experience provided another impetus toward defining radiology as a specialty. Prior to the war most x-ray work in military hospitals was done by someone with a number of other responsibilities. When the war started those people in the Surgeon General's Office responsible for setting up x-ray services had to make a choice. They might have continued to turn to surgeons and internists with interests in the x ray to do work on a part-time basis. Instead, in 1917 they turned to the American Roentgen Ray Society to set up schools to train people in roentgenology. In so doing, they gave additional force to the argument that those who ran x-ray machines ought to be specialists who worked as full-time radiologists.[74]

After World War I the Pennsylvania Hospital X-ray Department expanded rapidly. A new physician was employed as assistant radiologist in 1919. Bowen became the full-time radiographer in 1920, a year in which 4,005 patients were examined by x ray. The X-ray

Department at the New York Hospital also continued to expand, hiring new assistants and purchasing a portable x-ray machine.[75] The superintendent used the arrival of a portable x-ray machine in 1920 as a way to encourage attending physicians who admitted private patients to adhere to record-keeping standards. He informed the physicians that a portable x-ray unit was available and, at the same time, urged them to provide adequate documentation of each patient's history and physical examination, lest the house staff be called upon to do so.[76]

Although the x-ray machine was used more often by the 1920s, how important were its results for patient care? Was it still being used primarily for curiosity, or did the findings make a difference? Unfortunately, most hospital patient records do not contain a great deal of commentary about the results of the x-ray examination. Yet there are other ways of deriving answers to this question. One useful marker for the importance placed on x-ray use is the speed with which an examination was done. Consider, for example, the case of a man admitted to the Pennsylvania Hospital in 1902 complaining of "inability to walk after being run over by a horse."[77] A roentgenogram revealed that his leg was broken. This was not, however, an early diagnosis of fracture by x ray, at least not in any clinically significant sense. The plate was exposed only after two and a half weeks of uncomplicated hospitalization, during which the patient had been treated for a broken leg. Thus, the x ray was taken out of interest, not to improve patient care. This is the type of information that cannot usually be derived from sources such as annual reports and must be taken, instead, from an analysis of patient records. The lag of over two weeks suggests that the physicians who cared for this man, while they may have been interested in the x-ray results and could even have incorporated those findings into their decision making, did not see the x ray as providing them with critically important information for the immediate care of a person with a broken leg.[78]

More than for most tests, doing an x ray was a particularly complicated endeavor. Unlike a urinalysis, which could be easily done by a single person who was not a specialist, taking an x-ray image required some technological expertise. It required the use of machinery that was expensive and dangerous, to both patient and physician. It required the use of electricity, by no means a trivial consideration in an era when hospitals were only just starting to be systematically

Table 4.2   *"Lag" Time (in Days) between Entering the Hospital and Having an X Ray Done, for All Patients and for Patients with Fractures (fx)*

	Lag (mean)	Lag (median)	Lag-fx (mean)	Lag-fx (median)
		PENNSYLVANIA HOSPITAL		
1900	3.66 (1.83–6.56)	3 (0–7)	5 (2.40–9.19)	5 (3–7)
1909	12.54 (11.21–13.97)	2.5 (0–111)	1.89 (1.10–3.02)	1 (0–5)
1920	7.35 (6.75–8.01)	2 (0–64)	1.29 (.76–2.03)	1 (0–3)
1925	4.52 (4.11–4.97)	1.5 (0–65)	1.63 (.97–2.59)	0 (0–12)
		NEW YORK HOSPITAL		
1900	25 (18.56–32.96)	25 (4–46)	4	4 (1 obs)
1910	8.03 (7.08–9.06)	2 (0–44)	3.5 (2.17–5.35)	3 (0–9)
1920	3.09 (2.51–3.77)	2 (0–16)	1.2 (.44–2.61)	2 (0–2)

Note: 95 percent confidence intervals for means and range for medians are given in parentheses. The usual method of calculating confidence intervals assumes a normal distribution of the values, an assumption that clearly does not hold in this instance. Thus, the confidence intervals are calculated instead using a Poisson distribution.

wired for electric power. It required the use of expensive materials. It was, in other words, a "big deal," and a decision to take (or not to take) an x ray was probably made only after serious consideration.

Table 4.2 presents the time between a patient's admission and the taking of an x ray.[79] Having derived a series of values from the case record, each one being the number of days from admission to having an x-ray image taken, one can derive a number of ways of summarizing the central tendency of that period of time. The mean (or average) number of days is a useful measure, but it is susceptible to distortion from extreme values (as seen in this series). An alternative measure is the median number of days, which is the number of days for which there are equal numbers of cases of greater and fewer days.[80] The table gives both measures, and both paint a consistent picture. The first two columns give the mean and median for all patients who had an x ray taken; the second two columns give those values for those patients who had a fracture as well as the range of values.

For patients in general, those who had x rays taken tended to get them much sooner in their stay at the hospital over the course of the first quarter of the century. For both hospitals so few patients had an x-ray examination in 1900 that meaningful conclusions are difficult to draw about the length of time between admission and examination. The median length of time had fallen to two days by 1920 in both hospitals, indicating that, of those patients who were going to get x rays, over half received them within the first two days of their hospitalization. The number fell still more by 1925 at the Pennsylvania Hospital. The fall in the mean wait shows a similar picture. From 1910 to 1925 that value falls consistently and with similar values at each hospital: physicians elected to get an examination sooner and sooner during the hospital stay, suggesting that they placed increasing value on the information that could be obtained from it.

Not surprisingly, the length of time to get an x ray taken was usually shorter for people with fractures. As we have seen, the x ray was thought to be particularly useful for the diagnosis of broken bones. Patients with broken bones usually were admitted as a result of trauma and were quickly attended to. As the table shows, by around 1920 not only did most people with broken bones have an x-ray image taken; they also had it done fairly quickly. This was in part a decision by physicians that the images were important enough to be obtained in a timely fashion and in part the fact that the X-ray Department was able to accommodate their requests. In 1916 the New York Hospital X-ray Department began to be open seven days per week.[81] (It was open for a wide range of cases, not only trauma; for example, the department made provisions for starting a stomach series six days per week.) In 1920 patients at the New York Hospital waited, on average, less than two days to have an examination done for a possible broken bone. The same was true at the Pennsylvania Hospital. By 1920 the x ray had become a regular routine for patients with broken bones.

X RAYS, ELECTROCARDIOGRAMS, AND
THE HOSPITAL AS A DIAGNOSTIC CENTER

Another major diagnostic technology introduced into hospitals in the early twentieth century was the electrocardiogram. Unlike the sudden and dramatic discovery of the x ray, the development of the ECG followed many earlier attempts to record the electrical action of the human heart.[82] Willem Einthoven's 1902 description of the ECG machine did not provoke the dramatic public reaction that followed the discovery of the x ray only seven years earlier. Hospitals did not rush to buy this machine, as they had done for x-ray machines. The New York Hospital was given an ECG machine in 1914.[83] For a decade before the Pennsylvania Hospital purchased the machine, in 1921, the occasional patient who required an ECG was sent elsewhere to have a tracing made. When an ECG machine was purchased in 1921, arrangements were modeled on those for the x ray.[84] The Pennsylvania Hospital Board of Managers quickly approved the same 75 percent–25 percent split of fees for the "electro-cardiographer" as they had earlier for the radiographer. Electrocardiograph reports appeared on patients' charts within the year, usually for patients with irregular heartbeats. A separate room was set aside to house the ECG machine. In 1924 the New York Hospital adopted a very similar split of fees: two-thirds of the fees to go to the physician, one-third to the hospital.[85]

By 1925, although it was not as widely accepted as the x ray, the ECG was well on its way to becoming a routine part of patient care. The machine was used intensively enough at the Pennsylvania Hospital to require that a part-time technician be employed by the ECG laboratory. Attention and money were directed to heart diseases: a heart clinic attracted large numbers of patients, and a fellowship in cardiac diseases was established.

The Pennsylvania Hospital X-ray Department, like the ECG laboratory, was rapidly expanding. It performed 6,621 examinations during 1927 in a brand new, twelve-room, $21,000 suite that had been the featured topic in the 1925 annual report. The department also boasted a stereo unit to examine the lungs, reports within the same day for 95 percent of cases, and, with three transformers, the ability to handle even emergency cases. Examinations for possible fractures were done at the time of admission, even when there was a low suspicion that a fracture was actually present, and almost every patient diagnosed as having a fracture had an x ray taken.

In 1927, however, there was an even more significant transformation than the increased number of patients receiving an x ray or ECG. For the first time patients entered the hospital specifically "for study." This new indication for admission to the hospital marks a distinct qualitative shift in its use. The Pennsylvania Hospital in the nineteenth century had been a home for the long-term care of the chronically ill, which gradually became a turn-of-the-century institution for the management of acute accident cases, as the community became increasingly hard-pressed to care for the sick at home. Only in 1927 did it start to function as a repository for complex diagnostic machinery. Why did this function not emerge until thirty years after the hospital originally bought an x-ray machine? Why did physicians in the hospital start to use the x-ray machine regularly some twenty years after its initial purchase?

Hospital Organization and the Use of Medical Technology

One explanation, appealing in its simplicity, might be that technical improvements in diagnostic tools led directly to greater clinical utility. Clearly, a combination of new tubes, improved power supplies, and a moving grid improved the quality of x-ray pictures and made the x ray a more useful clinical tool.[86] Comparison with the ECG reveals a somewhat different story. Early ECG machines produced tracings of quality comparable to the best obtained today, albeit with considerably more difficulty. Yet the ECG, unlike the x ray, was of very little clinical value in the 1920s.[87] The primary treatable arrhythmia, atrial fibrillation, had already been well described on clinical grounds, without any instrumental aid. Its management was simple: enough digitalis to slow the pulse, which could be easily palpated at the bedside. The diagnosis of myocardial infarction (heart attack) was starting to be made with electrocardiographic aid, but there was little specific treatment for the disease.[88] The electrocardiogram's rapid integration into hospital management by 1927 cannot be explained simply by assuming that technical improvement with resulting clinical utility dictates how a machine will be used.

A better explanation may come from looking at changes in the hospital structure. In the late 1890s, when hospitals purchased their first x-ray machines, there was no structure into which such a diagnostic tool could fit: there were no physicians performing tests for fees; there were no forms for reporting results of any kind. Starting more than a decade later, in 1912, the Pennsylvania Hospital employed a physician specifically to take x rays. A growing base of private patients allowed this specialist to augment his income substantially by retaining 75 percent of all fees. By 1921 the x ray had become an accepted part of the hospital routine. When the Board of Managers of the Pennsylvania Hospital purchased an ECG machine in that year, they could easily adopt the same institutional procedures for the ECG which they had developed for the x ray. Having already established a mechanism for sharing reimbursement with the physician-operator as well as a format for reporting test results from special units, the hospital could incorporate a new technology with relative ease. The routines were already in place, as was the ideology that made it desirable to take precise, quantitative measurements with machines. By 1921 the hospital's experience with the x ray had provided a structure into which a new machine such as the ECG could be easily inserted.

Figure 4.2 demonstrates another way to look at the relationship between acceptance of the x ray and the ECG. Annual x ray and ECG receipts are displayed in constant 1914 dollars.[89] Both the figure and patient records reveal a substantial delay between the purchase of the x ray in 1897 and its widespread application by the late 1920s.

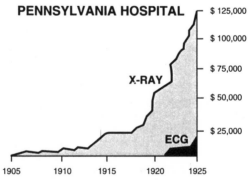

Figure 4.2   *X-ray and ECG receipts, Pennsylvania Hospital, 1900–1925 (in 1914 dollars).*

Receipts for x rays rose sharply in 1914, following the appointment of a half-time radiographer. After 1919, when the radiographer became a full-time employee and hired an assistant, receipts rose again. The ECG, a less clinically valuable tool, found rapid acceptance after the machine was purchased in 1921.

Complex Hospitals

Hospitals were becoming complex institutions and the decision regularly to use x-ray machines, as well as the decision to reimburse practitioners for their work with the machine, added to that complexity in two very important ways. First, the machines required special training to operate. No longer could a single superintendent confidently assert control over every decision about how a hospital was run. There were nearly constant changes in the types of x-ray equipment available, or needed, and the plea for more, better, bigger, more powerful x-ray equipment is found throughout the minutes of hospital governing boards over the first few decades of the century. The discussions reveal a growing gap between the technical sophistication of the person who used the equipment and the board that governed the hospital. The decision to establish a separate x-ray unit, run by a physician with special technical skills, was consistent with the increased complexity of the structure of U.S. business in general.[90] The technical complexity was also true for clinical laboratories designed to examine pathological specimens, but the x ray was a much more prominent technology.

Second, the x-ray machine generated formal reimbursement for services performed within the hospital using hospital equipment. Used in that way, it added to levels of authority and accounting within an increasingly more complex institution. The field of cost accounting had only been invented in the late nineteenth century. First applied in factories, cost accounting techniques were rapidly adopted by hospitals as well, as described in chapter 2, thus allowing hospital administrators to identify which units of the hospital were profitable and which were not. The new accounting techniques made it possible to identify the precise financial situation of the expensive but potentially profitable X-ray Department.

X-ray departments were themselves new inventions. Together with the hospital administration, and in the general spirit of the times, X-ray Department administrators such as New York Hospital's Archibald Busby tried to make the department as efficient and systematic as possible.[91] The department sought to be efficient in the management not only of information but also of the very images upon which their diagnoses were based. Plates were valuable, bulky, and difficult to store, and, if adequate care was not taken, they could very easily be misplaced.[92] Just as hospital administrators looked explicitly to industry for help in organizing financial accounts, so, too, x-ray administrators looked to commercial photography companies for help in deciding how to organize their x-ray plates.[93] The choice to use the photographic industry represented one arm of an ongoing tension between seeing the x-ray plate as a photograph and seeing it as analogous to medical evidence that was more clearly within the narrow domain of medicine.

THE ROLE OF THE RADIOLOGIST: CONSULTANT OR TECHNICIAN?

The rationale by which people who took x rays were paid was more important for them than for other groups. Pathologists, who were often the ones to run clinical laboratories, had long enjoyed a reasonable status in the medical world. On the other hand, those who took x-ray images were in a very precarious position in the early years of the twentieth century. Were they technicians, photographers, paid to run a machine that could produce pretty pictures? Or were they, instead, physicians, consultants, who used the machine as one means of establishing a diagnosis? Many physicians who used x-ray equipment wanted to establish themselves as specialists in the production and interpretation of x-ray images.[94] But those physicians who sought to establish the legitimacy of radiologists as specialists who not only took but also interpreted images were particularly concerned about what they saw as two major threats to their legitimacy. First, whereas people would often choose the physician or surgeon they wanted to care for them, they would rarely do so for the radiologist. Thus, the status of the radiologist as an integral member of the health care team was not widely appreciated. When they worked within the hospital setting, as many did, radiologists needed to voice continually the importance of their work to the hospital superintendent, in order that he or she would always be aware of the amount of work that was passing through the department. One way to do this was to have the superintendent sign each requisition card for an x-ray examination.[95]

The second concern had to do with payment arrangements for people who ran x-ray machines. Any system in which people were buying an x-ray plate risked looking like one in which people were buying a picture, much like going to a photographer. Better, from the point of view of the radiologist, if the person were paying for an expert opinion, a consultation.[96] Allowing the radiologist to see "private patients" while using hospital equipment enhanced the standing of the radiologist as a regular member of the medical staff, rather than as a fancy hospital photographer.

Those who took x-ray images addressed this problem on their own. One easy way of emphasizing the fact that patients bought a consultation, not a photograph, was simply to refuse to show the pictures to patients. The pictures were only part of a means to an end, went the claim. Patients got advice, not images. (The implications for the patient-physician relationship of withholding the image from the patient's view are discussed in chap. 5.)

Dealing with other physicians was different. One could hardly refuse to show another physician an x-ray image of a patient. On the other hand, once physicians had seen a few images, they might decide to buy a machine and take the images themselves. Many physicians suffered from the "childish but natural delusion that roentgenography differs little from photography" and would, unless stopped, continue to talk about "x-ray pictures" and thus diminish the stature of the true expert.[97] Here radiologists needed to use their expertise and special training to emphasize their role as consultant for other members of a medical staff. For example, if a physician wishing to make a diagnosis of acromegaly asked for a radiograph of the head, the radiologist could, and should, be able also to examine the hands and feet, knowing, as perhaps those less well trained in the art of x-ray diagnosis did not, that the hands and feet could provide valuable diagnostic information.[98] Being not merely a photographer who took pictures of whatever body part was requested, the person who ran the x-ray machine was a physician who served as a consultant for other physicians and was there to answer a clinical question.

An episode from the early days of the x ray illustrates one way in which the x-ray picture was at one time seen in a very different light than has become the case a century later. In New York City in the spring of 1896 Dr. Leopold Stieglitz, suspecting that his patient suffered from kidney stones, sent the patient to Dr. William James Morton to have an x-ray examination. Morton reported back that "the x-ray shows plainly that there is no stone of an appreciable size in the kidney" and that "the region of the kidneys is uniformly penetrated by the X-ray and there is no sign of any interruption by any foreign body." What is particularly noteworthy about this episode is the discussion of the appropriate fee. First is the amount of the fee. Morton wrote, "My usual charge to radiograph the entire body is $100." For 1896 this is quite an astounding sum.[99] Also interesting is the fact that Morton felt it quite natural to charge a different fee depending upon whether he saw a kidney stone. He wrote: "Like all physicians' services a negative result is harder to charge for than a positive one. If we had found the stone in the kidney it would have been worth that money—but we didn't. I think therefore it would be fair to say $75."[100] Obviously, somewhere over the ensuing decades the idea that physicians ought to base their charge for diagnostic services upon whether or not an abnormality was found has gone by the wayside.

Forms

The way information was reported within the hospital underwent a dramatic change from around 1900 to 1925. By 1925 quantitative results of diagnostic tests were usually reported on separate, standardized forms. These forms often depicted information with graphs, and physicians' increasing familiarity with visual, graphic, and quantitative reports produced by special units of the increasingly bureaucratic hospital in turn promoted the use of medical machines. Test results went from being handwritten by the intern to being laid into the chart in a patchwork fashion to finally being typed on a standardized form and signed by a specialist.

Forms emphasized the increasingly specialized nature of the knowledge produced by machines and, when signed by the director of a particular unit, reinforced the need for specially trained experts to interpret the results.[101] Having a form marked "Roentgen Ray Laboratory," signed by the director, guaranteed that everyone who received that form would know that the x-ray machine was no longer being run by some overgrown house officer who had no other job opportunities available but, rather, by a specialist who had chosen to devote his or her career to the field of radiology.

Forms could also be used to symbolize the scientific nature of early twentieth-century medicine. The meaning of *scientific*, as discussed in chapter 2, was partly embodied in the large-scale move toward using standardized forms. X-ray departments were at the forefront of those units that elected to use such standard devices to report the results of their diagnostic images. The form used to report gastrointestinal x rays at the Pennsylvania Hospital, shown as figure 2.5, was typical of the types of forms used to report gastrointestinal x rays in many other places around the country. Physicians were encouraged to use the available labels to define the radiographic nature of their patient's gastrointestinal tract. Certainly, they could choose to write in a different phrase, but it was a great deal easier to simply choose from one of those that was already available.

The standardization of forms clearly made reporting of x rays more systematic. It may have implicitly served to standardize patients as well. One can see this standardization of information about patients in the way that physical examination findings were recorded, first using drawings and later anatomical stamps. The drawing in figure 4.3 represents the physical findings obtained by a house officer who examined a nine-year-old schoolgirl admitted to the Pennsylvania Hospital on December 17, 1912, with a productive cough and a fever. Upon examination she was found to have pneumonia. The house officer drew a sketch of the patient's back and indicated that a specific area was dull to percussion and had faint breath sounds as well as a combination of other findings which together served to confirm a diagnosis of pneumonia—specifically, that the right lung's lower portion was infected and partially solidified. (The patient went home, cured, soon after the new year.) This type of visual presentation of information is consonant with the increasing use of the x ray during this period. One cannot be certain the extent to which knowledge of and experience with the x ray informed this house officer's decision to draw a picture. Yet consider that he did have other options available to him; he might have recorded his examination findings in words, perhaps by noting that "the right lung base is dull, has faint breath sounds," etc. His decision, instead, to draw the patient's back allows him to convey a

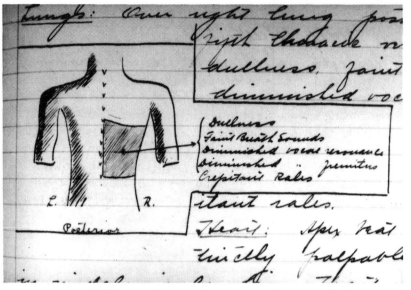

Figure 4.3 *Hand drawing of a patient with pneumonia. From Pennsylvania Hospital Case Records 196 (1912): 3165.*

much more spatial meaning to his description as well as to indicate, although the patient did not have such a picture taken, something like what an x-ray image of that region would look like.

The use of drawings (and stamps) also interrupted the flow of the patient record. It broke up what had been a narrative description of events and replaced it, along with all of the other forms and graphs, with a series of related descriptions. As a result, not only the intellectual construction of patients and their diseases but also the physical construction of the charts started to become fragmented.

A decade later a very different kind of a depiction was being made. Then, instead of a freehand drawing of a person's back, house officers were using a stamped, anatomical chart on which to draw their findings (see fig. 4.4).[102] All patients' thoraxes, despite their obviously different sizes and shapes, were to be represented by a single stamp. The patient's body had thus become standardized. The person recording the physical examination could not use his or her judgment about how to represent the patient; whoever made the stamp got to control how the person was to be depicted in the chart. This shift was similar to other changes going on in the gathering of

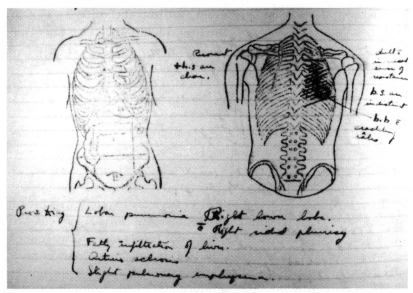

Figure 4.4   *Stamp used for denoting physical diagnosis. From Pennsylvania Hospital Case Records 396 (1917): 1054.*

information about patients. Recording the daily amount of urine put out by a patient or his or her intake of food was very different from hearing about symptoms or making general assertions about diet. This change in the perception of the patient was consistent with the scientific ideology of controlled, reproducible experiments. Viewing test results in only a few, sharply defined ways deflected attention from differences between individual patients and focused, instead, on similarities in the particular organs under investigation. Thus, in the name of efficiency people started to become organs; symptoms, diseases.

Technology and Hospital Medicine

The placement of x-ray machines in hospitals has been used to explain, in part, the rapid growth of hospitals in the early twentieth century.[103] This study suggests the importance of other factors. Although the Pennsylvania and New York hospitals purchased their first x-ray machines in the nineteenth century, it took two decades before the technology was routinely utilized and three decades for such technology to draw patients into the hospital. The mere existence of a diagnostic technology did not dictate how or where it would be used; both hospital and machine had to change before the x ray or any other machine could significantly influence hospital care. At least in this instance, health care technology was not autonomous.

Historical analysis should give us pause as we attempt to predict, using unequivocally rational and logical criteria, just how new machines will be applied. The x ray was first used in an exploratory, experimental fashion, and pictures were taken of patients with many different conditions. Only after the social system in which it was applied had changed did specific indications for its application become accepted. The lesson of this study for contemporary technology assessment is that changes in both organizational and conceptual systems are critically important, albeit difficult to predict, in determining how technology will be used.

5

THE X-RAY IMAGE
Meaning, Gender, and Power

From the very start the x-ray machine was used to create images of a wide range of bodies: some were of women and some of men; some were healthy and some were held to have various diseases. How did people learn to think about these pictures? What meanings did they create for these strange, other-worldly shadows? Thomas Laqueur has suggested that, "instead of being the consequence of increased scientific knowledge, new ways of looking at the body were . . . new ways of representing and indeed of constituting social realities."[1] Although Laqueur was not talking specifically about the x-ray machine, his statement is no less germane for images created by that new device. For the meanings of the x-ray image did not exist, waiting to be found, already preordained in the laws of physics which, in the late twentieth century, we have come to believe govern the creation of the image.[2] Rather, before images could become a part of the larger practice of medicine they had to be interpreted; meanings had to be assigned.

Recent work on the social construction of diseases has shown that medical definitions are informed by a wide range of cultural features.[3] Although historians have carefully examined the social construction of conditions such as mental illness or diseases of sexuality, the social nature of the knowledge produced by medical machines has heretofore escaped much critical analysis. Too often information derived from machines is taken implicitly to be a privileged form of information, even within otherwise sensitive discussions.[4] While we should not privilege the information derived from machines, neither should we ignore it.

One construction that informed the reading of machine-generated information is gender. X-ray images were read (and continue to be read) by people—physicists, physicians, and the public—who existed in a society in which gender was (and remains) a central defining feature, perhaps *the* central defining feature, of one's own body image, one's personhood, but also that of all other people in the world. Moreover, the x ray produced not a number but an image, something not to be counted or measured but, rather, to be looked at.[5] Hence, it is not at all surprising that people viewed the x-ray image in ways that were informed by their preexisting ideas about the differences between men's and women's bodies.

To explore the role of gender in medical technology it would be ideal to look for the ways in which gender informs interpretations of *both* male and female images. Otherwise, one runs the risk of treating male as the universal state and female as the "other." One would like not to be constrained to examining only conditions that are unique to women, such as pregnancy, childbirth, and menstruation. Moreover, any analysis of how viewers constructed the x-ray image should attempt to take into account not only gender but also a wide range of social definitions, including race, class, and ethnicity.

In this chapter, after an overview of the social response to the invention of the x ray, I shall examine responses to using the x-ray machine for men and women. I shall then ask if use of the x-ray machine differed for male and female hospitalized patients, using case records from the Pennsylvania and the New York hospitals. The influence of gender on the decision to take an x-ray image was different in these two institutions. Finally, I shall speculate on the ways in which interpretation of the x-ray image may have both contributed to and reflected a fin de siècle change to a masculine, technology-centered view of medicine and medical care, one that has persisted to the end of the twentieth century.

THE NEW RAYS

Near the end of 1895, dazzled by the scientific achievements of the past few decades, some observers thought that the ultimate limits of science were fast being reached. The dramatic invention, however, of a startlingly new machine, the x-ray machine, led to renewed hope that, through science, literally anything might be possible.[6] The invention provoked an extremely broad and intense reaction, not only within the medical community but also among the public at large. Anyone who simply glances through newspapers, magazines, and other items intended for popular consumption during the first few months of 1896 will soon become aware of just how quickly and intensely the idea of the x ray permeated public awareness.[7] Few publications managed to avoid prominent discussion of the machine and its pictures.

The intense public reaction to seeing within the body with x-ray machines was largely a result of how that knowledge was made widely accessible. The x-ray image represented, not just for physicians but also for the public, a very different and very new way to look inside the human body. The interior of the human body had not, of course, been previously unknown to medical practitioners: surgeons had long looked into the human body. Yet most members of the public did not have access to those surgical views. They were not invited to stand and watch within the new hospital operating rooms that were being built in the late nineteenth century. Moreover, the very nature of the surgical view limited even indirect public access. Images of surgery were difficult to reproduce, because of both the detail and the accurate color needed for verisimilitude. Merely looking at textbook illustrations did not in any sense prepare the budding surgeon to be able to read the interior of the human body.[8] Thus, for the case of surgery Ludmilla Jordanova is quite right when she describes medical images as not being accessible to the public.[9] That was probably true up until the moment that Frau Röntgen's hand appeared throughout the world.[10]

But the x-ray image changed everything. It was perhaps the first medical image to be widely accessible, in similar (if not identical) form to medical and lay observers alike.[11] There were several reasons why this was the case. First, x-ray images were not particularly detailed. Yes, there were certainly subtleties to be appreciated. But, as compared to other medical images, an x-ray image was quite simple. The interior of the human body as seen by a surgeon was more complex: fascia looked like nerves; oozing blood obscured vision even in the best of circumstances. On the other hand, the x ray was a much cleaner image; it was, after all, merely a shadow and, as such, required only a limited amount of detail.

Second, the x ray was itself a photograph. It was static, unchanging. It was not a representation of some other, more privileged view, as was the case for drawings done by people who were observing medical care. The x-ray image was *itself* the evidence that needed to be interpreted, to be read, whether by the public or by physicians.

Third, the x ray, unlike surgery, was experienced by all viewers in black and white. Around the time of the x-ray machine's invention, improved technology enabled easier printing of black-and-white images.[12] Old and new magazines took advantage of the newly created opportunity to publish better illustrations than had ever before been possible; many of the illustrations were of people. Although some of the magazines used this technology to publish pictures of "women in discreet stages of undress," many also used it to publish pictures of x-ray images (see fig. 5.1).[13]

Finally, unlike surgery, the x-ray image was itself two-dimensional. Any reproduction did not have to attempt to enable the reader to imagine a third dimension, depth. All of these features combined to make the x-ray image one that could be easily reproduced for widespread consumption, in ways that lost very little of the original image.

Viewing the New Pictures

The x-ray machine's inventor, Röntgen, took a picture of his wife's hand and reported that "the realism of this weird picture simply fascinated all who beheld it."[14] The *New York Times* proclaimed: "Hidden Solids Revealed."[15] The discovery was widely reported in popular newspapers.[16] The x ray became central for social events. X-ray machines were easy enough to make and to use that nonmedical people could produce and view their own x-ray images. Exhibits were set up at town halls and other public settings. People lined up for up to one-hour sittings to see their bones; there was a coin-operated machine in Chicago to let them get a glimpse of their hands and a demonstration in the Lawrence, Kansas, opera house, with reserved tickets available at the Santa Fe train station.[17] X-ray pictures of everyday objects became popular.

And the pictures were popular for aesthetic as well as for novelty

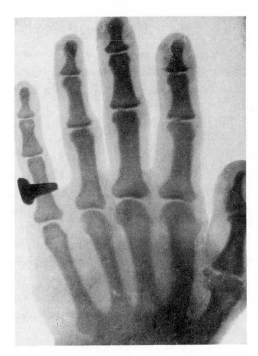

Figure 5.1 *"Hand of a Living Person." From "'Photographing the Unseen': A Symposium on the Roentgen Rays," Century Illustrated Monthly 30 (May–October 1896): 123.*

value. High-class New York women had pictures taken holding hands with their betrothed. People were pleased and amazed at the sights of their own interiors, giving pictures to their friends and lovers. One woman's full-length portrait was "as coquettish as an X-ray picture may be." Another woman exclaimed, upon seeing a picture of her bones, "This is really the dearest picture, altogether and in every way, that I ever had taken."[18] Hans Castorp, in Thomas Mann's *The Magic Mountain,* is enamored of the x-ray image of his beloved. "He drew out his keepsake, his treasure . . . a thin glass plate, which must be held towards the light to see anything on it. It was Claudia's X-ray portrait, showing not her face, but the delicate bony structure of the upper half of her body, and the organs of the thoracic cavity, surrounded by the pale, ghostlike envelope of flesh . . . How often had he looked at it, how often pressed it to his lips."[19]

A Picture of Death

The x-ray image revealed not only beauty, however, but also death. The dominant feature of many x-ray pictures is bones, and the idea of the skeleton as a harbinger of death is quite old.[20] Early in *The Magic Mountain*, when Hans Castorp looks at an x-ray image of his own body—specifically, again, his hand, also with jewelry—"he looked into his own grave":

> The process of decay was forestalled by the light-ray; the flesh in which he walked disintegrated, annihilated, dissolved in vacant mist, and there within it was the finely turned skeleton of his own hand, the seal ring he had inherited from his grandfather hanging loose and black on the joint of his ring-finger—a hard, material object with which man adorns the body that is fated to melt away beneath it, when it passes on to another flesh that can wear it for yet a little while. . . . [H]e gazed at this familiar part of his own body, and for the first time in his life he understood that he would die.[21]

The hand was a favored organ for x-raying in the early days because it is thin, convenient, and easy to manipulate. Images of the hand were a prominent feature in descriptions and demonstrations using the new rays. Upon first developing an x-ray plate of his hand, one early x-ray user noted, "As the skeleton fingers came gradually forth from the blank plate, he felt a sort of creepy sensation, as though it was some ghostly hand beckoning to him from another world—and it was another world; a new scientific world."[22] The point is for now the unpleasant sensation upon seeing his hand with the new device (we will return later to the idea that it was a particularly scientific view). The noted inventor Thomas Alva Edison, who worked extensively with early x-ray apparatus, exhibited an X-ray room in 1896, at which one person, upon seeing skeletal hands, was so amazed and frightened that he exclaimed, "Oh my God!" and ran from the room.[23]

Popular literature took up the "x ray as horrendous invention" theme. An 1896 short story, "Röntgen's Curse," described the horrors of having one's eyes assume x-ray powers.[24] The tale of that protagonist, one Herbert Newton, provides some insight into the way in which the x ray was originally seen as not only potentially dehumanizing by its actions but also as being derived from a fundamentally flawed view of the world.[25] Herbert Newton had heard about the x rays, as had everyone: "The whole world of scientific men felt that they were on the verge of a great event. Every magazine had an article on so-called photography of the invisible. . . ." In a foolish attempt to invent a substance that would enable him to have x-ray vision, Newton neglects his wife and children to spend endless hours in his laboratory. He first attempts the experiment on his trusting dog, his "one faithful friend." His method works: the dog is able to see with x-ray vision—but the sights are terrifying. Even the powerful bond between Newton and his dog will not suffice to comfort the animal. The dog runs into a thicket, where he "perished miserably from fear and famine."

Newton, obsessed with the seeming allure of the new vision, fails to heed the obvious warning provided by his dog's portentous experience. He applies the experiment to his own eyes. The result is a "ghastly and sickening sight" when he looks at himself and "grotesque horror" when he beholds his wife and child. He soon realizes that "everything in the outer world which had given [him] pleasure and happiness had gone from [him]." He would rather go blind than live with x-ray vision.

Newton's wife calls in a physician, a distinguished acquaintance from London, who, "like many of his kind . . . took little interest in anything that in his view did not lead to some practical end in his profession."[26] He advises Newton to remain in bed and sleep as much as possible. Eventually, the effects of Newton's potion spontaneously pass, and he regains his normal sight.

The story tells us a great deal about immediate literary reaction to the x-ray machine. The discovery was seen as distancing people from humanity and the medical profession as relatively uninterested in the device. More to the point of this chapter, the danger of the x ray in this depiction is derived from science and is distinctly masculine. The only feminine element in the story, albeit a central one, is Newton's wife, who at the end saves her husband by throwing away all of his laboratory equipment. She realizes that the knowledge to be gained by this new way of seeing is not worth the cost.

Newspapers took up the theme of "Röntgen's Curse." Writers called the idea of being able to see through the body repulsive and said the discoverers and items needed to make the rays should be sunk in the ocean: "Let the fish contemplate each other's bones if they like, but not us."[27] For a time after its invention some reacted to the x-ray image with fear and revulsion.

A Threat to Privacy

Although part of the concern about the x-ray image may have come from an association with death, part may have been simply a general disinclination to be seen in too much detail, combined with fear that the x ray would penetrate formerly private areas. Photographs themselves, only recently having become a common part of daily life, were bad enough: they could make public that which was private, and they were already invading "the sacred precincts of private and domestic life." By 1890 they served as a warning for scholars who were afraid that new "mechanical devices" could further invade what was being defined as a new right to privacy.[28] Five years later these fears were realized with a new device, the x-ray machine. Coming close upon the heels of the telephone, which could ring people up in the "very bosom of their families," and the phonograph, which could register and reproduce "the most intimate of domestic confidences," the x ray could be viewed as "uncompromisingly evil" in its ability to "render privacy a mere tradition of an unscientific past."[29] Its rays could pass through "all fleshy disguises as easily as light does through glass."[30] As a poem in *Punch* put it:

> We do not want, like Dr. Swift,
>   To take our flesh off and to pose in
> Our bones, or show each little rift
>   And joint for you to poke your nose in.
>
> We only crave to contemplate
>   Each other's usual full-dress photo;
> Your worse than "altogether" state
>   Of portraiture we bar *in toto!*[31]

Invasion of privacy need not be a curse, however, especially if the person whose privacy was being invaded was a "bad person." Consider an 1898 short story entitled "A Debt to Science," in which a scoundrel is identified by an x-ray image of a bullet.[32] The story centers on Jack Leslie, a self-made man. He once came afoul of a scoundrel named Jose Tandil, who was caught cheating at cards in Rio. During the ruckus that followed the discovery of an ace up his sleeve, Jose was shot in the shoulder, where the bullet remains. Sometime later Jack visits in South America, where he discovers that his cousin is engaged to a wealthy South American millionaire named Christobal Queretaro. Jack, of course, soon recognizes that the smooth-talking and smart-dressing Christobal Queretaro is really the previously wounded scoundrel, Jose Tandil. But Christobal has already used his considerable social skills to charm not only Jack's cousin but also everybody else. How can Jack prove that Christobal is really Jose?

Enter Jack's friend, who carries with him his roentgen ray apparatus ("You know it's my pet hobby, and I take it about with me everywhere"). The machine was in 1898 not yet professionalized; it was still the toy of wealthy amateur photographers. The story implies, however, that the x-ray machine is fairly widely known, at least among proper members of society, a group that does not include Tandil. Jack's friend predicts that Tandil won't recognize the apparatus: "It's more than likely that he has never heard of Roentgen Rays. The ignorance of some of these fellows is absolutely phenomenal." The machine is demonstrated to an audience before Queretaro shows up one evening, and it amazes the crowd; they completely forget about the scheduled dance. Eventually, Queretaro arrives. He is persuaded to stand for an x-ray image, which shows the bullet and proves that he is, indeed, Tandil. Tandil leaves town, and fair womanhood is protected.

This story was published within two years of the invention of the x-ray machine, when the ability of the x-ray image to show a bullet within the body was still held to be amazing; the author of the story saw no need to introduce fancier ideas for dramatic effect. By invading the privacy of Jose Tandil, the new science did good things—hence the title, "A Debt to Science." The x-ray machine also, perhaps, enhanced the quality and interest of the fictional account.

Political cartoonists showed how the x ray could reveal important hidden truths, such as a German observer using Röntgen's discovery in January 1896 to find that the English empire's backbone was of "unsuspected size and strength."[33] Literary observers suggested other possibilities for using the x-ray machine for dramatic effect, perhaps by being able to see through walls.[34]

But the x ray could penetrate walls for both bad and good purposes. Entrepreneurs advertised their x-ray services for use in divorce cases.[35] Cartoons showed how x rays could reveal to a nosy landlady what was going on behind a closed door.[36] Experiments purported to show that one could use x rays to read the contents of a letter enclosed in its envelope: the solution was to wrap the letter in tinfoil.[37] The x ray was thus a device whose implications for privacy were more often feared than desired.

The most consistent fears had to do with personal privacy, and many of these concerns appear to have implicitly focused on women more than men. On February 19, 1896, Assemblyman Reed, of Somerset County, New Jersey, is said to have introduced a bill into the State Legislature, at Trenton, to prohibit "the use of X-rays in opera glasses in theaters or other public places." The suggestion is said to have been greeted with a loud laugh.[38] There is no record of the bill's passage; in fact, there is reason to doubt whether the bill was ever actually introduced.[39] Nonetheless, the alleged legislative proposal warrants attention, if for no other reason than the fact that the story became, almost instantly, a part of the standard lore of the x ray. Told and retold in the history of radiology literature, a literature primarily written by (and for) physicians, the tale carries a number of messages. It emphasizes the foolishness of allowing lay people to attempt to manage new medical technology: they simply cannot understand it and will say (and perhaps do) foolish things. A second message is to emphasize the distance we have come and the achievements we have achieved.

The alleged 1896 bill may have been merely a joke. Serious or not, it says a great deal about public awareness of the amazing new rays and their possibilities, possibilities that seemed for a time to include the frightful thought that everyone's innermost secrets would be laid bare to "every fiend with a camera."[40]

Yet women didn't need simply to accept this assault on their privacy. Firms advertised x-ray-proof underwear to guard against up-to-date Peeping Toms with a "picture" showing two women, one of whom wore the protective dress interlining and one of whom did not.[41] (It is interesting to note that the illustration shows that the dress's lining somehow prevented the x rays from penetrating not only her thorax and abdomen but also her whole body, including her head.) These undergarments afforded "an impenetrable shield against the mortifying possibilities of the surreptitious use of this new photographic wonder." Lest one doubt the veracity of the merchant's claims, the advertisement included a telegram from a New York City electrician attesting to the fact that the textile buckskin was "impervious to the Roentgen rays."

A number of questions appear to the reader of several decades hence, not the least of which is the question about why (or how) the offending x rays could penetrate through a woman's clothes and somehow, in a manner most convenient for the voyeur, stop at the skin. (Otherwise one would simply see through both cloth and skin to the bones beneath.) This question appears not to have been asked. Whether or not one could actually use x rays in opera glasses to see through the clothes of women who gathered to see the latest theatrical production is an interesting question—the answer is almost certainly "no." But it is not the most important issue to be addressed here. In order to understand how x rays were perceived, we need to know about what people *thought* they could do. Some entrepreneurs went to the trouble of putting advertisements in papers and, presumably, would have *something* to sell individuals who responded. Perhaps not. Even so, whoever introduced the special women's underwear designed to block the new rays was responding to a perception that x rays were a threat to feminine privacy, a perception that informed public attitudes at the turn of the century, no matter what we may now think of such speculation.

Ample additional evidence supports this conclusion. Waiting to be viewed by the new rays, women asked to see one another's bones but "not below the waist."[42] Poems reflected the invasive potential of the new rays:

> The Roentgen rays, the Roentgen rays
> What is this craze?
> The town's ablaze
> With this new phrase
> Of X-ray ways.
> I'm full of daze
> Shock and amaze,

> For nowadays
> I hear they'll gaze Thro' cloak and gown—and even stays!
> Those naughty, naughty Roentgen rays![43]

The "naughty" nature of the rays became fair game for artists. Some of them, such as Francis Picabia, alluded to their lascivious nature. Others, such as Marcel Duchamp, seem to have used x-ray images to stimulate a series of progressively transparent images of women.[44]

More than merely showing the physical exterior, the rays were thought to reveal the truth about a woman's inner feelings, as in the poem "To a Fickle Miss" in 1896 (cathodic rays are the same as x rays).[45]

> Not worth your while
> That false sweet smile
> Which o'er your features plays:
>
> Thy heart of steel
> I can reveal
> By my cathodic rays.

Feminine, superficial appeal is undone by the cold, objective rays. This (presumably male) suitor will not be fooled. Similar feelings are expressed in "An Idyl of the Roentgen Rays," in which Strephon, rebuffed by the unfeeling Chloe, convinces her to sit for a picture with the roentgen ray. The picture shows that they are the same, except:

> The only difference lay in this:
> Something attracted the beholder
> Just between Chloe's ribs and shoulder.
>
> Chloe observed it with surprise,
> And scarcely credited her eyes,
> "Why Strephon," rashly she begun
> "I have a heart and you have none."
> Strephon, now certain of his aim,
> Replied, "The case is not the same.

Mine was by nature soft, you knew it,
And with your eyes made holes all through it;
So to the X-rays it can give
No more resistance than a sieve.
But look at yours; how well defined,
How clear, how sharply 'tis outlined!
I always guessed, what now is known—
Your heart, fair Chloe, is a stone."[46]

The x-ray beam could pierce through the artificial, false exterior, whether it was a person's manner or dress, and discern the reality beneath, the inner person, which was assumed to be the "true" person.[47] The x-ray beam was also used as a metaphor for intensive scrutiny, to warn those trying to achieve a certain social status that they must be careful about how they present themselves, as in the 1896 bachelor who was warned to take excellent care of his belongings as he would be subjected to "the X-ray of criticism."[48] Yet within a few months of its invention the x-ray metaphor of searching beneath the surface was already coming in for a share of criticism, as a device that, while it might see "the invisible on the other side of a stone wall," might miss things as clear as glass which were even more important.[49]

By looking beneath the skin, the x-ray image could help eliminate distinctions between human beings, or it could serve to intensify them. The x-ray image could provide evidence of the grotesque nature of some of the artificial affectations of the upper class. It demonstrated that the tight lacing popular among some classes of women, supposedly to improve their outer appearance, in fact distorted their inner body by unnaturally compressing their ribs.[50] Take away the lacings and the outer trappings, and, it was suggested, all skeletons look basically the same.[51]

Others disagreed. Some insisted that class differences were quite clear, that "a laboring man or athlete's muscle [is] far more resistant than those of a person of sedentary habits" or that "there is quite as much difference in the hand of a washerwoman and the hand of a fine lady in an X-ray picture as in reality."[52] Some of the difference was in the bones; some was in the external ornaments, which could also be examined by the beam. Women had x rays taken of their hands covered with jewelry, to show that "beauty is not altogether of the flesh." Perhaps so, but, if beauty was not of the flesh but of the jewels, then it was only accessible to those people who could afford the jewels. And those would not include people who heretofore had been able to fool gullible friends with costume jewelry, for the x-ray image could demonstrate that supposedly rare gems were fake.[53] Through the all-seeing eyes of the x ray only the truly rare, truly valuable gems were beautiful.

The x ray's ability to generate and detect secrets was thought to vary for different types of people: "Babies and young women are the most easily photographed. A person who has a great deal of red blood, a strong robust person like a laboring man, is more difficult for the X-ray to penetrate."[54] Thus, it was thought to be easier to take x-ray images of women than of men, and public x-ray images tend to be those of women's bodies.

There is more going on here, however, than a mere difference in the technical ability of the x-ray beam to take pictures of men and women. A central theme had to do with the potential for the invasion of privacy, and that threat, for reasons that have to do with more than simply a difference in body mass, was a more serious concern for women than for men. Yet for certain kinds of examinations of women concerns about privacy could actually provide reasons to use the new x-ray machine.

FEMALE ORGANS

The x-ray beam could "see" within the body. It could reveal not just bones but also internal organs, including those found only in women. Its use for that purpose has to be understood in terms of the general issue of (mainly) male physicians examining women, a subject that was seen very differently from male physicians examining other men. The difference was a result of both gender and sex. The social construction of "femaleness"—gender—had a great deal to do with how physicians and other health care providers were to look at women, but so too did the actual anatomy.

Examination of the female genitalia was often done with special tools. Foremost among these tools was the vaginal speculum, which was known in ancient Greece but thereafter lapsed into disuse.[55] In 1810 it was revived and was used by the Parisian police who, during the nineteenth century, forced prostitutes to undergo examinations with the device. As an instrument of control, it was far more than a useful tool for doing physical examinations; it was a means of exploration and domination. Physicians described the speculum using the metaphor of being a "conquering and colonizing hero."[56] It was, both literally and metaphorically, the expression of male physicians' desire to open up and see deep within the female body.[57]

But which female's body? Certainly not all. Perhaps on account of its recent usage, the speculum was thought not to be appropriate for indiscriminate use in the nineteenth-century United States. It was held to be "unjustifiable on the grounds of propriety and morality" for the examination of most women because it involved looking at the female genitalia.[58] The moral issue was not physical but, rather, visual contact: there was no problem with a male physician examining the female genitalia, even breaking down the hymen with a finger, so long as he did not look. In the United States in the late nineteenth century the gaze was a far more potent cultural symbol of eroticism than was the touch. The gaze was what young lovers shared across a crowded room. Unlike the touch, it could not be easily controlled or even accurately located.[59] Male clinicians who intended to take care of respectable women needed to learn to operate without the gaze, to operate by touch, and look only in an emergency. "Catheterism, vaginal exploration, delivery by forceps, can all be performed by a competent man as well without the eye as with it."[60] It was better that women, particularly middle- and upper-class women, should suffer "extreme danger and pain" than waive decency. Physical examination, when necessary, should be done only after considering "the feelings of the patient."[61]

The dangers of having men examine women were especially acute during childbirth, as women were thought to be particularly prone to succumb to medical men at that time: "In the submission of women to the unnecessary examinations of physicians, *exposing* the secrets of nature, it is forgotten that every indecency of this kind is a violent attack against chastity. . . . Some women are attended by half a dozen different doctors. How much "affection" is left for the poor husband?"[62] Perhaps not surprisingly, in light of the male-dominated nature of the prevailing discourse, the expressed concern was not about any threat to the women's sensibilities but, rather, a threat to her husband's future access to her affections. At the extreme, following introduction to the pleasures of "instrumental sex," as the medical historian Ornella Moscucci has called it, women were never the same, reduced to the mental and moral conditions of prostitutes, upon whom the speculum was first employed, seeking to give themselves the same indulgence by means of solitary vice, forever seeking medical practitioners to examine their sexual organs.

Given the general disapproval of men looking directly at women's sexual organs, the x-ray beam could be more than a threat to women's privacy. It could also be simultaneously a protector of women's privacy, if it could allow medical men to examine women without having to look directly at their genitalia.[63] The x ray might be particularly useful for examining women before and during childbirth.

Issues of privacy are stated explicitly in the first description, in 1896, of using x rays to visualize the fetal skeleton. The author, a clinical professor of obstetrics at Jefferson Medical College in Philadelphia who had recently been named chair of the department, paid careful attention to the issue of female exposure to the male gaze. He noted that the eighteen-year-old patient had her abdomen covered by a sheet and that a nurse was in attendance.[64] Although the author did not emphasize this aspect of the woman's preparation, the fact that he chose to include the details of who was in attendance and how the patient was covered is unusual. Such descriptions are not usually found in medical reports about men undergoing an x-ray examination.

The woman was told that the rays would be used to ascertain the position of the fetus. The first exposure of one hour did not show the fetus. (Although the people who did the study did not think in our present-day terms, by not long after this experiment contemporary observers had conceptualized several reasons why a long exposure was necessary. There is a considerable thickness of the woman's and fetus's body which needed to be penetrated, and the fetal skeleton is less ossified than that of an adult.[65] Also, the fetus moves, which blurs the image. In addition, early x-ray machines were not particularly powerful nor were x-ray recording media particularly sensitive. Another problem arose from the hardness of the x-ray tube that was used, given the need to use either static electricity or batteries to power the tube.) Another exposure of an hour and fifteen minutes gave an image, but it was not sufficient to allow the examiners to tell the fetal position. The woman and fetus thus received a total of two hours and fifteen minutes of radiation. We have no record of the eventual outcome of the pregnancy.[66] The authors are quite clear about the value of the examination in terms of protecting the woman's privacy. They noted in their report that the procedure "requires no exposure of the patient, no vaginal manipulation." Of course, at the same time that the woman's privacy was being protected, the physicians' reputations were also being protected from charges of invading such privacy.[67] Thus, in this early description the x-ray machine acted to protect rather than to compromise a woman's privacy.

Visualizing a fetus with the x ray could make the diagnosis of pregnancy, a task by no means easy late in the nineteenth century. The absence of menstruation could have many causes. A swelling in the lower abdomen might indicate pregnancy, or it might denote something else, such as a tumor. A wrong diagnosis of pregnancy could be devastating, particularly for a single, "respectable" woman. In one instance an erroneous diagnosis of pregnancy was made, and, in that case, it was reported that the woman "belongs to a highly respectable family and will always feel the effect of a wrong diagnosis."[68] Perhaps the x ray would help make a diagnosis of pregnancy: "Should such a thing become possible it certainly will be practicable, as it may be carried on with the intended mother well covered in bed, the clothing offering no obstacle to the ray." Thus, one could dissipate "scandalous reports originated and circulated by venomous gossip-mongers."[69] Until the mid-1920s laboratory tests to diagnose pregnancy were not available, and, it was thought, images of the fetus might provide the most definitive evidence of pregnancy possible, short of childbirth.

But the differences between treatment of men and women who were being x-rayed extended beyond simply diagnosing pregnancy or examining female organs. There was a marked difference in the way men and women were to be treated for more general examinations. In a highly practical guide to taking x rays practitioners were advised that, for gastrointestinal, chest, or genitourinary examinations, "all clothing is removed." If, however, the patient were female, "a white washable gown [was] slipped on."[70] No mention is made of the need for a gown if the patient were male. Thus, men need not have had attention paid to their possible exposure during the procedure, whereas women did. Advertisements for public demonstrations of the x ray noted that "a lady assistant is in attendance," implying some sensitivity to the all-seeing nature of the rays.[71] The privacy issue is very clear in other discussions of how to take x rays of women, some of which emphasize the need for trained nurses who can give "support of feminine presence."[72]

One can also see gender differences in advice given to physicians about how to take x-ray images while inflicting minimal emotional upset upon the patient. "Tension and fear" were impediments to obtaining adequate images, as these emotions would "cause bones to quiver, which destroys detail."[73] The problems caused by fear were held to be greater for women than for men. There was general concern about a woman's emotional response to having an x ray taken. One physician noted that x rays were a new experience: "The patient . . . usually has in mind all the possible dangers she has read about in the newspapers. Her nervous condition can bring about an increased pulse rate, a nervous diarrhea, vomiting, and even a headache."[74] A *New York Times* article entitled "Her Latest Photograph" takes pains to point out in the headline, as well as in a subheading, that "women are not afraid," at least not after they have been assured that there is no danger.[75] Women were held to be weaker than men, and pregnant women were held to be particularly frail. In addition to the difficulties already noted, x-ray images of pregnant women were thought to be further limited because pregnant women could not lie still for any length of time. On the other hand, the authors of the initial report of x-ray visualization of the fetus noted that the mother was not perturbed, and, in fact, "she seemed rather to be soothed by the constant sound of the apparatus."[76] There is an interesting gender issue here. Pregnant women are certainly not the only group of people of whom x-ray pictures were being taken who might find it difficult to lie still for any length of time. A man with a broken leg or a kidney stone would have a great deal of difficulty remaining immobile. Kidney stones were one of the early types of objects visible on an x-ray examination, and they were also held to be more common in men than in women. They were also thought, then as well as now, to be excruciatingly painful; when the ureter was obstructed it would cause "agonizing pain," "nausea," "vomiting," and "collapse."[77] Yet one does not find admonitions about the difficulty in immobilizing male patients, only female. Nor does one see any great concern about male emotional reactions to the x-ray apparatus.

THEORY AND PRACTICE: DIFFERENCES BETWEEN X-RAY EXAMINATIONS OF MEN AND WOMEN

Thus far the discussion has focused on the ideas expressed in the popular and medical press. It may be useful to shift attention back to patient care. How were these ideas expressed in medical practice? How did gender inform the practice of using x rays to make diagnoses? Were male physicians more inclined to take x-ray images of women as a means of obtaining information without having women take off their clothes? Or as a means of exerting their power? Or because women had less red blood and it was therefore easier to obtain images of their bodies? Or, alternatively, were physicians less inclined to take x-ray images of women, perhaps concerned that the frail nature of women would make them more susceptible to the deleterious effects of the rays? Or concerned that they would be somehow inappropriately invading women's privacy?

How did patients react? Figure 5.2 shows a prominent early worker with the x ray (who later died from exposure to the rays) examining a woman's chest. How did she feel about being "looked into" in this way? Were women afraid of the new machines? Did they feel comforted that they were receiving the very latest in medical care? There has been some discussion of the very different ways in which physicians and pregnant women experience the imaging of a fetus late in the twentieth century.[78] It would be useful to know more about the feelings and perceptions of the first women and men who experienced the new imaging technology of the x ray, particularly those who did not leave a written record of their experience: the poor, the illiterate, and the otherwise disenfranchised. Perhaps we could understand how ethnicity and class informed a patient's experience.

We are restricted in our ability to answer such questions by a lack of sources. Unfortunately, patients did not (usually) keep diaries, and physicians did not systematically record their reasoning for each patient on whom they decided to take an x-ray picture. Yet, informed by the published literature, we can use existing hospital patient records to gain some insight into practice patterns, which we may then use to inform speculation about the reasoning and rationale of how x rays were used. When we do so we will find that the results are quite different for the New York and Pennsylvania hospitals.

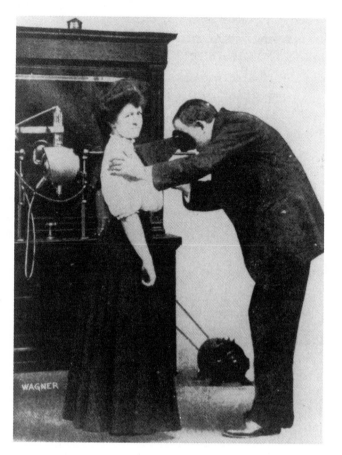

Figure 5.2   *X rays being used to look at the chest of a woman; Rome Wagner using the fluoroscope. Courtesy Nancy Knight, Center for the American History of Radiology.*

As a first step, one might simply compare how often physicians obtained x rays of men and women who were admitted to the hospital, with any diagnosis. This could move us away from a focus on diseases and conditions of women and allow us to examine how gender informed the taking of an x ray for whatever reason. At the Pennsylvania Hospital between 1900 and 1925 women were less likely to be studied with an x-ray image than were men.

Table 5.1 shows that, whereas almost 15 of every 100 men admitted to the hospital had an x-ray examination done, fewer than 10 of

Table 5.1   *X-ray Use at Pennsylvania Hospital, by Sex, 1900–1925:*
Totals and Percentages

	No X Ray	X Ray	Total
Males	847	148	995
	(85.13)	(14.87)	(100.00)
Females	568	59	627
	(90.59)	(9.41)	(100.00)
Total	1,415	207	1,622
	(87.24)	(12.76)	(100.00)

Note: Pearson chi-square (1) = 10.3160.   Pr = 0.001.

every 100 women had one done. Standard statistical techniques indicate that this difference is unlikely to be due simply to chance. The difference between the use of x rays for men and women is statistically significant.[79]

Yet this raw data does not adequately tell us why women received fewer x-ray examinations than men, though several reasons might explain why this was so: the age distribution of women admitted to the hospital was different than that of men; there was a different proportion of Americans and people of other nationalities; this analysis combines the entire first quarter of the twentieth century, and ideas about x rays may have changed differently for men and for women between 1900 and 1925; and, perhaps most important, we know that women and men did not enter the hospital for the same reasons. Men were more likely than women, for example, to enter the hospital as a result of trauma, and this might have contributed to the greater percentage of men receiving an x ray. As discussed in chapter 4, by 1920, almost everyone with a broken limb had an x-ray image taken before he or she left the hospital. Not surprisingly, given the traumatic nature of such disorders, more men than women entered the hospital with broken limbs. Of all men who were admitted, 5.63 percent had fractures, as compared with 2.07 percent of women.[80]

Statistical techniques to account for variation in diagnosis, as well as other variables, have been well established for use by health services researchers in the late twentieth century. (The term now used is *case-mix adjustment,* or *age adjustment.*) Obviously, practitioners at the Pennsylvania Hospital between 1900 and 1925 did not use such techniques. Thus, by themselves these statistical techniques cannot answer questions about the causes of behavior. Nevertheless, they enable us analytically to separate gender difference from other types of differences among patients who entered the hospital.

Using this technique, logistic regression, one estimates an equation to predict whether or not a given patient would have had an x-ray image taken. One can also include in the equation variables for other factors which could also have influenced the decision. In this instance I have corrected for the age and race of the patient, the patient's nationality (American or foreign), the year, and the diagnosis.[81] This analysis has the advantage that it includes all types of diagnoses, not just those of women, and thus captures behavior with respect to disorders not specifically related to sexual anatomy. One can then ask: Having corrected for age, race, diagnosis, and year, was the likelihood of a person having an x-ray examination still different for men and women?

At the Pennsylvania Hospital the answer is yes: women would still be significantly less likely to have had an x-ray image taken. (The detailed results of the analysis are provided in the notes.)[82] This difference was not a result of differing diagnoses on admission or of differences in ages. Interestingly, once these other factors were taken into account, neither race or nationality appeared to make a difference.

Statistics offers correlations, not explanations. We are left to speculate about why women had an x-ray image taken less often than men. By 1920 and 1925, when most of these x rays were taken, physicians may have started to perceive increasing dangers associated with x-ray use and may have been more hesitant about sending women for an x-ray examination. Perhaps they believed women to be more susceptible to the deleterious effects of the rays or more likely to become upset at the process of having an image taken. Perhaps physicians feared lawsuits more if women were injured than men. Awareness of that potential may have been heightened by a 1920 case in which a woman, the sister of a judge, was burned by the x rays.[83] Following the incident the radiologist, David Bowen, visited the home of the unfortunate woman, to explain that burns were an unfortunate, but not uncommon, complication. Evidently, Bowen felt that it was more important to explain the situation to the woman's husband than to the woman herself, an unsurprising assumption in 1920. Bowen was frustrated in his mission in part because the woman insisted that her husband not be informed of her condition, thus making it impossible for Bowen to discuss the matter frankly with him. The medical staff concluded that Bowen was blameless. Nonetheless, he described himself as being placed into a "humiliating position."

Another incident occurred three years later. A woman brought her daughter to the hospital to have an elbow injury evaluated. The mother was asked to hold the "little girl's" arm during the taking of the x ray. "The technician allowed one of the wires to be too close to the patient and her mother and a spark from the wire slightly burned both mother and child and knocked them both down. In the fall the mother sprained her ankle. At the present time [twenty days after the episode] the burns are healed and the sprained ankle is much better."[84] One must wonder about the intensity of the spark necessary to knock the mother down! The Board of Managers was relieved that neither the woman nor her husband had displayed any intention to pursue legal action against the institution. The impact of these episodes on the decision to use x rays on other women must remain a matter of speculation, but they may have sensitized physicians at the Pennsylvania Hospital to potential hazards of the x ray.

Even if it did not result in injury, the act of going to receive an examination was rather unpleasant. X-ray machines were not particularly comforting to be around. One person described watching such a machine at work: "A spark about a foot long leaped between the end of two horizontal lightening rods on the top of the machine, crackling like fury and supercharging the atmosphere with ozone."[85] Perhaps physicians were more concerned about how women would react than they were about men. On the other hand, perhaps for some the reasoning was less kind. If the x ray were seen as an important tool for aiding a patient's recovery, men may have been more likely to be tested with the tool because they may have been perceived as more important. We do not know.

We can compare findings at the Pennsylvania Hospital with those at the New York Hospital, for which we see a different type of pattern. Here the results are in the opposite direction and are also statistically significant.[86] Women were more likely to receive an x-ray examination.

Table 5.2 *X-ray Use at New York Hospital, by Sex, 1900–1920:*
Totals and Percentages

	No X Ray	X Ray	Total
Male	529	31	560
	(94.46)	(5.54)	(100.00)
Female	317	33	350
	(90.57)	(9.43)	(100.00)
Total	846	64	910
	(92.97)	(7.03)	(100.00)

Note: Pearson chi-square (1) = 4.9921.   Pr = 0.025. (In thirty cases the sex of the patient could not be determined.)

Again, one can do a logistic regression to correct for differences in diagnosis, age, year, and nationality. (Race cannot be used because it was recorded in less than 10 percent of cases in the New York Hospital records.) Here correcting for case mix changes the conclusions. The difference between men and women is no longer significant. At the New York Hospital the observed difference between the use of x rays for men and women was due to differences in the diagnoses that first brought men and women into the hospital. (The note provides the full analysis.)[87]

Why the difference between the two hospitals? One might speculate about factors that would explain the difference in findings as a result of variations in data collection rather than behavior. For one, the data from the New York Hospital does not include cases from 1925, and it is possible that by 1925 the fear of the x ray causing injury had increased enough to influence physicians' willingness to subject women to possible ill effects. By not having data from 1925 at the New York Hospital, the impact of this change may be obscured. Because race was infrequently recorded at the New York Hospital, it could not be used in the analysis. Although at the Pennsylvania Hospital race was not an important predictor of x-ray use, it may have been at the New York Hospital, and failure to have that information may have obscured a real difference between the way men and women were treated.

Or there may simply have been a difference in the local culture at the two hospitals, with differences in gender having an impact on x-ray use at one hospital and not the other. If there were no high-profile, untoward incidents involving x rays and women at the New York Hospital (and I could not locate any record of such events), as there were at the Pennsylvania Hospital, physicians may have been less hesitant to send women for studies. Perhaps there are other reasons as well. Without information from other hospitals we have no way of knowing which, if either, of these two hospitals was typical of U.S. medical practice between 1900 and 1925. Even so, this finding suggests the importance of controlling appropriately for case-mix differences in historical analysis. It also shows how gender mattered in deciding whether to obtain x-ray examinations in at least one institution, and not in another, and emphasizes the importance of considering gender in the analysis of imaging technologies.

Whose New World?

In order to understand how the early-twentieth-century meaning of the x-ray image was constructed, it may help to consider some relationships between the new machine and various groups of people, particularly physicians, a group who worked hard to claim authority over the new machine. For both within the hospitals and outside of them a central question was: Who was going to control the x-ray machine?

I shall first discuss this debate in light of the rise in status of American physicians and the relationship of that status to the authority of the x-ray image and those who read it. Second, I will note how the x-ray machine was defined differently among medical sects. Finally, I will consider how x-ray images played into the relationship between mechanizing the body and making the study of medicine an apparently objective, scientific, and, perhaps, masculine enterprise.

American physicians in the nineteenth century were not held in particularly high regard. Most health care was delivered in a patient's home, often by lay providers, often women. Few people perceived any direct linkage between science and medical practice. That impression began to change with the microbiological revolution, though the much-praised identification of the organism responsible for tuberculosis probably did not have any immediate effect on mortality and morbidity from the disease.[88] The following years were filled with the identification of many other microorganisms that were assigned roles in causing human disease. Thus, when it appeared, the x-ray image was seen as one more marker of a new, scientific medicine—recall that the x-ray image of the hand appearing in the developing tank was a coming from a new world, a new "scientific" world.[89] Partially as a result of the scientific efficiency craze, partially as a result of the fruits of the microbiological revolution and the reform of medical education, appeals to science started to carry more weight. They did so in a social context in which other, related concepts—psychoanalysis, cubism, the theory of relativity—changed the ways in which people thought about the world; all were concepts that we now think of as based on a scientific worldview.[90]

Like science, the appeal of technology was broadly based. During the late nineteenth and the early twentieth centuries an increasing number of machines—the telegraph, telephone, automobile, and airplane—had an enormous impact on everyday life. These innovations had implications for changing cultural ideas about machines. Having made an appointment using a telephone and driven in a car or taken a form of mass transit to the doctor's office, it seemed natural to be measured and imaged by a mechanical device, to acknowledge the implicit authority of the machine. One could hear easily phrases such as: "The skiagraph [x ray] is never wrong. When error exists it lies in the interpretation."[91] Other physicians simply asserted that "shadows do not lie."[92] The dominance of machine-generated knowledge persists to this day.

If the x-ray machine helped provide a more authoritative, more scientific voice for diagnosis of disease, who was to lay claim to the authority produced by the machine and its images? For whom? Technology in general is used by those in power to assert their positions of power.[93] Medical technology is no different; the images medical machines produce and the uses to which they are put reflect choices among a number of possible options, and those choices often reflect the professional goals of the people who are in control of the machines. Part of the reason to use x-ray images was to make medicine scientific, as a way of gaining professional power, not for the sake of inanimate machines that made x rays but, rather, for people who could claim special expertise in their use. Medical specialists attempted to use the technology in order to increase their status among both the public and other medical specialties.[94]

But there was a problem for physicians wishing to use new, scientific technology to assert their power through machine-generated information. The machines were easy to make, and the images appeared to be easy to read. Foreign bodies, such as a penny stuck in a child's esophagus, were obvious on an x-ray image. So were broken bones. Such pictures had appeared widely in the popular press as well as in medical publications. At least for a time there appeared to have been general agreement that lay people could derive some meaning from an x-ray image.[95] The fact that x-ray images were easy to understand made the x-ray machine a more useful device in some ways. Clinicians could use it to convince their patients to follow medical advice. If patients were worried, but in the opinion of the physician quite well, the physician could show them an x-ray image to demonstrate that they (or their organ) were indeed healthy.[96] Conversely, the physician could show a sick person, perhaps an alcoholic, the ravages of his or her disease in order to convince that person to stop drinking. Moreover, the actual test result, the x ray itself, was something people could hold in their hand, could carry about with them, and could look at without special equipment, anywhere there was a source of light. Useful though this might be for patient education, if the x-ray machine and the image's meanings were accessible to all viewers, this presented a problem for those wishing to become authorities. How could they assert control over the new technology?

One important way was by taking possession of the image itself. The x-ray plate was, basically, a photograph. In fact, the hospital photographer was initially called upon to run the x-ray equipment at many U.S. hospitals, including some quite prominent ones.[97] Yet physicians using the x ray did not want to be classed as "photographers and picture makers."[98] They feared that soon patients might start calling to make appointments for a sitting.[99] Therefore, medical practitioners who worked with the x-ray machine took pains to distance themselves not only from other physicians, as discussed in chapter 4, but also from photographers, whom they wished to portray as people of lower stature and ability, judged on their ability to make an attractive image more than their skill in arriving at a difficult medical conclusion. One way physicians could differentiate themselves from photographers was to emphasize that the patient paid for an opinion and that the practitioner, not the patient, owned the plate. This issue of ownership was firmly established by the Pennsylvania Hospital's Board of Managers, who, when they started charging outpatients for x-ray examinations, gave each patient a card that read, in part, that "the charge for x-rays . . . does not entitle the patient to any plates, prints, or reports for use outside the hospital."[100] This statement left no doubt about what, precisely, one was purchasing from the hospital, and it was not an x-ray plate: it was a medical opinion.

Another approach that could help differentiate physician from photographer was simply not to show a patient the image. The public had quickly become familiar with x-ray pictures through reproductions in the popular press, such as that in figure 5.1. Clinicians contended that familiarity need not imply the ability to make medical judgments, that the x-ray image was not, as it might at first appear, an easily interpreted picture. Rather, it was a complex piece of scientific data and, as such, deserved to be treated like other kinds of clinical scientific data. Physicians would not "consider it proper to exhibit to the patient such diagnostic evidence as a slide of a urinary sediment or a blood smear."[101] This would never occur to them; after all, the urinary sediment and blood smear required specialized expertise and equipment to interpret. Similarly, "the patient ha[d] no more right to expect or demand an X-ray print than . . . to receive a photomicrograph or pathological slide from his pathologist."[102] Subtleties of the x-ray image, heretofore not properly recognized (or so it was claimed), demanded that medical practitioners provide patients only with the information that could be derived therefrom. Patients could not on their own derive information from the x ray and would only be confused. Physicians should withhold not only from the patients' possession but also from their sight the actual, physical image.

If an image is perceived as being valuable or useful, ownership of that image creates power. By controlling the x-ray image, physicians forced patients to come into the medical practitioner's office as supplicants, not only with less knowledge initially but also with less access to the medical information that was to be gleaned about them. Defining most forms of medical knowledge as privileged information for the health care provider became much more common in the early twentieth century, and the trend has continued. This was, and has continued to be, defended as a necessary consequence of the increasingly technical nature of medical care. In the case of x-ray images, however, the inequities of power which flowed from differential access to the images that provided such power were, to some extent, actively and artificially created by those who had the most to gain. Thus, the x ray was used as a means of gaining knowledge and power for medicine in general. Similar observations have been made about other elements of medical care; the x-ray image was neither the first nor the last example in which members of the medical profession defined some forms of knowledge as inaccessible to the layperson.

It is not at all clear from a late-twentieth-century vantage point just how easy (or difficult) it was for early-twentieth-century patients to make sense out of x-ray images. Showing such images to lay (nonmedically trained) audiences in the 1990s—including both patients in the clinical setting and historians in the seminar room—has yielded decidedly mixed results in terms of their ability to make sense of the shadows. Some lay people have quickly grasped meaning from the images; some have been unable to perceive any information without considerable explanation. Patients who have had the opportunity to view many x-ray images of their own body over long periods of time, such as patients confined to hospitals or sanatoria with chronic diseases, are often able, quickly and accurately, to identify the key radiological features of their own shadows, sometimes more quickly and accurately than their medically trained caregivers.[103]

It was perhaps inevitable that those people in the early years of the twentieth century who viewed x-ray images most often would, through experience, gain greater expertise. Yet, prior to 1895, no one had any expertise in interpreting x-ray images. At least for a time x-ray images were part of popular culture, appearing in mass-market magazines alongside explanations of what was revealed by the shadows. But the x-ray image gradually became mystified; it became located within the province of the physician. Other technical representations of the material world have remained part of the lay universe—such things as maps and timetables. The x-ray machine is perhaps worthy of particular note due to its prominence, the way that it served as the model for so many other imaging devices, and the fact that it was, for a short period of time, perceived as being part of the public sphere.

Physicians in the early twentieth century were a heterogeneous lot. Medical licensure laws had been generally eliminated during the nineteenth century, and the new licensing laws of the early twentieth century divided responsibility among various sects.[104] Allopathic physicians, those who are now the holders of M.D. degrees, were only one of many alternative medical sects. Examining ways in which some other sects looked at the new machine may help us see other ways of thinking about the x-ray machine, other ways it could have been used.

Chiropractic practitioners, for example, at first refused to use medical technology in general and derided those who "wasted valuable time" looking at tissues under the microscope. But chiropractors had various attitudes and displayed a range of reactions to the x-ray machine. While some of the more orthodox practitioners resisted the interposition of anything between the patient's back and the examiner's hand, by the 1920s most chiropractors had come to accept use of the x rays in some form, and some of them did extensive research using machines as sophisticated as those available anywhere.[105] When they did accept use of the x-ray machine, it was specifically targeted to fit with diagnosing the essential chiropractic disorder of vertebral subluxations.[106] Thus, x-ray images were used to reinforce the central tenets of the chiropractic system.

Homeopathy was a much more important and powerful sect in the 1900s than it is in the 1990s, constituting about 10 percent of all American physicians and competing effectively for seats on state licensing boards.[107] Rather than striving for scientific objectification, the essence of the idea of science for the allopaths, homeopaths held that attempts to standardize x rays were fruitless: "All these mathematical and physical and chemical methods are dangerous because they do not take into consideration the biological and personal equations. Every roentgenologist of experience knows that young and old, the sick and the well, the anemic and hyperemic, the brunette and blond, the Caucasian and African, react differently."[108] This statement was meant to be read in opposition to the perception that those practicing allopathic medicine were starting to think about patients in purely biological terms and not as social beings. Homeopaths ascribed the x ray's healing powers not to the rays but, instead, to the patient's own body.[109] These attitudes reveal a very different approach to the machine. Similar to their use of dilute concentrations of drugs, homeopaths practiced a style of medicine which was very attentive to their patients' specific circumstances.[110] The individual patient was at the center of attention, rather than the machine.

Yet, instead of chiropractic, homeopathy, or any of the several other sects that we could have wound up with, allopathy, for better or for worse, has become the dominant medical sect in the United States. Over the course of the twentieth century allopathic medicine has become increasingly reductionist and scientific.

Allopathic medicine has also, like most other formal medical systems, been controlled primarily by men. Although women were initially banned from most medical schools, a combination of progressive admission practices and new medical schools specifically for women led to a surprisingly high number of female physicians by the turn of the twentieth century. Around 20 percent of Boston physicians were women in 1900 as well as almost 6 percent of those in the United States.[111] From 1900 until midcentury the proportion of female physicians constantly declined. To the extent that there are gender differences in relation to the ways that physicians practice medicine, the masculine nature of U.S. medicine may be related to the use of technology. This observation in not new. Even in the 1900s popular fiction often portrayed modern doctors as technology based, treating people as machines, obsessed with time management, utterly uninterested in the empathetic aspects of medical care, and clearly, unambiguously male.[112] As the percentage of female physicians fell, medicine became more technology based. The idea that health and disease are defined by technology, and in ways that are inaccessible to the patient, may in part reflect a male rather than a female view of health care, one associated with the fact that most American physicians are men.[113] Whether the increasing numbers of female physicians entering medical practice near the end of the twentieth century will effect a change in the nature of medical care remains to be seen.

Art can provide a useful expression of reactions to technology as well as give insight into social ideas about the human body. The 1926 etching and aquatint by the American artist John Sloan (1871–1951), presented in figure 5.3, gives a particularly telling interpretation of how one patient perceived the ways that the x-ray machine could distance physicians from patients. Sloan was himself a patient as

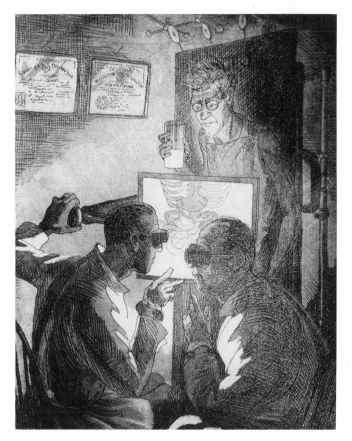

Figure 5.3   X-rays, *by John Sloan (1926).*

well as an artist who prided himself on his skills at looking behind the obvious.[114] He underwent a series of investigations to determine the cause of his maladies. The way that he depicted his relationship with his physicians and the technology that they used provides an interesting window into one person's experience with medical technology.

Sloan shows himself drinking barium while x rays are passed through his body from behind to create an image of his gastrointestinal tract. Two people, presumably physicians, look intently at the glowing screen. Diplomas on the walls mark them as experts, probably specialists, not merely opportunistic entrepreneurs who happened to purchase a new machine. The artist has accentuated the physicians' distance from their patient in several ways. The scene has been altered: physicians would usually wear the goggles only when the room lights were on; here they wear them even though the room is in darkness, which highlights how much Sloan felt separate from his physicians.[115] The goggles also emphasize the physicians' alliance with the machine: the goggles make them look as though they are almost part of the machine or at least an extension of the machinery. The physicians appear to be pointing down not only at the gastrointestinal tract but also, perhaps, at the patient's genital area as well. They look aggressive as they crouch and peer into the body's image on the screen; the patient appears passive and distant, both physically and emotionally. It appears that the patient would like very much to look at the image himself, to join in the discussion, but that is clearly not an option. The physicians are not interested in talking to the person but would rather examine his organs. The artist has chosen to highlight the physician, while leaving the patient in a secondary position on the other side of the screen. The x-ray screen here serves to emphasize not only the mechanical nature of the human body but also how the machine separates the patient from his physicians. In Sloan's case this separation is no less intense because Sloan is male, not female.

Some have suggested that medical machines inevitably distance patients from their physicians, as Sloan has depicted. It is by no means clear that this must have been the case. Machines were central to the efficiency movement, and with them physicians could make better use of their time. If machines could permit physicians and their patients to obtain the same clinical results in less time, physicians could have used the time saved by machines to spend more time talking with their patients. There is no reason inherent in the technology which would have prohibited them from using the extra time in that way. But such was not the case for Sloan and is not the case today. That machines now symbolize a distancing of patient from physician reflects our societal ideas about medicine more than it does the physical artifact of the machine.

Machines are associated with fundamental thoughts about the nature of the human body. Ideas about the mechanical nature of the human body are very old. There are obviously other ways in which one could conceptualize the body. One could use metaphors having to do with nature, for example, or with heat and light. The machine metaphor was particularly central to U.S. medicine in the early twentieth century, precisely the period when the x ray was having such an impact on popular ideas about the human body.[116]

X-ray pictures provided a stimulus for artists to make the mechanical features of the body more visible as well as providing a reason for visual artists to reevaluate their assumptions about how to create their images.[117] In so doing, gender once again informed the creation of new ideas and models. As the historian Lana Rakow has observed: "Technologies both constitute and express a model of social relationships. The contemporary meaning and experience of gender does not exist somewhere outside of and distinct from technology; gender is articulated through it."[118] Thus, technologies did not create the ways in which we choose to conceptualize male and female; they reflected those ideas. In a world in which physicians were already starting to think of themselves as analogous to engineers, it seemed more natural than ever to see the body as a machine.[119] X-ray images could define what was different about women, the other, and help to label them as reproductive vehicles.

These images were reflected in various works of art. In a painting titled *Mechanized Maternity* the noted Mexican artist Diego Rivera portrayed the female body in ways that are reminiscent of the x ray's ability to "open up" the human body and which evoke the perceived relevance of science not only for the human body but also for engineering and for factories (see fig. 5.4).[120] The interior of the woman's body is taken up by machinery; it appears that the primary purpose of that machinery is reproduction. Her body is split into two parts; the top and the bottom are not connected. The internal reproductive machines are distanced from the rest of her body. They are no longer sexual; they are no longer social; they are simply mechanical. The flowing, organic nature of the traditional female form is contrasted with the sharp, angular nature of her internal machinery. The externalization of her "inner" organs evokes some of the work—and, indeed, the life—of Rivera's wife, Frieda Kahlo.[121] In commentary on *Mechanized Maternity* Rivera stated that he wished to critique how capitalist society used machinery to exploit people; he simultaneously provided a critique of how women are treated as reproductive vessels, using for both messages an image of an opening up of the female body.

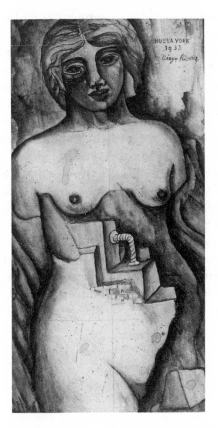

Figure 5.4   Mechanized Maternity, *by Diego Rivera (1933). Courtesy of the Dolores Olmedo collection*

The x-ray image could be used to objectify the body. Using it, one could look at the body without being overtly sexual; one could look at the body as a scientist, without having to deal with emotions. One could thus look through the body surface to the inside, without having to deal with external issues. The x-ray image thus helped to bring the meaning of the body out of the social sphere.

Were the x ray's images and ways of looking at the body, the idea of objectivity and focusing on the eye, particularly masculine? Vision creates a distance between the viewer and that which is being viewed. The emphasis on the x-ray image as a privileged way of knowing may be part of a male dominance of the whole enterprise of scientific medicine, along with a diminution of the importance of an affective understanding of illness, which has traditionally been the realm of female understanding.[122]

What difference does it make that the x ray was used in a male-dominated world of science and medicine? Would the machine have been thought about differently, or applied differently, had women been able to control and define the imaging device, rather than only be seen by it? We cannot know the answers to these questions. We can only point out the ways in which the x-ray image was defined in terms of a larger social world and assume that other medical devices, likewise, are defined and used in ways that reflect broad social assumptions about relationships among human beings.

The use of the x-ray machine and ideas about the images that it created reflected both social and biological aspects of being male and female. The images were interpreted in ways that reflected social ideas about women and men, and the images were incorporated into much older debates that reflected broad cultural ideals. The x-ray machine and its images both were and are shaped by and shaping of the ways that we look at the body.

6

BLOOD AND BLOOD COUNTS
Ideas and Instruments

At the turn of the twentieth century, the x-ray beam provided new and exciting pictures about what was going on inside the human body. At the same time as the x ray was becoming part of a scientifically oriented medical world so, too, were a whole host of other laboratory tests, which also helped to define U.S. medical care as being based on science. In chapter 3 we addressed how an old test, the urinalysis, was transformed into a different type of test, albeit still called a urinalysis. We now consider a set of laboratory tests that were seen as much newer: those done on the blood.

Ideas about what makes up blood have a long history. As early as 1673, the Dutch naturalist Antoni van Leeuwenhoek used the newly invented microscope to describe globules in his own blood as well as in that of various animals.[1] His primary concern was discovering where and how the blood was made, not caring for sick people. But in the seventeenth century, as always, blood was often a prominent feature when people were ill. Both patients and their caregivers doubtless wondered about whether useful diagnostic or prognostic information could be derived from the blood's appearance, either with the naked eye or, for those few practitioners who had access to the necessary tools, microscopically.

During the nineteenth century caregivers in the United States frequently treated patients by bleeding them. Partly because of the widespread use of bloodletting, partly because of the common appearance of blood in both intentional and unintentional incisions into the human body, the sight of blood was common; indeed, observers noted that "no fluid of the body is more open to inspection than the blood."[2] Physicians became familiar with the gross appearance of the blood. Some attempted to draw conclusions from what they could see with their unaided eyes. As the practice of bloodletting became less popular over the last portion of the nineteenth century, direct observation of the blood became less of a factor in diagnosis and prognosis. Nonetheless, physicians' earlier experience with examining blood provided some precedents for using it to read diagnostic information. For example, when blood drawn from a vein was allowed to clot, it would sometimes display a grayish crust, or buff. This appearance, also called corium phlogisticum, was often seen in patients with violent inflammation and was interpreted as indicating the need for more aggressive bleeding. The buff that coated the blood was called the "buffy coat." It was originally thought to contain only an inert material known as fibrin, and the thickness was believed to correlate with the severity of the infection. The term *buffy coat* persisted even after the coat was shown microscopically to be made of white blood cells.[3]

Even as the practice of bloodletting declined in popularity, the use of laboratory aids for diagnosis was starting to become more prevalent. Prompted in part by the burgeoning German school of laboratory medicine, physicians and scientists in the United States and England attempted laboratory examination of blood in a variety of ways. In the remainder of this chapter I shall explore various ways of examining the blood, considering the implications for a physician's practice of adopting certain methods as well as the effect that blood drawing might have had upon the patient. The next chapter will address the use of blood counts in more detail for three specific diseases: pneumonia, typhoid fever, and appendicitis.

BLOOD: TECHNIQUES

For purposes of discussion the many instrumental techniques that were proposed may be divided into two general categories: those that included various ways of looking at the blood through a microscope and those that involved measuring properties of the blood in some other way.

Looking At and Counting the Blood

First, there was the possibility of looking directly at solid elements in the blood through a microscope. One of the most prominent of the nineteenth-century European physicians who described the microscopic appearance of blood was the French physician Gabriel Andral. Andral considered the properties that were visible without instrumental aids to be unreliable. In 1843 he described the appearance of blood corpuscles under the microscope.[4] He went on to carry out a range of chemical studies of the blood, faulting those who had promulgated what he considered to be inferior theories for having not examined the blood themselves.

In 1852 the German physician Karl Vierordt described a method for counting red blood cells. His method was accurate but difficult; it was said that he was able to accomplish only one cell count per week.[5] This technique would hardly be practical for routine clinical use. Others attempted to devise more reasonable methods for counting the cellular elements in blood.

In 1877 the English physician Sir William Richard Gowers published a brief article in which he described a method for the "Numeration of the Red Corpuscles."[6] Rather than making his grid a part of the microscope, as had been the case for earlier devices, Gowers made his counting grid a part of the slide (the slide with a counting chamber was called a hemocytometer; see fig. 6.1). Using this special device, an observer could count the cellular elements of the blood, including the two major types of cells present in the blood—what were termed red and white blood cells. Because the grid was part of the slide, it could be removed when the microscope was used for other purposes. As early as 1880, two physicians working at King's College Hospital in London counted the red blood cells of patients with a variety of conditions, attempting to correlate blood counts with clinical diseases.[7] Gowers's device was soon used as well by a handful of American physicians.[8] Several modifications were proposed on the ways that one could go about counting both red and white blood cells, with differences ranging from the type of slide to use, the site and style of the ruling, the type of pipette to use, to many other possibilities for technical variations.[9]

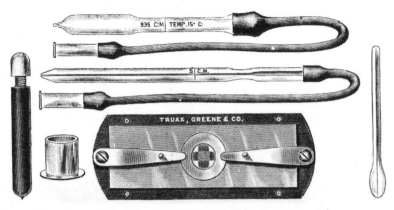

Figure 6.1 *Gower's hemocytometer. From Charles Truax,* The Mechanics of Surgery *(Chicago: Hammond Press, 1899), 42.*

Measuring the Blood

Counting the cells was difficult, perhaps too difficult for routine work. Another possibility was not to count cells at all but, instead, either to measure the volume taken up by some blood cells or to measure some characteristic property of those cells. This was not possible for white cells, which make up a very small minority of the cell population in the blood (though a very interesting and important minority, as we shall see). But for the far more numerous red blood cells some means other than microscopic enumeration could be used. One possibility involved the pigment that was known to make the red blood cells appear red, a molecule called hemoglobin. Perhaps one could measure the amount of hemoglobin in the blood. In 1878 Gowers followed up on his earlier blood-counting invention by demonstrating an apparatus that allowed physicians to compare the color of blood with the color of a known standard. Using this device, one could estimate the amount of hemoglobin in the blood and thus, indirectly, the number of red blood cells. As with methods for counting cells, innumerable variations and enhancements were proposed on methods for visually estimating the amount of hemoglobin in the blood, along with an equivalent number of debates over which was the better method.

Another method for evaluating the red blood cells was to measure the amount of the blood they occupied by spinning a blood sample in a small tube using a centrifuge, possibly the same centrifuge as was used for a urinalysis. This compressed the red cells at one end of the tube, and the percentage of the total blood volume occupied by red cells could thus be ascertained. A numerical value, called the hematocrit, could be obtained in only about ten minutes, without the need for special expertise. These methods worked, in part because red blood cells were numerous and, in part, because they contained an easily measured pigment.

WHITE BLOOD CELLS

Looking at the blood with a microscope, nineteenth-century scientists could see different types of cells in the blood, red and white blood cells. One of the major problems, however, was how to tell them apart. Pathologists had described differences between red blood cells and white blood cells from their work on solid tissues.[10] But the white blood cells, also known as leucocytes, were far less numerous than the red and did not contain a distinctive pigment. Other differences between the two types of cells made assessment of white cells in the blood even more difficult. All mature red blood cells are the same basic type of cell,[11] but there are several different types of white cells found in the blood of both normal and ill individuals, a fact that had been known to pathologists for some time.

Even telling white cells apart from red cells in blood preparations was not easy. Some suggested adjusting the microscope while examining blood so that the image was slightly out of focus. Within the blurry image the white blood cells were larger than the red blood cells, and they would thus stand out; this method, it was observed, was quite trying to the eyes. Others proposed a reagent that would destroy one cell type but not the other. Still others suggested that differential stains would help.

Because the blood contains relatively few white blood cells, physicians at first believed that the cells did not play an important function, but two observations at the end of the nineteenth century combined to draw attention to white cells.[12] First was the discovery of leukemia, a disease characterized in some cases by a strikingly large increase in the number of white blood cells. Second was the realization that tissue inflammation of many causes was associated with an emigration of white blood cells from the tissues into the blood.

Two basic goals drove investigators to study the different types of white blood cells. Pathologists described the cells as part of a program of "pure" pathology, attempting to understand the meaning of the different types of tissues that make up the human body. Clinicians had a different goal in mind: they sought ways to identify disease in their patients. Clinicians wondered if the changes in the blood could provides clues to help identify tumors, diseases of the blood, and, most important, infections—diseases that were known to alter the number of white cells in the blood. They also knew, however, that the total number of white cells changed as part of normal life, in response to events such as eating a meal or becoming pregnant. In order for the white cells to provide useful information to guide medical care, clinicians needed to be able to differentiate a normal from an abnormal white blood cell picture.

The most common diagnostic problem arose when the white cell count was found to be higher than normal. Although a high white cell count could indicate the presence of infection, sometimes a person who had a high white cell count was found at autopsy to have suffered not from an infection but, instead, from leukemia. Conversely, even when the total white cell count was normal, abnormal types of cells in the bloodstream could indicate the presence of disease.[13] A number of different methods were proposed to differentiate between a normal and a pathological elevation in the white cell count or to detect abnormalities even when the total number of cells was normal.

Iodine Reaction

Although now long forgotten, the iodine reaction was once regarded as a useful way of differentiating a normal from a pathological increase in the white blood cell count, or leucocytosis. The test was quite easy to do: it was performed by "exposing a dried but unfixed blood film to the vapour arising from iodine crystals in some closed jar for about half an hour. The film is then examined [under a microscope] with oil immersion and there may be seen in some of the leucocytes (the majority of which stain light yellow or not at all) a brownish discolouration or brown granules."[14] The iodine reaction was seen as proof positive of disease, particularly infectious disease, which could cause sepsis: "In other words, no septic condition of any severity can be present without a positive reaction."[15] The Boston physician Richard C. Cabot, whose writings on examination of the blood had the greatest impact of any writer of the period, chose to include that same quotation in his textbook.[16] The use of iodophilia appears to have been widely accepted; it was included in textbooks well into the 1920s, but, for reasons unclear, it eventually fell from favor.[17] Perhaps one reason was that it did not enhance general understanding of white blood cells. Although one could empirically correlate the iodine reaction with the presence of infection, it was more difficult to put it into any kind of broader theoretical understanding. The test also did not fit into any preexisting basis for understanding white blood cells, certainly not in the way that the differential count did.

Differential Count

Another method for distinguishing different types of changes in the white cell count came from examining morphologically the different types of cells. In 1879 the German medical scientist Paul Ehrlich used a triacid stain to distinguish five different types of white blood cells.[18] This classification of white cells continues to be the basis for our understanding near the end of the twentieth century.[19] It was seen as valuable for at least two reasons: it served as a tool to understand better the different types of cells, quite apart from any clinical significance; and it was seen as helping physicians evaluate an abnormal white blood cell count.

Ehrlich's staining method attracted attention from U.S. physicians, one of whom in 1893 saw it as a way of studying the "much-neglected white blood-corpuscle."[20] The newly recognized importance of white blood cells in the body's reaction to infection suggested that Ehrlich's method could be useful in differentiating the various types of white blood cells in the peripheral circulation.

A formal counting of the percentage of the different types of cells in the peripheral circulation produced what was called a differential count, which attracted increasing attention in the U.S. medical literature starting around 1905–6, sparked by a report by the New York surgeon Charles Gibson on his use of the differential count in eight thousand cases in private practice. Gibson's article, along with one by F. E. Sondern, had significant impact, at least in the medical

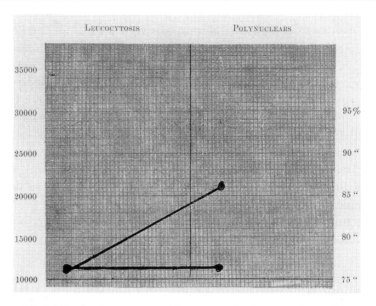

Figure 6.2   *Gibson's leucocyte graph. From Charles Langdon Gibson,
"The Value of the Differential Leucocyte Count in Acute Surgical
Disease,"* Annals of Surgery *43 (1906): 485–99.*

literature, perhaps because each claimed to be written based not on
academic theorizing at the laboratory bench but, rather, on clinical
experience obtained in private practice.[21] Gibson announced that
"the differential blood count and its relation to the total leucocytosis is today the most valuable diagnostic and prognostic aid in acute
surgical diseases that is furnished by any of the methods of blood
examination."[22] The leucocyte count alone, without knowing the
percentage of polymorphonuclear leucocytes, was of little value.
Gibson felt that the clinician needed to count the percentage of
those cells that were polymorphonuclear leucocytes, the cells
thought to be most directly responsible for fighting infection.

The evidence, characteristically for the Progressive era, was to be
evaluated in graphic form. For each count Gibson advised the clinician to prepare a chart similar to the one shown in figure 6.2. On the
lefthand side was listed the number of leucocytes, or white blood
cells. On the righthand side was listed the percentage of polymorphonuclear cells. The clinician was instructed to draw a line con-
necting the two values. If the line was straight, as was the case for

the lower line in this example, it indicated that the body was re-acting adequately to the infection. If the line ran upward from the leucocyte side toward the polymorphonuclear side, that indicated less resistance and a poor prognosis. A line running down, conversely, indicated good resistance. This information helped the physician to make a diagnosis as well as to formulate a prognosis. Such a chart was most valuable in the more complex and perplexing cases and, it was claimed, would "hardly ever lead us astray."[23] Graphs based on Gibson's ideas were widely reproduced, appearing in not only the major, predominantly East Coast medical journals but also the smaller, regional ones.[24]

As with other technologies, the role of the differential count was not immediately accepted by all. Gibson noted that it took some time to be able to appreciate fully the value of the white cell count for medical care. In 1910 a New York physician recalled that "five or six years ago one of our surgeons of at least national fame and of truly scientific bent, opened an abdomen filled with pus and then sneered at the laboratory report of leucopenia in that case." A differential white blood cell count would explain the apparent paradox. Having found pus, evidence of massive infection, in the abdominal cavity, the surgeon expected that the white blood cell count should have been elevated. But it was normal or, perhaps, low. The surgeon con-cluded that the white cell count had been misleading, as it failed to provide evidence of infection. Yet, as the authors of the 1910 report point out, although the total count was low, it was markedly abnor-mal. This is what, by 1910, those who understood white counts would expect to find in a patient who had severe infection but low resistance.[25] In fact, the patient in this case died.

We shall now examine some practical aspects of what it meant to do a blood examination from around 1900 to 1925. In chapter 7 I shall return to the issue of specific uses of the blood count to diag-nose disorders such as abdominal infections, including the use of differential blood counts at the New York and the Pennsylvania hospitals.

WHAT IS A BLOOD EXAM? PRACTICAL ASPECTS

How should medical practitioners examine the blood? While choos-ing among many alternative methods, they considered not only theoretical discussions but also practical concerns. Those decisions had consequences in terms of what a "blood examination" would mean. The differences were key for practitioners, in terms of the time required to do the test, the expense in acquiring the necessary tools, and, perhaps most important, the time needed to learn how to do the test.

Reports of blood counts written for practitioners frequently discussed how long it would take to do an exam. Busy clinicians wanted to obtain the maximum of practical information but in the shortest possible amount of time. Doing a lengthy blood examination cost the practitioner time that could be spent seeing more patients, and thus making more money, a significant consideration in an era when the practice of medicine was not as lucrative as it would later become. It could also cost time that delayed potentially life-saving treatment, particularly in the case of appendicitis, as will be discussed in chapter 7.

If the test could be relegated to an assistant, the physician's time would not be as large a factor. This was one appeal of the hematocrit, which could tell us "inside of five minutes, at slight strain of the muscles of the arm—and it might just as well be the arm of an untrained assistant—practically what we may learn from the haematocytometer in an hour at the least, with much eye-strain, and necessitating either personal attention or the services of a well-trained, sharp-sighted, and thoroughly conscientious assistant."[26] In other words, if you believed this commentator, counting the cells with a hemacytometer was arduous and difficult. On the other hand, measuring the hematocrit was easy and could be relegated to an untrained (and therefore, presumably, low-paid) assistant. Some physicians believed that the hematocrit was as valuable as the red cell count for assessing the number of red blood cells. None, however, thought that the hematocrit could provide information about the white blood cells.

To learn about the white blood cells one needed to count them. Around the turn of the twentieth century leading practitioners, such as the Chicago physician James Herrick, exhorted their fellow physicians to learn the techniques necessary for blood examination.[27] But their fellow physicians' nineteenth-century medical training had not included instruction on how to do a blood count. These busy practitioners had already completed whatever formal training they might have had. When they thought about learning the new tech- niques, it was obviously important to them how much time they were going to need to invest in order to learn how to count blood cells. Some claimed that the techniques were easy to learn. Per- haps even assistants could be trained to count leucocytes.[28] Others claimed that to become adequately skilled took up to three months of practice. A study of students at Johns Hopkins University sug- gested that the techniques were difficult to learn and easy to forget. Physicians required constant practice to remain proficient in look- ing at the cells; even a few weeks' vacation took its toll on accu- racy.[29] Such a result was not surprising for a high-status, elite training program that no doubt prided itself on its educational pro- grams and wished to suggest that its students left the university with a level of expertise that was difficult to obtain elsewhere.

Once they were convinced that it was worthwhile to learn how to do a blood count practitioners wanted to know how long it would take them to actually do a count as well as how much the equipment would cost them. They could find little agreement in the literature. Some physicians claimed that a leucocyte count could be done in five minutes and that "two complete blood examinations [could be done] in about 45 minutes."[30] Others said that a count might take fifteen minutes, others said thirty, while still others said it could take up to an hour and a half.[31] Clearly, the difference between five and ninety minutes was significant to the busy practitioner, particu- larly if he or she took seriously the advice to make counts on almost all patients. If nurses could help physicians prepare smears for anal- ysis, this could save physicians considerable time.[32] Similar differ- ences of opinion held about the expense required to do acceptable counts. A physician could start with twenty-five dollars worth of equipment, though, if interested, he or she might wish to spend up to one hundred dollars.[33]

Where should that equipment be? Some practitioners set up labo- ratories in their offices. Within hospitals laboratories were starting to be set up on the wards, but in the early twentieth century much of medicine was still practiced by general practitioners in their patients' homes—and the blood count was seen as particularly im- portant for general practitioners. After all, it was these physicians, rather than specialists, who saw patients early in the course of their ailments and who thus would have the opportunity to intervene in illness before irreversible harm was done. Toward that aim the general practitioner needed to know that "the examination of a patient can no longer be considered thorough or complete that leaves out the examination of blood."[34] But what might have been feasible in an office laboratory was quite difficult "on the road." Perhaps physicians should carry devices for counting blood around with them in their coat pockets, like they already did with a thermometer or a hypodermic syringe. They could then make smears at each patient's bedside and stain them in their offices.[35] Others devised aids to doing counts "when at the bedside and far from a microscope" which could give results "as good as could be obtained from a microscope."[36] Nonetheless, as long as physicians had to carry *all* the necessary equipment to the patient's home (including equipment not only for blood counts but also for anything else that they might wish to do), it was going to be difficult routinely to examine the blood of each of their patients.

The most extreme position to take was to deny completely any need for instrumental aids. Perhaps no equipment was necessary. Although the knowledge gained by use of blood-examining devices was valuable in the scientific, laboratory investigation of blood diseases, this fact need not imply that the clinician must use those instrumental devices in medical practice. Such a stance was one way of resisting the apparent need for instruments and machines to care for patients. Those who took such a position did not, in general, tend to deny that scientific instruments could provide useful medical information. Nor were they harking back to the era of bloodletting and wishing for more of that. Rather, they tended to believe that the inconvenience and expense of the instruments was greater than the added precision such techniques could bring.

To a certain extent this position was taken by those who were simply unfamiliar with the new techniques and who had no desire to invest the time and money (and some of each was clearly required) to learn how to use them. But there were also elite physicians, quite comfortable with the use of tools for investigation, who simply saw instrumental devices as inappropriate for day-to-day clinical use. Thomas Lewis and James Mackenzie, two leading practitioners with regards to heart disease, had made that point, strongly, in reference to use of the electrocardiogram. They felt that, while the electrocardiogram provided a useful tool for training the unaided senses better to measure the pulse, skilled clinicians could gain all the useful information needed for patient care at the bedside without the need for any tools besides their unaided senses.[37] Similarly, some felt that, whereas blood counts were useful for scientific studies, clinical information could be obtained without instrumental devices. By putting a drop of blood on a handkerchief and observing the color, one could obtain a useful estimate of the hemoglobin. Others argued that leukocytosis could be seen in fresh blood.[38] It was said that a trained man looking at a fresh blood specimen would "guess at a blood-count and hemoglobin percentage and get it closer than a less experienced man can with a counter and hemoglobinometer."[39] Someone who was "*thoroughly* trained in laboratory work" could tell at a glance whether a full leucocyte or differential count was necessary.[40] Moreover, as patients would have to pay for any counts that were done, it was wrong to ask them to pay for tests done only for the sake of completeness and scientific curiosity. Proponents of blood exams felt obliged to respond to such claims. One replied that it was "utterly impossible to count the number of blood corpuscles in a cubic millimeter of blood without artificial aid."[41] Late in the twentieth century most U.S. practitioners would probably agree.

One issue came from the difference between simply estimating whether the total white cell count is high or low and producing an accurate differential count of the various types of white blood cells. Many commentators were quite content with the notion that one standard of accuracy was necessary for publication-quality work while another would suffice for routine clinical care. Part of the question had to do with the value of blood counts in the practice of medicine, as distinct from its scientific study. As early as 1900, one practitioner declared: "A few years ago we knew little or nothing about the blood; now, too much is expected from blood examinations."[42] The careful, detailed work of scientific investigators studying blood and its diseases had produced an expectation of accurate, precise blood counts. The technical needs of medical practitioners, most of whom had no intention of making great discoveries, were much more modest.[43] Instead of accurately counting the number of white cells in each box of the counting chamber, one could simply observe several fields of blood and note if there tended to be many white cells.[44] That process of observation would indicate if the count was normal or abnormal, which, some claimed, was all one needed to know. Others pointed out that even the best examiner would be imperfect and that clinicians needed to know by how much they should expect their blood counts to be in error. This could be done, in true Progressive-era style, by keeping accurate records.[45]

Medical historians have emphasized that most of the methods proposed for measuring the blood were rather unreliable.[46] The issue of accuracy was as much a feature of early-twentieth-century debates as it is of historical interpretation. Medical articles and books paid a great deal of attention to the technical details of precisely how to do a count. This detail had two messages: one was simply the account of precisely how to do the procedure, written for an audience that had not learned the techniques during whatever formal medical training they may have had; the other, implicit, message was to define as a proper "blood count" whatever method the author chose to use, to define the test implicitly rather than explicitly. There was no better way to establish one's own method as superior to an alternative method than to claim that it was more accurate. To a certain extent, however, these debates were also about how to define what constituted the "best" blood test in terms other than accuracy. Decisions about which test to use were also based on how much skill it took to do a test, how much time, and how precise the results needed to be in order for the caregiver to find them clinically useful.

Central to many of these discussions was the microscope, used in a variety of ways. Those who talked at length about the microscope as the defining characteristic, or who simply labeled it implicitly as the marker for blood tests, were doing more than merely making it a random symbol of the laboratory. Were that the case, other laboratory tools, such as the centrifuge, would have sufficed. The microscope was, in fact, a device for distinguishing between two ways of seeing the blood picture as important.

Learning and Looking: The Meanings of Microscopic Exams

Whether one chose only to estimate the red and white cells, to count the total number carefully, or to do a full differential count, a fair amount of technical skill was required to perform a microscopic examination of the blood. The physician needed to obtain the specimen (either locate a blood vessel, puncture it, and withdraw the blood or prick a finger or an earlobe, all without causing the patient too much pain or unease), to smear it on a slide (not too thick, not too thin), perhaps to stain it (just the right amount of dye), and only then to interpret the findings as seen through the microscope. A major concern was the possibility of introducing artifacts during preparation of the slide or of misinterpreting the microscopic findings. Misinterpretation of visual evidence was a problem not confined to blood smears; similar concerns were expressed for the interpretation of all images, such as those produced by the x-ray machines. (Concern about proper interpretation of images led to a different kind of debate than that over the interpretation of numbers, such as those produced by blood pressure measuring equipment or machines to estimate the hematocrit.) Simply put, the problem was that people could see things that they do not understand, particularly in blood. An 1890 editorial in a Philadelphia medical journal commented: "The border lines between disease and health are probably more faintly traced in the blood than in any other tissue in the body. . . . The mere preparation of a blood specimen may give rise to alterations in the corpuscles, which simulate most closely those universally regarded as morbid."[47] An "inexperienced" observer could easily be fooled and might mistakenly label a healthy person as being diseased.

This message drew the attention of a young physician who would soon become one of the most prominent physicians of his day or any other. William Osler responded, perhaps aware of a change in the terms of what constituted being a good physician. The terms were starting to be based more on appropriate use of the self-consciously scientific clinical laboratory and less on the acquisition of experience at the autopsy table, at which Osler had gained the kinds of skills that would make him a leader among physicians.[48] Osler suggested that blood examination was actually not all that ambiguous to a skilled observer and that only a "tyro," someone lacking practical knowledge and the skills of clinical observation, could possibly be confused.[49]

Osler, like most high-status physicians of the late nineteenth century, trained as a pathologist. He stood for years by the autopsy bench, peered through a microscope at endless tissue sections, attempting to discern what *really* happened to a patient. Osler's response suggested that blood tests *could* become a part of pathology's grand tradition, if they were fundamentally based on the visual interpretation of microscopic evidence. If that was what blood tests were all about, they could be accepted into an already established tradition.

But blood counts could also threaten Osler's image of the good physician, opposing, as they might, the traditional view of pathology. Blood tests threatened to make a definitive diagnosis possible while the patient was still alive and to render objective data, all based on only a few drops of fluid. Moreover, they could do so in a way that would devalue the skills that pathologists, and the physicians that many later became, had worked so hard to acquire. These were skills of the precise differentiation of subtle clinical signs, skills that could only be acquired through experience.[50] If the blood examination were a mere technical skill, a mere enumeration of easily distinguished cells, those experiential skills would be devalued. Moreover, if the blood exam produced merely a number—the number of red cells, perhaps—and if that number were produced by simply whirling some blood through the air, as in the spinning of a hematocrit, perhaps by an untrained assistant, then pathologists' skills would be even less important.

There was, however, a way out. The visual evidence supplied by *looking* at a specimen under a microscope held a certain power in the older tradition, a power that numbers of red and white cells could not totally eclipse. If the observer were examining an object, rather than counting it, the old traditions might still hold. This possibility had been open from the start. In what was probably the first photomicrograph of blood, an 1844 photograph of a frog's red blood cells, the French photomicroscopist (and later physicist) J. B. L. Foucault observed that "the object itself . . . will be placed before the eyes and in the hands of the audience."[51] If examination of the blood were examination of a tissue—a liquid tissue, yes, but a tissue nonetheless—then visual skills, particularly the pathologists' skills at interpreting morphological images, would continue to be indispensable.

Some disagreed. Cabot, an influential figure in any discussion of blood, argued that to consider the blood as a tissue made little sense.[52] But Ehrlich, the German scientist whose staining methods had a great impact upon blood exams, explicitly linked blood examination with other, older, pathological traditions by calling his book *The Histology of the Blood.*[53] Pathologists saw "the microscope as authority."[54] Microscopic anatomy—or histology, as it came to be called—had played a key role in the development of the elite pathologists and clinicians of the mid- and late nineteenth century.[55] Histology, and the story that it told through the microscope, were touted as a fundamental basis for late-nineteenth-century medical progress.[56] Any success at putting examination of the blood into the same terms as histology would thus link blood exams with a respectable part of medicine's heritage.

THEORY AND PRACTICE

Theory was one thing; practice was another. How did ideas about blood counts gradually make their way into the clinical practice of medicine? When, and why, did practitioners actually start to use blood counts to care for patients? As early as 1893, George Dock, at the University of Michigan, was calling for the routine use of blood counts in clinical medicine,[57] and he was not alone. Guides for blood tests are found not only in literature aimed at pathologists and in clinical research publications but also in *vade mecums*, works intended specifically to be carried about by the busy practitioner or by the physician-in-training.[58] There is little evidence to suggest, however, that the calls for blood tests were quickly heeded. The published literature suggests, instead, that well into the twentieth-century blood counts were a distinctly unusual event. Although practitioners with a special interest in the new technique published numerous case reports and series, the occasional allusions to routine use of the blood count paint a picture of a technique talked about a great deal but used very little. For example, Louis Fisher of New York City commented at a 1900 American Medical Association meeting that, although many of the cases he saw would benefit from a blood examination, only one case in ten had a blood examination made.[59] The situation in the Midwest, George Dock notwithstanding, was little different. In Michigan W. K. West in 1902 noted that 90 percent of the general practitioners in the state did no blood work and did not have it done for them.[60] Yet others saw blood counts as valuable; they were part of some surgeons' armamentarium in 1901, used to reassure those caring for President McKinley after he was shot that there was no evidence of blood poisoning.[61]

By the turn of the century blood counts appear to have been used somewhat more commonly in teaching hospitals than in private, outpatient practice. This difference might have existed for at least two reasons. First, the hospitals may have been more inclined to be progressive in their clinical approaches. Such hospitals as the New York Hospital and the Pennsylvania Hospital, while not formal teaching hospitals of a medical school (at least not yet, in the case of the New York Hospital), were nonetheless fairly well connected with the world of academic medicine. Medical students and house officers were fresh out of medical schools, in which professors were increasingly seeing their role, in part, as being to contribute to new medical knowledge.[62] Thus, new tools such as blood exams might be more familiar to these physicians-in-training. Second, and perhaps more important, hospital work offered trainees both an opportunity to do laboratory work and a laboratory in which to do it. Many of the problems associated with trying to do blood counts for patients in their homes were nonexistent for the intern or clinician with access to an on-site, well-equipped laboratory. From the perspective of the attending physician, the time required to do an exam was also less of a factor. The attending physician needed only to ask his (and almost all were male) team of house officers and students to do the counts. The members of that team, being paid a salary, had no financial disincentive to spend their time that way. As a result, some interns around the turn of the twentieth century did several hundred blood exams per year.[63]

The introduction of blood tests into teaching hospitals is important for several reasons. Hospitals disseminated new medical ideas into the larger community.[64] Although hospital training had been a rarity for medical students in the nineteenth-century United States, early in the twentieth century it would become the norm. Those students who trained in hospitals would, eventually, make up the next generation of medical practitioners. Also, medical textbooks and journals increasingly were being written by academic physicians. Finally, apart from these two avenues, ideas from academic centers made their way into the practitioners' communities through practicing physicians who would spend time in a major center, such as the Johns Hopkins University, and return home to recount their experiences to the local medical society.[65]

Although blood counts were widely described in medical literature from the end of the nineteenth century as being an essential part of patient care, implementation of these ideas was somewhat different. At the New York Hospital less than 4 percent of all of the patients admitted in 1900 had a blood count performed. At the Pennsylvania Hospital that percentage was only slightly higher than 5 percent. But in both hospitals, by 1920, almost one out of every three patients admitted had a blood count done.[66] Another way of examining the perceived usefulness of laboratory tests is to examine how long after a patient was admitted that a test was performed. In 1900 the average number of days between admission of a patient and when a blood count was done was 5.93 days in the New York Hospital and 11.3 days at the Pennsylvania Hospital. Roughly a decade later that figure had fallen to 1.99 days at the New York Hospital and 1.27 days at the Pennsylvania Hospital.[67] In other words, when a blood count was done in 1900 the average wait was almost a week in one hospital and more than eleven days in another, suggesting that the decision to perform a blood test was not one that came early in the hospital stay. A decade later the mean wait was less than two days, suggesting that the decision to do a blood count was perceived as a more central part of the initial evaluation of the patient. Summary statistics suggest that the major change in the use of the blood count came between 1900 and 1910. Thus, the transition of the blood count from an interesting idea to a routine procedure cannot be attributed easily to the tremendous changes in understanding of the blood which took place before the turn of the century but must, instead, be explained by events that took place after the turn of the twentieth century.

PATIENTS' PERSPECTIVES ON TAKING THE BLOOD

Medical care was becoming based on laboratory tests, and the blood count was one of several possible diagnostic tests which the practitioner might use. Those who wished to see an increased use of blood tests turned to taking the temperature and doing a urinalysis, both established by late in the nineteenth century as routine diagnostic procedures, as possible models for examining blood.[68] As H. Miller Galt put it in 1913: "It seems strange that, while the examination of the urine has become a routine practice, the state of the blood has not received the attention it deserves. It is quite a mistake to assume that special skill and costly apparatus are necessary; the general practitioner will find that he can obtain in very many cases information of the utmost value with a minimum of effort. The apparatus is neither costly nor cumbersome, and it can be employed at the bedside with practically no discomfort to the patient."[69]

And discomfort to the patient was something with which examining the blood was, perforce, associated. In order to get blood out, patients needed, one way or another, to be poked, lanced, incised, or otherwise opened up. This was the case whether the blood was obtained incidentally to therapeutic purposes, such as bloodletting, or specifically for diagnostic purposes, such as a blood count. This interaction scared the patient. The incision or the puncture hurt, perhaps quite a bit.[70] It was messy and could get the clothes or bedding dirty. All in all, having blood drawn was not a very pleasant experience.

The very act of taking blood was therefore a major concern. Yes, there were precedents. Bloodletting had made several generations of patients and practitioners familiar, in general, with removal of blood from a person. But bloodletting's popularity was on the decline in the latter part of the nineteenth century, and few of the patients and practitioners from the early part of the twentieth century would have had personal experience with it. Moreover, bloodletting was a fundamentally different type of procedure than drawing blood for diagnosis. Bloodletting was done to patients when they were ill, usually quite ill. Those patients may not have cared a great deal what was being done to them—or even been aware of it. Blood counts, on the other hand, were being described as valuable for patients who felt relatively well, people who came to see a physician complaining only of a chronic ailment, people who might, in fact, not have a serious illness at all. Indeed, by the 1910s some were advocating routine blood tests as a screening test for people who were, in fact, quite healthy.

Patients of lower social status might submit easily to having blood drawn, feeling that they had no voice in any medical decisions that were being made about them. Other patients, however, might well object. William Savage's 1902 observation about English patients was doubtless germane as well for the American side of the Atlantic, that "patients, particularly for private practice, object to the deep puncture required."[71] But, if the operator were skilled, blood could be removed, or so Galt claimed, with no discomfort to the patient.[72]

How best to remove blood? If patients were to be induced to allow their physicians to do blood counts, this was a crucial question. The precise mechanism for getting the blood for laboratory tests differed somewhat depending upon the purpose for which it was intended. For microbiological studies, such as bacterial cultures, large quantities of blood were needed, as were usually obtained from a vein. For this, one needed to insert a needle into the vein and leave it there for a minute or two. For doing blood counts a similar technique could be employed. Or one might obtain a few drops from other sources, such as the finger or earlobe.

Each of these sources had certain advantages and disadvantages. The finger was easily manipulated. But if the patient were a child, or nervous, the earlobe—being out of sight of the patient—would work better.[73] The earlobe was also above the bedclothes as a patient lay sleeping. That it was seen as an advantage that the earlobe was accessible for obtaining blood even while a patient was sleeping suggests that physicians might initiate blood drawing without much, or any, discussion with the patient.[74] Another putative advantage of the earlobe—that it was particularly valuable for patients who refused "to submit their hand for puncture"—again suggests that sometimes force was used to obtain a blood sample.[75] Obviously, simply not asking a patient's permission was an effective way of dealing with the possibility that he or she might object. It is unclear to what extent patients in late nineteenth- and early twentieth-century U.S. hospitals were forced to undergo procedures or tests, such as having blood drawn. Certainly, late twentieth-century ideas about autonomy and informed consent would not have been obvious to practitioners of this period. A New York City hospital boasted in 1891 that patients were well treated because "no operation is performed on them without their consent." This suggests that in at least some (presumably other) institutions, consent for operation was not considered essential.[76] If consent was not thought to be necessary for an operation, it was probably not thought to be necessary for a blood count either.

Force was not needed for all patients. Particularly in the setting of private, office practice, in which, presumably, patients had the purposes of the test explained to them, having blood drawn could be a positive experience. Some of Cabot's patients were grateful for having their blood drawn and took pleasure in knowing the precise numbers that emanated from its examination.[77]

Examination of the blood was done in a laboratory, away from the patient. A Chicago physician, in an eminently practical account to the Chicago Medical Society on how to do "blood-examinations," noted, after preparing a smear: "We have now finished with the patient, who may be dismissed."[78] The patient's presence was no longer necessary for the diagnostic process to continue. Thus, the physical separation of the patient from the specimen set a blood count apart from a physical examination. Instrumental aids, such as the sphygmomanometer, used in taking the blood pressure, were applied at the bedside; the skill in doing a blood count was applied elsewhere. These blood counts could reinforce the clinical pathologist's skills, which could draw distinctions from fine morphological details. Or they could reinforce the ideas of Progressive-era reformers, who wanted a rational, numerical, graphic way to understand what the blood could tell a physician.

People came to see doing laboratory tests as part of their ongoing responsibility. These people ranged from interns to specialists in pathology. At first, performing the test was delegated to the interns, the least highly skilled members of the team.[79] Eventually, the blood count moved under the general umbrella of clinical pathology. I shall continue to focus on the blood count in chapter 7, approaching its use in the terms most familiar to physicians' debates, both to contemporaries in 1900 and to more recent observers of laboratory testing, by looking at the use of blood counts for diagnosing and monitoring specific diseases.

7

BLOOD AND DISEASES
Pneumonia, Typhoid Fever, and
Appendicitis

On which patients ought physicians to do blood counts? Perhaps blood counts were primarily useful for patients with diseases of the blood or of the blood-forming organs. As the medical historian Keith Wailoo has observed, even if one made this choice, it remained unclear what organ was to be seen as the actual site of blood disease.[1] Pathologists might see the location of blood diseases as the bone marrow; surgeons might locate the source of the disease of leukemia or anemia as the spleen. It was in the blood, however, that certain diseases made their most reliable and consistent mark. Perhaps the emblematic disorder associated with the blood was anemia.

Throughout the nineteenth century the diagnosis of anemia could be, and often was, arrived at on the basis of pallor alone. Into the twentieth century some authorities still argued that most cases of anemia could be diagnosed in the traditional way, based on clinical signs and symptoms. Only in certain, selected cases was a blood count needed to confirm a diagnosis.[2] Yet by early in the twentieth century medical wisdom had started to change, and progressive prac-titioners were turning to scientific laboratory examinations to make their diagnoses. Appearance alone was held be insufficient, for "all pale people are not anemic, neither are all anemic people pale."[3] The laboratory was now to be the touchstone for locating anemic pa-tients, and physicians who failed to heed the admonition to diagnose anemia on the basis of a blood count were said to be treating their patients inappropriately.[4]

A 1913 case report illustrates the problem that could befall patients who were labeled anemic without laboratory confirmation. A woman was treated for anemia for some time but failed to show the expected improvement. Finally, a blood exam was done, which showed that her problem was not anemia but, rather, leukemia.[5] This case report may be read in two ways: it was first a plea to physicians to make blood counts more regularly in patients thought to suffer from anemia. It was also an example of how many physicians did not, in fact, make blood counts regularly. Although it had been so advocated in the medical literature for some time, in 1913 a blood count was not deemed necessary in actual practice to make the diagnosis of anemia.[6]

One can read a similar story in hospital charts of the period. For instance, on March 10, 1900, a twenty-one-year-old Swedish woman, a carpet weaver, was admitted to the New York Hospital with anemia. She stayed but seven days and left without anyone checking her blood count.[7] Similarly, at the Pennsylvania Hospital a twenty-year-old Irish chambermaid was admitted on February 22, 1900.[8] Her chart notes that she "has often been on our ward before. Is a servant in the hospital and is rather anemic." She was discharged on March 4, with a diagnosis of anemia but without having had a blood count. One might wonder if, perhaps, enough blood counts had been done in the past so that another one was unnecessary. There is no indication in the chart of the results of any previous blood tests. But she did have a urinalysis noted, despite the absence of any symptoms or signs that would suggest the need to look at her urine. The urinalysis was in 1900 simply a routine test that was done without contemplation on almost anyone admitted to the hospital. The blood count, however, was still a good deal less routine.

Some blood tests were occasionally done on patients with blood diseases. A twenty-four-year-old Irish domestic worker with chlorosis, whose mucous membranes were noted to be "*very* pale," had her hemoglobin and red blood cell count checked twice.[9] Even as late as 1925, at the Pennsylvania Hospital, a thirty-eight-year-old woman could be assigned a diagnosis of anemia before a blood count, although it was noted that the "blood count verifies this."[10]

But anemia, though a prototypical disease seen to be rooted in the bloodstream, was still not all that common a problem, constituting well under 0.5 percent of admissions to either of the hospitals.[11] The annual reports of each hospital confirm the low prevalence of the diagnosis. It is hard to generalize from the few cases that were seen in the two hospitals. More important, it is unlikely that most American physicians and patients would have had their primary encounters with blood counts over the issue of anemia.

THREE DISEASES

To begin to understand when and how blood counts made their way into the routine practice of medicine, we must turn to some of the most common diseases of the turn of the century; these diseases were primarily infectious.[12] Malaria was still a common disease in most of the United States.[13] Charles Louis Alphonse, a French army surgeon, demonstrated the malaria parasite in red blood cells in the late nineteenth century, a discovery that made a striking impression on a wide range of physicians. Although the disease was characterized by a specific temperature curve, the definitive diagnosis was made in the laboratory. At some elite institutions the diagnosis of malaria was not made without a microscopic demonstration of the parasite.[14] The demonstrated value of microscopic examination of blood in making a specific diagnosis of malaria also encouraged attention to the general value of blood examination.

But it was not only for malaria that blood was useful for making a diagnosis. White blood cells could give clues to illness even in the absence of a clearly visible organism, and white blood cells soon came to occupy the most intense interest of physicians wishing to use the blood count to diagnose infectious diseases. I shall now consider the use of blood counts for diagnosis of three specific infectious diseases: pneumonia, typhoid fever, and appendicitis. I have focused my attention on these three diseases for two reasons. First, they were common diseases; they were common outside of the hospital and within the hospital, both within U.S. hospitals in general and within the two hospitals I have selected for detailed study.[15] Second, these three diseases were important beyond their numbers. They were emblematic of medical practice at the turn of the twentieth century. Pneumonia soon surpassed consumption as the "captain of the men of death," a common and feared cause of death for both young and old.[16] Typhoid fever was the "exemplary disease," according to the noted medical historian Lloyd Stevenson.[17] Appendicitis provided the opening for a new, aggressive, surgical approach to medical care. In all three diseases the role of the blood count was intensely debated. Situating this analysis in terms of each of the three diseases will clarify the issues that framed the use of the blood tests for individual patients.

Pneumonia

Near the end of the nineteenth century pneumonia was one of the most widespread of acute diseases. In 1892 it accounted for approximately 2–3 percent of all hospital admissions, and by 1901 the incidence of admissions to a hospital for pneumonia had almost doubled.[18] These national estimates are consistent with the cases sampled for this study, in which pneumonia accounted for 5.5 percent of the admissions to the Pennsylvania Hospital and 5.1 percent of those admitted to the New York Hospital.[19] Not only a common cause of hospital admission, pneumonia was a common cause of death; at the turn of the twentieth century almost one person out of every five hundred died from pneumonia in any given year.[20] According to the noted American physician Sir William Osler, "Among diseases there is not one which requires to be more fully and carefully presented than pneumonia—the most common as well as the most serious acute affectation of this country."[21] More than merely a common cause of death, the disease had pedagogical value beyond its numbers: pneumonia, Osler told his students at Johns Hopkins, was "the most important acute affectation you will be called upon to treat."[22] He called upon them to make systematic records of all patients with pneumonia admitted to their care; these records included the number of leucocytes. As the incidence of typhoid fever, the other major medical infectious disease, declined during the first few decades of the twentieth century, the attention paid to pneumonia increased. Osler's enormously influential textbook of medicine was succeeded in 1928 by a new work, with a new editor, in which the introductory section on typhoid fever was replaced by one on respiratory infections, including pneumonia.[23]

Pneumonia thus drew the attention of anyone wishing to study a new diagnostic technique. New techniques could be valuable for two reasons: first, they could aid in making a diagnosis, which could guide treatment, both by warning against inappropriate treatment and by guiding active intervention when so indicated; second, the test could aid in providing a prognosis. At times devalued by medical historians, prognostication is one of the more important tasks performed by health care providers. Whether or not anything specific could be done to treat disease, being able to predict a fatal or a benign course was of more than casual interest to the patient and his or her family.

Richard Cabot, who was later to write the most widely acclaimed book on blood counts of the period, in 1893 published a brief report of his first clinical studies on the white blood cells in pneumonia, performed while he was serving as an intern at the Massachusetts General Hospital. His technique was crude by the standards that he would later support, for he did not actually count the white blood cells but merely estimated whether their overall number was high or low. He found that in all five cases in which leucocytosis was absent—that is, the white count was normal—the patient died.[24] The next year Cabot submitted a much more detailed account of his findings. Based on 332 blood counts, Cabot traced the findings in a wide range of conditions, concluding that the counts were valuable in typhoid and pneumonia. A high white count was an unusual finding in typhoid fever. In a presumed case of typhoid, or suspected typhoid, a high white count should lead one to doubt the diagnosis and suspect instead a deep-seated bacterial infection. A high white count was expected in pneumonia; this finding could lead physicians to suspect pneumonia before any physical signs were evident. In addition, Cabot confirmed his earlier report on the white count's value in prognosis, as a low count predicted a poor outcome.[25]

Also in 1893, a young New York physician, James Ewing, published his results on leucocytosis and pneumonia. Seen as an important study by contemporaries, his paper was frequently referred to for at least the next two decades.[26] The study also warrants attention as an example of the type of interest that blood counts attracted in the late nineteenth century and the role they played in one physician's career. Ewing had graduated from the medical school at Columbia in 1891, and he continued for several years to work with T. Mitchell Prudden, who had developed at Columbia one of the first required laboratory courses in a U.S. medical school.[27] On January 1,

1892, Ewing started his tenure as a medical intern at the Roosevelt Hospital in New York City. Imbued with the desire to use his laboratory skills to carry on research, he promptly started to investigate the utility of laboratory tests for patients with pneumonia. He first studied the behavior of urinary chlorides, although that work never resulted in a published paper.[28] The study of leucocytosis in patients with pneumonia followed. It was Ewing's first investigative paper, his second overall.[29] Although it did not turn out to be obviously central to his later intellectual development, Ewing always remembered this piece of investigation; it was the only paper that he chose to mention at a testimonial dinner given for him thirty-eight years later.[30]

Ewing started his 1893 paper on leucocytosis in patients with pneumonia by summarizing the state of knowledge regarding leucocytes. The white blood cell count went up in pregnancy and digestion, and it could also go up in a variety of "cachectic" and "febrile" conditions, of which pneumonia had thus far received the most attention from physicians. After reviewing the available literature, he then stated in a remarkably clear and straightforward manner the hypothesis he wished to test: "In order to test the truth of the statement that a large increase in the number of leucocytes in the blood offers a favorable prognosis in lobar pneumonia, the writer examined the blood in a hundred and one cases of this disease occurring in Roosevelt Hospital during the first five months of the year 1893." Thus, Ewing stated a hypothesis, including the direction of the change he expected to find, and described the cases from which he attempted to derive a conclusion. Because he doubted if the blood examination could become a part of routine care if several measurements were required, he limited himself to a single observation made during the height of the disease, which he termed a "practical procedure." Ewing was therefore attempting not only to establish the presence or absence of a biological phenomenon but also to evaluate the practical, clinical utility of a new laboratory test in hospital practice.

Ewing published full results from all 101 patients with pneumonia as well as 14 others with "miscellaneous" diseases. He listed the patients by name and included their age, the site of the pneumonia, their highest body temperature, the character of the infection and of the reaction (these two items were clinical measures of disease severity), the presence of any complications, the eventual outcome, and the leucocyte count. Thus, Ewing, though displaying somewhat less regard for patient confidentiality than would be considered appropriate a century later, did a reasonable job of providing a detailed list of the cofactors that might have altered the leucocyte count. Part of the reason for this detail may have been Ewing's realization that summary statistics would not have been readily accepted by his contemporaries; by providing enough detail, he could perhaps enable readers to imagine each individual patient, which might permit his message to be better received.

Ewing concluded that blood counts could provide useful information about patients with pneumonia. The absence of leucocytosis in an otherwise severe case of pneumonia was a grave sign. Its presence was a valuable aid in differentiating between pneumonia and typhoid fever but was not helpful in identifying empyema (a collection of pus in the chest cavity) which would require surgical drainage for recovery to take place.

This study was important for a number of reasons. It was widely cited in the published literature and doubtless influenced others to attempt to use blood counts in their clinical practice. It also was important in the career of James Ewing. Ewing next studied leucocytosis in another infectious disease, diphtheria.[31] This second study of leucocytosis shares some of the features of his study of pneumonia, in that Ewing paid careful attention to the covariants that could influence the white count, and he gave full details on each of the fifty-three cases on which he reported (omitting, this time, patients' names). The study, however, displays the beginning of a shift in Ewing's career, back to a more traditional, morphological type of pathology. He discussed at some length the staining reactions and the appearance as well as numbers of white cells. Indeed, Ewing was to return quickly to a morphological approach to disease.[32] He went on to write a well-received text on examination of the blood in 1901,[33] emphasizing that in order to view pathological changes in the blood one needs experience at the autopsy table as well as experience with viewing the microscopic examination of diseased tissue. Ewing treated the blood as just another bodily tissue, susceptible to study by the usual means that were well-known to pathologists.

Neoplastic diseases came to be the focus of Ewing's later attention. As professor of Pathology at Cornell, he was instrumental in

Table 7.1 *Pneumonia, Blood Counts, and X Rays at the Pennsylvania and New York Hospitals, 1900–1925*

Year	No. of Cases	Patients with Pneumonia Who Had at Least One Blood Count (%)	Patients Who Had a Differential Count* (%)	Patients Who Died (%)	Patients Who Were Examined with X rays (%)
		PENNSYLVANIA HOSPITAL			
1900	27	3.7	0	30	0
1909	25	76	0	36	0
1920	21	90	0	14	4
1925	17	100	24	30	47
		NEW YORK HOSPITAL			
1900	13	8	0	46	0
1910	23	74	100	26	4
1920	12	83	100	33	42

*When a blood count was done.

introducing cancer radiotherapy as well as in the decision by the Memorial Hospital in New York City to make its mission the treatment of patients with cancer. Perhaps the early study of leucocytosis in pneumonia was only a transitional phase in Ewing's career, a brief flirtation with a new laboratory tool before moving back to traditional anatomic pathology. Physicians eventually were to accept the use of blood counts in the diagnosis of pneumonia, although it would take over a decade after Ewing published his discussions.

A few years later William Osler weighed in with his observations on the blood corpuscles in pneumonia, commenting that the red cells showed little change, while the white cells were generally more numerous than normal—a slight leucocytosis indicating a less favorable prognosis.[34] By 1898 numerous observations had been made regarding the number of leucocytes present in cases of pneumonia. There was general agreement that a high white count gave a good prognosis and a low white count gave a grave prognosis.[35] The count helped to differentiate pneumonia from other diseases, such as typhoid, malaria, and sometimes influenza.[36] Moreover, once pneumonia was confirmed, a persistently high white count could lead the physician to suspect empyema.[37] It was said that the two common diseases from which one gained the most from a white blood cell count were typhoid and pneumonia, and the number in each goes in the opposite direction[38]: in other words, in pneumonia the white count tends to increase, whereas in typhoid fever it tends to decrease. Yet neither of these generalizations always holds.

Table 7.1 illustrates that pneumonia was a common and serious disease at the Pennsylvania and the New York hospitals, with a substantial mortality rate. The death rates at these two hospitals are similar to the rates reported for other institutions.[39] Two clear patterns emerge from this data, both of which are meaningful and statistically significant. First, a consensus about the need for the routine use of blood counts in patients with pneumonia was formed between 1900 and 1910. In 1900 only 3.7 percent of the patients at the Pennsylvania Hospital and 8 percent of the patients at the New York Hospital with pneumonia had a blood count done. A decade later 75 percent did, and that number continued to increase at both hospitals. Thus, whatever reason one might invoke to explain this specific change in medical practice must explain changes taking place between 1900 and 1910. The increase in x-ray use occurred a decade later, showing that what happened was more than a general change in attitudes toward the diagnostic investigation of people with pneumonia.

Perhaps in 1900 house physicians simply did not have the necessary expertise to do a blood count, whereas by 1910 most house physicians had obtained such skills. The primarily elite medical schools that house physicians at the New York Hospital and the Pennsylvania Hospital had attended were, by early in the twentieth century, probably teaching the laboratory examination of blood. But physicians at the two hospitals were far from identical in the ways they used blood counts; in fact, the differences are striking. A second pattern in this data is that patients at the New York Hospital were far more likely to have a differential count. I will consider those differences later, as part of a general discussion on the use of differential counts.

The white count in patients with pneumonia was most valuable in making diagnoses. For example, a twenty-five-year-old man who arrived at the Pennsylvania Hospital on January 28, 1920, was initially given a diagnosis of influenza.[40] He did not do well, however. When the white blood cell count was found to be elevated, at 19,600, his diagnosis was changed to lobar pneumonia, soon revised to include, specifically, disease affecting the right upper and lower lobes. After a stormy course, during which the patient was noted to have become "restless and irrational," he recovered and was discharged on February 21. Here the high white count enabled the diagnosis, and the prognosis, to be changed from the somewhat benign one of influenza to the more grave one of multilobar pneumonia. The diagnosis was not changed entirely on the basis of the blood count; traditional diagnostic methods also played a role. Yet the blood count indicated a more serious illness than had originally been suspected, leading the patient's physicians to search for a cause for the elevated count.

The white blood cell count could also be used to suggest a less serious disease. For example, a twenty-two-year-old woman, a warper, was admitted on February 1 with a provisional diagnosis of pneumonia and was discharged ten days later, her diagnosis changed to influenza. Her clinical course was benign, a finding that may have been presaged, for the physicians taking care of her, by a white blood cell count of only 12,600.[41]

The information that physicians obtained from a blood count in patients with pneumonia was generally prognostic. It did not usually serve to guide action on the part of the health care team. In typhoid, however, despite the fact that this was another "medical" (as opposed to surgical) illness, the blood count could be useful in guiding the course of therapy.

Typhoid

Even though it was starting to become far less common, typhoid fever still played a major role in U.S. medical thought at the turn of the twentieth century. Near the end of the nineteenth century scientists in the midst of the microbiological revolution had succeeded in identifying an organism that was seen as the cause of typhoid fever. William Osler elected to start his magisterial 1892 textbook of medicine with more than forty pages on typhoid fever and eventually wrote seventy-two papers on the subject. At the turn of the twentieth century typhoid was the most common reason for admission to some city hospitals.[42] But the death rate in the United States fell sharply soon thereafter, from 31.3 per 100,000 in 1900 to 7.8 per 100,000 in 1925, largely because of public health improvements, with urban areas showing a far greater decline than rural areas.[43] Osler lived to see the day when there were no longer enough cases in Baltimore even for teaching purposes.[44] Still, at the turn of the century typhoid's protean manifestations, coupled with newfound scientific understanding of the disease, made it a natural target for any new laboratory technology.[45]

The clinical picture of a patient stricken by typhoid fever was classic: a dull, expressionless face, a musty odor, a coated tongue, a large spleen. The course of the disease lasted approximately four weeks. Patients would start with an insidious febrile illness, with the temperature gradually rising over the first week, at which time—if the diagnosing physician were lucky—characteristic skin lesions called rose spots might appear on the patient's abdomen and chest. During the "febrile plateau" of the second and third week the patient would appear to be the most ill, with a high fever lasting most of the day. In the final week the temperature would gradually fall, by lysis rather than by crisis.

Yet the clinical course was not always so smooth or so easy to

diagnose.[46] A febrile patient without rose spots could have pneumonia instead of typhoid. Even when characteristic cutaneous lesions
were present, experienced, distinguished clinicians, such as George
Dock, could still mistake smallpox for typhoid fever.[47] Other infectious diseases could also confuse the issue, such as tuberculosis,
influenza, typhus, or acute articular rheumatism.

The onset of abdominal pain could pose additional diagnostic
problems. Pain in patients with typhoid could be due to inflammation of infected glands in the abdomen, a self-limited condition
that required no specific medical attention. On the other hand,
abdominal pain could also be due to perforation of the bowels, the
dreaded complication of typhoid fever, for which the only practical
cure was immediate surgical intervention. If so, speed was of the
essence. As one practitioner put it in 1899: "The diagnosis of intestinal perforation in typhoid fever is at times one of the most difficult
problems that is presented to the physician for solution. At the same
time, early operation, before collapse symptoms have developed,
affords, in the majority of instances, the only chance the patient
has of recovery."[48] Or, perhaps, the pain could be due to some other
disease entirely, such as appendicitis. Whenever a patient with
known typhoid fever complained of stomach pain, a clinical dilemma started to unfold.

The basic clinical decision centered on whether and when to call
on the surgeon to operate. For early in the twentieth century there
was little doubt that surgical medicine held sway as the branch of
medical practice seen as most progressive, most scientific, and most
influential. Some experts advised routine blood examinations to
help decide when surgical consultation was necessary in a case of
typhoid fever.[49] A falling red blood count could indicate internal
bleeding, not otherwise obvious (yet) at the bedside, and suggest the
need for immediate surgical intervention to stanch the flow of blood.
The white count could also help. Typhoid fever was usually associated with a normal or low leucocyte count. In cases in which the
diagnosis was not clear, students were taught that the absence of
leucocytosis suggested typhoid fever, while a rising white count
suggested something else, such as appendicitis.[50] Conversely, a normal or low white count could stay an inappropriately raised knife. In
a case thought initially to be appendicitis but found to be typhoid:
"The microscope decided the line of treatment."[51]

Blood counts offered only indirect guidance for the diagnosis of typhoid fever. Obviously, the most direct means of diagnosis was to isolate the typhoid bacillus itself from the body. Early observers had difficulty consistently isolating the bacillus from blood, in part because they used small quantities of blood or unsuitable culture media.[52] Other types of laboratory tests were devised with which to search for typhoid fever.

In 1882, Paul Ehrlich described what he called a "diazo reaction," in which chemical solutions, when mixed with urine, were said to produce a carmine color if the patient had typhoid fever.[53] The test was the object of much controversy, as it was said to be positive in a variety of febrile diseases, including not only typhoid but also tuberculosis and malaria. Even though it was often done, it appears to have not been given much weight by clinicians attempting to differentiate typhoid from other diseases.[54] That certainly was not true of another type of test, one based on observing the agglutination of typhoid-causing bacteria.

In 1896 Max Gruber described an agglutination test for typhoid fever, a test that came to be better known for the name of the investigator who also worked on it, F. J. Widal. They each observed that the blood or serum (the part of blood that remained liquid after a clot had formed) from a patient with typhoid fever would exert characteristic effects on typhoid bacilli. A culture of typhoid bacilli would first lose its motility and then become agglutinated in masses. Serum from noninfected people had no effect on the bacilli. Moreover, the test was not simply positive or negative. If positive, the strength of the reaction could be easily measured, by observing at what dilution one could still observe the effect. If serum at a dilution of 1:100 still produced agglutination, that was a more positive reaction than if serum at only a 1:5 dilution would cause a reaction. The test, though promising, had a major limitation: it did not become diagnostic until after the first week of the illness. This left clinicians to resort to other means of diagnosis during the early phase of the disease. Nonetheless, the suggestion of a definitive blood test for typhoid fever quickly attracted attention from people who thought it could help solve a variety of diagnostic dilemmas.

The so-called Widal reaction was widely discussed and applied in U.S. medical practice.[55] Although initially done using a microscope, as was the case for blood counts, there were quickly those who

Table 7.2 *Typhoid, Blood Counts, and Widals at Pennsylvania and New York Hospitals, 1900–1925*

Year	No. of Cases	Patients with Typhoid Who Had at Least One Blood Count (%)	Patients Who Had a Differential Count* (%)	Patients Who Had Widal Reaction Done (%)	Patients Who Died (%)
		PENNSYLVANIA HOSPITAL			
1900	30	17	0	93	20
1909	26	85	0	93	4
1920	6	83	0	50	33
1925	1	100	0	100	0
		NEW YORK HOSPITAL			
1900	6	33	0	100	17
1910	14	100	100	85	0
1920	0	—	—	—	—

*When a blood count was done.

claimed that one could just as well apply the test by observing the reaction with the naked eye.[56] Two methods were described, a microscopic one, in which the clumping or a lack of motility was observed with a microscope, and a macroscopic one, in which the sedimentation of bacteria was observed at the bottom of a test tube. An 1897 American Medical Association session on "Serum Diagnosis in the Practice of Medicine" was able to draw on four thousand cases of typhoid diagnosis in the literature and to claim a 95 percent success rate for the Widal method of diagnosis.[57] In 1900 the test was in routine use at the University of Michigan, where George Dock used the dilution at which the test was positive as an indication of the confidence in the diagnosis.[58] By 1904 almost one thousand studies had been published on the subject.[59] Not only useful for making the diagnosis, the Widal reaction could also help guide the clinician away from thinking of typhoid fever and toward other diagnoses. For example, in one instance the Widal was negative, but the urine suggested an infection; thus, the diagnosis was changed to an infected kidney (a "pus" kidney), which called for a very different therapy.[60] The Widal reaction was seen at the time as part of a general pattern of blood tests and was discussed in the same books as blood counts.

As was the case with pneumonia, the practice of doing a blood count on patients admitted with typhoid fever to the New York and the Pennsylvania hospitals changed most dramatically between 1900 and 1910 (see table 7.2). In 1900 few patients at either hospital had a blood count done: 33 percent at the New York Hospital and 17 percent at the Pennsylvania Hospital. By 1910 all of the patients at the New York Hospital, and 85 percent of the patients at the Pennsylvania Hospital had a blood count done. The number of cases of the disease dropped rapidly after 1910, reflecting a general decline in the incidence of the disease.

The experiences at the New York Hospital and the Pennsylvania Hospital confirm findings in the medical literature which suggest that the Widal reaction was quickly adopted for clinical care. The Widal reaction was different from the blood count. Rather than being a general guide to health, or to the presence of a nonspecific infection, its supporters claimed that it was diagnostic for a specific disease. Together with the less specific leucocyte count, it was found useful in distinguishing typhoid fever from other diseases.[61]

Consider, for example, a twenty-two-year-old Italian woman admitted to the Pennsylvania Hospital on May 7, 1909, complaining of abdominal pain.[62] She had delivered a child twelve days before coming to the hospital, but the child had lived for only four days. Physicians in the receiving ward considered the diagnosis of typhoid fever. They noted the absence of rose spots as well as the absence of a palpable spleen. On admission her physicians drew blood for both a white count and a Widal reaction. The leucocyte count was 9,900—low, consistent with typhoid fever—but the Widal reaction was negative. The patient gradually improved and went home seventeen days later, with a diagnosis not of typhoid fever but of puerperal sepsis, an infection of her uterus. Sometimes the blood examination led physicians away from a diagnosis of typhoid fever in other ways, as by observing in the blood both a negative Widal and parasites consistent with malaria.[63]

Even if characteristic skin lesions were present, physicians still felt obliged at times to use laboratory aids to make a diagnosis. On January 7, 1902, a thirty-two-year-old male machinist was admitted to the Pennsylvania Hospital after a two-week course marked by languor and malaise. He had been nauseated and had retched but without vomiting; he was also constipated. On admission he was febrile to 104 degrees. He had a palpable spleen and numerous rose spots on his abdomen and back. A Widal reaction was done and was positive, and a diagnosis of typhoid fever was made. Over a month later, on February 14, after a total of fifty-five sponge baths, he was discharged. Seven years later, on March 29, 1909, another thirty-two-year-old man, this time a driver, was also admitted. This time the skin spots were described in great detail in the chart: "numerous erythematous spots, some of them slightly raised above the surface and all disappearing on pressure and distinctly circumscribed."[64] These were the rose spots characteristic of typhoid fever. Nonetheless, a Widal reaction was done, which showed "good clumping" at dilutions of both 1:50 and 1:100. A white blood count also revealed a count of 3,100, low, and quite suggestive of typhoid fever.

Although there appears to have been a consensus by 1910 about the need for a Widal test and a blood count in patients with typhoid fever, there is, again, a marked disparity between the New York Hospital and the Pennsylvania Hospital over the issue of doing a differential count. At the New York Hospital *all* of the blood counts in 1910 included a differential; at the Pennsylvania Hospital *none* did. The differential count was thought to be most useful when there existed the possibility of an occult bacterial infection, often in the abdomen, which could only be cured by surgical drainage. That situation was often found when the differential diagnosis included appendicitis. One of the main diagnostic dilemmas for physicians at the turn of the twentieth century was to tell the difference between typhoid fever and appendicitis.

Appendicitis

The history of acute appendicitis is often written as though it began and ended with Reginald Heber Fitz's famous June 1886 presentation to the Association of American Physicians: "Penetrating Inflammation of the Veriform Appendix, with Special Reference to its Early Diagnosis and Treatment." But the history of surgery for acute appendicitis is a good deal more complex than an event at a single moment in time.[65] At the end of the nineteenth century the disease was seen as new, and exciting, and as posing problems in diagnosis and treatment.[66] More than simply the recognition of some previously misunderstood intestinal inflammation, by a decade or two into the twentieth century many Americans saw the surgical treatment of appendicitis as signifying one of the most glorious triumphs of modern medicine, and many Americans, not only surgeons, saw it as an indicator of the surgeon's dominant role in those triumphs. It is thus not a surprise that the value of the blood count, a progressive and scientific technique, in the diagnosing of appendicitis, a new and quite prominent disease, would be the subject of intense and prolonged debate, one that is important not only for what it tells us about appendicitis and blood counts but also for what it tells us about the process by which new techniques such as the blood count were placed into the context of medical practice.

One place to start to analyze that process is at the 1901 annual meeting of the American Surgical Association in Baltimore. On the afternoon of the first day of the meeting, May 7, 1901, the sixty-one people in attendance heard an impassioned debate over the importance of blood counts in cases with appendicitis. John Chalmers Da Costa, Jr., was invited to present some remarks. Da Costa came from a noted Philadelphia medical family.[67] He attended Princeton

University and went from there to Jefferson Medical College, in Philadelphia, from which he graduated in 1893. Shortly after his graduation from Jefferson, Da Costa started to focus his attention on internal medicine. He served in a variety of positions at Jefferson and, in addition, worked as a hematologist at the German Hospital of Philadelphia (now Lankenau Hospital). There he had the opportunity to study 118 patients with appendicitis. In 1901, the same year in which his textbook on hematology was first published, Da Costa stood before the American Surgical Association to report on his findings.[68] He apologized for bringing up in his discussion of blood counts a topic "already familiar to all surgeons" but felt that he nonetheless had something to add.

What Da Costa added was unabashed enthusiasm for the new technique combined with evidence for its usefulness. He saw both the red blood cell count and the white blood cell count as valuable, both for diagnosing appendicitis and for guiding the surgeon's hand in its treatment. Da Costa thought that the red cell count, and the related laboratory test, the hemoglobin, could identify those patients who could safely undergo an operation. He felt that because blood loss was a common feature of appendicitis, it "seems sufficient to call for a routine haemoglobin test in all patients [who are] to be treated surgically." A low value might indicate some reason to delay the operation, although Da Costa carefully pointed out that in his experience even the cases with the lowest values had recovered uneventfully.

But it was the white count that attracted the most attention. A high white blood cell count indicated the presence of pus. "It is obvious that a decided increase in the number of leucocytes, if correlated with other clinical symptoms, may serve as a diagnostic sign of definite value." On the other hand, a low count did not necessarily mean that pus was absent, and "the fact cannot be emphasized too forcibly that an absence of leucocytosis, except in conspicuously septic patients, signifies nothing." Da Costa argued for a broad interpretation of the value of blood tests: They were not only important as aids in making the decision to operate but also as indices of the patient's postoperative course. The surgeon might remove an inflamed appendix and all of the pus he or she could find, but it was not uncommon for a significant collection of pus to remain, undetected, in the abdomen. If not removed, this pus would eventually lead to peritonitis (a generalized abdominal infection) and, probably, death. Thus, Da Costa argued that counts should be made daily after an operation. A high white blood cell count could detect the presence of residual pus and indicate the need for a life-saving re-operation. Da Costa saw the total white blood cell count as most important and would only do a differential count in exceptional cases. Thus, in a very public forum Da Costa advocated the routine use of blood counts for patients with appendicitis.

To listen only to Da Costa, however, would be to miss a tension that must have permeated the distinguished surgeons' springtime Baltimore meeting. For another physician stood squarely in opposition to Da Costa. John B. Deaver also had a distinguished pedigree and was on his way to an illustrious career. Deaver graduated from the University of Pennsylvania in 1878. He had written a treatise on appendicitis in 1896, the same year that he had been named the chief surgeon at the German Hospital of Philadelphia.[69] Later in his life Deaver returned to the University of Pennsylvania, as the John Rhea Barton Professor of Surgery. Deaver was an intensely charismatic teacher, whose public surgical demonstrations routinely drew overflow crowds. He shared others' high opinions of his own surgical skills and operated on his own children because "he felt he could do it better than anybody else."[70] He was an "evangelist" for the "newfound resources of surgery," a hard worker who performed as many as eighteen to twenty-four operations a day.[71]

While in the operating room, Deaver had no more favorite organ in his sights than the appendix. He was well-known for his inclination to remove it in a wide range of situations; his entry into a party was once greeted with one guest's admonition to the others there to "hold onto it, gentlemen, hold onto it."[72] Deaver's name became inseparably associated with his personal skill at removing inflamed appendices. He was, perhaps, even more important for his role in convincing others to do likewise, through tirelessly preaching the value of appendectomy. It was said that "many owe their lives to his skillful surgery, but many more to his powerful advocacy of the early operation."[73] He felt that, above all, the surgeon must be bold and be quick; he was fond of saying, "What these cases need is the aseptic scalpel at the earliest possible moment."[74]

Deaver was one of the "earliest and most valiant champions of immediate appendectomy for acute appendicitis," at a time when such an approach was far from universally accepted. In advocating early operation for acute appendicitis, Deaver was hardly a traditionalist; rather, he "was regarded as a *radical* in his early years, and he was proud to maintain this reputation to the last."[75] But the meaning of radicalism changes, and Deaver, as has often been the case for radicals, eventually found himself defending a frontier line that was no longer at the cutting edge of the surgical battleground.[76]

The title of Deaver's 1901 presentation left no doubt about where he stood on the subject of blood counts: "The Examination of Blood in Relation to Surgery of Scientific but Often of No Practical Value, and May Misguide the Surgeon."[77] Deaver thus immediately distinguished between the scientific and the practical value of the new laboratory test. As he continued his talk, his rhetoric made his reasoning clear: "In the past few years there has crept into the profession a tendency to replace the bedside by the laboratory as the point from which to make the diagnosis; to substitute the highly magnified but extremely limited field of the microscope for the broader view of the eye of the physician." This is a very telling metaphor. Those who look through the microscope are not clinicians: they espouse a narrow outlook, in the interest of science. Clinicians, on the other hand, use a broad outlook for their patients' best interests.[78]

Deaver continued: "This we regret, for in the majority of instances the diagnosis must be made at the bedside without the aid of the microscopist, and any man who has no confidence in diagnoses made without the aid of the laboratory limits his usefulness." Deaver here implies that someone else will do the microscopy. Moreover, he sees the use of the microscope as an index of lack of self-confidence in one's abilities, and self-confidence is precisely what the surgeon needed in order to go into the abdomen and save a patient's life. Laboratory tests, said Deaver, provide "opportunities for inaccuracies without number." Most important: "The secret of life-saving surgery is promptness in diagnosis and operation, and often the time lost in awaiting the confirmation of our opinions by the laboratory can be ill afforded by the patient." The surgeon, unlike some other varieties of physicians, is able to cure the patient, not merely to provide palliation. But to accomplish this goal the surgeon must do the operation early, in the first few hours of the attack. Don't wait, don't count; rather, cut and cure. Laboratory tests were not only useless; they were dangerous and could actually prevent the patient from being cured.

The Da Costa–Deaver debate appears to have been more than merely a couple of passing presentations that were soon forgotten. Instead, both Deaver and Da Costa were quoted widely, sometimes with approval, sometimes not.[79] Given the attention that this controversy received from contemporaries, it behooves us to try to understand what it was that made their disagreement so compelling to their colleagues.

This debate is all the more interesting when one realizes that the two protagonists were talking past each other, that they disagreed less in substance than their rhetoric would suggest. Both agreed that blood counts were not determinative and should only be used in conjunction with a careful clinical evaluation. Deaver was most concerned that the blood count could dissuade a surgeon from operating when surgery appeared to be the appropriate course based on clinical grounds. To some extent, Da Costa would see this as a possibility, particularly if the hemoglobin were low. On the other hand, Da Costa took pains to point out that, among the 118 patients with appendicitis on whom he reported, even when the hemoglobin had been low the patient had survived surgery and done well.[80] Moreover, Da Costa felt that a high white count might indicate the need for operation. Da Costa did not feel that one ought to use a low count as a signal not to operate. Thus, Da Costa was hardly attempting to still the surgeon's scalpel in the heavy-handed way that Deaver implied.

Finally, much of Da Costa's discussion had to do with using blood counts to follow a patient's recovery after surgery. After an abdominal operation there existed the possibility that not all of the infected material had been removed. If the white count remained high, according to Da Costa, that would be a reason to go back in and clean out more pus, to do *more* surgery rather than *less*. In other words, Da Costa's rationale for using the blood count was far more interventionist, far more as an indication *for* rather than *against* surgery, than Deaver's response would suggest. So, one wonders, why Deaver's fervent, sustained opposition to blood counts?

To some extent, that opposition stemmed from Deaver's generalized fear that someone, probably an internist, would prevent him (or some other surgeon) from saving the life of a patient. His confrontational tone made him the dominant figure opposing the routine use of blood counts.[81] He complained that sometimes the physician may want to wait for another attack, once the acute one has subsided: "Unfortunately, the medical man and not the surgeon, is too often the consultant in acute appendicitis; as unfortunate perhaps as having the surgeon and not the medical man the consultant in cases of typhoid or scarlet fever. . . . For every death from appendicitis someone is to blame."[82] Late in his life he declared: "The battle is not yet entirely won and will not be until the nine-lived procrastinator finally disappears. Not until then will surgery enjoy the complete triumph of having added at least one to the list of curable diseases."[83] The blame could, thought Deaver, be laid at the feet of those internists who insisted on letting the blood count influence their decision about whether or not to send a patient for an operation.

But it would be a mistake to dismiss the argument between Deaver and Da Costa as only a stereotypical internist versus surgeon confrontation, although there was certainly a good deal of conflict between the two groups. According to one writer: "The surgeon usually claims that blood examinations are good only for the medical man, and the medical man protests that all cases brought to the surgeon should have an examination in order to arrive at a correct diagnosis; and in either case, even if an operation is required, a better prognosis could be made."[84] In some ways, this was also a confrontation between two schools of elite surgeons. Deaver was trained in the "old," pre-microbiology, pre–laboratory tests school of surgery. The new school of surgery could be exemplified by the uncle of John Chalmers Da Costa, Jr., John Chalmers Da Costa,[85] who had chosen to open the first chapter of his textbook of surgery with a discussion not of surgical anatomy but, rather, of bacteriology. Indeed, the book's first illustration is of the tetanus bacillus.[86] His initial contribution to the massive, multivolume, multiauthor textbook of surgery edited by William Keen, the "Bible of American surgeons" in the first few decades of the twentieth century, was on an infectious, microbiological disease: surgical tuberculosis.[87] John Da Costa thus linked himself with the new, progressive school of scientific surgery. His nephew, John Da Costa, Jr., had contributed a chapter on surgical hematology to that same textbook.[88] In it the junior Da Costa did not retreat from his earlier claim that the leucocyte count could help the surgeon, particularly in cases of appendicitis. Here, as elsewhere, Da Costa continued to emphasize that the blood count must always be understood as part of a broader clinical picture. Keen's decision to ask for a chapter on the blood count in appendicitis for his surgical text indicates the desire to include the blood count among important topics to be covered.

Deaver, on the other hand, was not a strong champion of the laboratory. Although he used infectious diseases as part of the reason to justify going into the abdomen, he was much more a student of the old school of anatomy. In his 1896 treatise on appendicitis he followed a historical introduction with a discussion of anatomy, the subject (rather than bacteriology) on which he had earlier published a massive tome and in which he now chose to ground his discussion of appendicitis.[89] It is interesting that he discussed the etiology of the disease by starting with the anatomic lesions that may predispose a person to appendicitis, only later turning to the exciting causes, as it is "probable" that appendicitis is caused by microorganisms. Later in life Deaver recalled: "The more I see and hear [of changes in medicine], the greater is my conviction that the royal road to surgery still begins and ends in the charted route of the dissecting room."[90] The first attribute of a good surgeon, Deaver continued to insist, was a sound knowledge of anatomy.[91]

To the extent that Deaver wished to use a laboratory it was in the older sense of the pathological museum, with the diseased appendix itself, preserved in formalin, providing the scientific evidence. By 1905 Deaver had assembled a collection of over a thousand appendices at the German Hospital, to be used for pathological studies and demonstrations. Each of the appendices was carefully cataloged, with a card listing the details of the operation and the outcome of the case.[92]

Deaver based his surgical prestige not on laboratory investigations but, rather, on clinical skill. Early in his career it seems that the "magic number" at which he felt a conclusion was warranted was one hundred operations. This was the case for his early publications on the radical treatment of hernia as well as an early paper on appendicitis, both of which opened with a claim for authority based on his experience.[93] The basis for his book on appendicitis was experience in the treatment of over five hundred cases. Deaver emphasized the importance of his surgical experience by noting, twice, the number of cases he had treated, on both the first page of the preface and the last page of the book. He reemphasized the primary importance of his personal surgical skill, rather than the experience of others, by choosing not to include any references to other authors in his book.[94]

By the time he revised his classic book on appendicitis for the fourth and final edition, in 1914, Deaver had modified his original views but little. Some of the confrontational language with regards to physicians (internists) is gone, and Deaver had inserted a chapter on "The Blood in Appendicitis." Nevertheless, his conclusion was the same as in 1900. He condemned the use of the white count, with or without differential, as "pernicious and dangerous." It should be made explicitly clear that Deaver, as with many others who opposed the routine use of blood counts, did not do so out of lack of skill or lack of availability of such laboratory techniques. Deaver was quite willing to report fully on the blood picture when he wrote up a case for presentation.[95] Moreover, by 1914 physicians in Deaver's clinic did counts daily, including differential counts.[96] The issue, rather, was whether such tests ought to become a part of *routine* care of patients by most physicians. Deaver continued to feel strongly that the count should almost never be a determinative factor in the decision about whether or not to operate. The only exception he made is that a very low white blood cell count in the presence of overwhelming infection could indicate a bad prognosis and might be a reason to delay operation.[97] His lifetime's lesson for the care of appendicitis was simple: early operation. As he recalled of another Da Costa in 1920, J. M. Da Costa, who had said, "It seems to me, if we take this view a person with appendicitis will go to bed not with the sword of Damocles suspended over his head, but with the scalpel of the surgeon already on his abdominal wall": "Today the person with appendicitis does indeed go to bed with the scalpel of the surgeon already on his abdomen, and unless he does so, the sword of Damocles actually is suspended over his head in the shape of recurrences, if not death."[98]

The debate over the use of white blood cell counts for patients thought to have appendicitis brought several issues to the fore in the interpretation of laboratory tests. First was the distinction between medicine and science in the interpretation of the data. Scientists, who were looking to discover general trends, could find rough statistical associations useful. Medical practitioners, on the other hand, needed to deal with individual patients. Moreover, they often had to deal with single data points for those individual patients, and the absence of any knowledge about the time trend of a blood count could lead to erroneous conclusions.[99] Trying to diagnose an internal abscess had been noted as a difficult diagnostic dilemma for some time, and any assistance offered by the white count would be most welcome.[100] A high white count could be used as a marker of acute abdominal inflammation. Yet it was well-known that the white blood count went up and down with a variety of normal events, ranging from pregnancy to eating dinner. Such variation led one physician to declare in 1900: "We are taught to expect pus when the count is high. It may be true on the average, but we are dealing now with individuals."[101] James Ewing had expressed similar concerns when attempting to prognosticate the outcome in pneumonia. But the stakes were a bit higher in the case of appendicitis, and the increased stakes may have sharpened the debate. Rather than merely predicting a happy or a morbid outcome, the blood count was being asked to guide the surgeon's hand, to determine whether or not to attempt a dangerous but potentially life-saving operation. Medical practitioners were acutely aware of the difference between scientific and practical value. They had a different set of priorities than did scientists; they were attuned to the peculiarities of individual patients.[102] So long as the results of blood counts were seen as too variable to be useful for the care of individual patients, they would not be part of routine patient care.[103]

One could attempt to eliminate the variation, or one could attempt to understand it. One could eliminate it, perhaps, by better laboratory tests. One could understand it by graphical methods, such as Gibson's chart, which enabled the practitioner to interpret the white blood cell count better by counting the different types of cells. Yet another response, one much more to the liking of practitioners such as Deaver, was to allow the physical examination to supersede the laboratory test, to allow the clinicians' five senses to take over. "There is nothing as yet," said Deaver, "that can even partially take the place of detailed knowledge of the phenomenon of disease as gained by the use of the five senses."[104] That knowledge would help make the decision about whether to operate. As Deaver said again and again: "The degree of abdominal tenderness is much more decisive than the degree of leucocytosis. This, of course, demands experience and a light touch which is so valuable an asset to every surgeon."[105] This experience was presumably obtainable only through surgical training.

Part of Deaver's concern about laboratory examinations was that they would diminish trainees' appreciation of the clinical skills of older physicians: "To a proper respect for Nature and her healing power should be added a respect for your seniors in practice. If you are inclined to patronize old Dr. X because he had never seen a tubercle bacillus until you showed him one under your new microscope, you will do well to observe how much he will learn from feeling a pulse and after he has made a diagnosis from a facies which did not strike you as in any way peculiar, your self esteem may suffer a marvelous diminution."[106] Older physicians were, even in the early decades of the twentieth century, thought to be especially skilled in the art of medicine and, perhaps most important, in the art of physical diagnosis.

Discussions about laboratory tests and appendicitis should also be seen in terms of where patients lived and where surgeons worked. The success of urban surgeons, such as Deaver, created a problem for the emergency care of patients with acute appendicitis. By soon after the turn of the century most physicians agreed that acute, localized appendicitis required an immediate operation.[107] But there were not enough skilled surgeons to go around, especially in rural areas. The lack of surgeons was exacerbated by difficulty in transportation. Often the only way to move a seriously ill person was on the back of a horse. The automobile, when available for patient or physician, had to deal with unpaved (and, in northern winters, unplowed) roads.[108] The operation itself was more difficult than most of the other operations of the day, and it was one that many practitioners who were otherwise surgically inclined would hesitate to undertake.[109] The deficit in the supply of adequate surgeons would take time to remedy. In the meantime, those rural practitioners with whom patients first came in contact needed to be able to make a diagnosis of appendicitis more quickly, so that patient and surgeon could meet before the appendix burst and the more serious condition of peritonitis ensued. Far too often, however, they failed to do so, and people died.[110] Poignant stories are common, as, for example of a boy living in the Maine woods who died because of the delay in getting surgical treatment.[111] Appendicitis continued to carry a high death rate through the 1920s because, it was claimed, many cases were atypical and general practitioners had a hard time making the diagnosis.[112]

Discussions of the time were quite sensitive to the paradox that confronted the general practitioner. General practitioners were held to have less surgical training and experience in recognizing appendicitis than surgeons; they lacked the "experience and light touch" that Deaver noted as an asset of the skilled surgeon. Yet general practitioners were precisely the ones who most needed to be able to make an early diagnosis of appendicitis. Whereas surgeons would usually be called to the bedside when the diagnosis of appendicitis and the need for an immediate operation was clear, general physicians would see the patient earlier in the course, when their abdominal pain could be caused by many lesions, most less serious than acute appendicitis. They were more accustomed to waiting and observing. How could they get help in deciding when to pursue a more invasive course?[113]

The very success of surgeons such as Deaver could support a strong argument for general practitioners to use blood counts to diagnose appendicitis, as a crutch to make up for their lack of clinical experience and skills. Seen in this way, the laboratory test could be seen to produce "real," scientific evidence that disease was present. Some felt that the test required neither complicated apparatus nor a great deal of skill, at least less skill than was required for a bedside exam.[114] In fact, blood counts could serve an educational purpose. If general practitioners did white blood cell counts, they could recognize appendicitis more readily.[115] There were vivid examples of cases in which the clinical setting may have been somewhat unclear but in which laboratory tests, and the blood count in particular, led the way toward a life-saving abdominal operation.[116]

The meaning of the blood count as a technology was thus twofold. On the one hand, it was a mark of scientific progress, a technique using microscopes, creating numbers and graphs, and defining the practice of medicine as scientific. On the other hand, it was a crutch, a means to make up for the absence of other, more subtle clinical skills. Cabot argued for a synthesis of these two opinions, for the use of laboratory tests as personal data, for he felt that, just as one could not interpret the results of blood (or urine) examinations unless one were doing such examinations oneself, neither could one interpret the results of the examinations without also caring for the patient.[117]

The issue was eventually resolved by clinical pathology and a system in which blood counts were routinely done (or, at least, supervised) by physicians other than those directly involved with bedside patient care. These people, who came to be known as clinical pathologists, had to fight for status. They laid claim to an old tradition but felt the need to assert with some regularity that they were, or ought to be, of the same rank as the internist or surgeon.[118] One way of doing so was by claiming that only physicians should draw blood from patients.[119] This would keep the position of the laboratory expert—by the 1930s, the clinical pathologist—at the bedside, along with other high-status professionals. Although such a stance might seem logical, particularly when expressed in the inaugural volume of a journal written explicitly for clinical pathologists (who, one might think, had the most to gain from making the practice of blood testing as professional as possible), that position would eventually falter when the sheer volume of blood counts made it more practical, and profitable, for the clinical pathologist to become the supervisor of many technicians drawing blood and doing blood counts, rather than doing them directly. Eventually, the debate over the status of those physicians who did the blood counts became moot, as clinical pathologists came to direct technicians, run laboratories, and operate as independent consultants.[120] In the meantime, to see the use of the blood test as a "crutch" nonetheless encouraged its use, as an aid for the clinically less skilled general practitioner to identify those patients who needed to be seen by a specialist.

The eventual use of blood counts in appendicitis came at the end of a long process of change, after reasoned, significant opposition to its use. Surgeons such as Deaver were hardly old when the debate started—Deaver was only forty-six in 1901—nor were they necessarily traditionalist. Deaver was, in the spirit of the times, a radical surgeon. His reaction was more in response to what blood counts symbolized than to the actual counts themselves.

Deaver appears to have been very fond of telling stories about his cases. This appearance is partly a consequence of the fact that the bulk of Deaver's personal papers have been preserved and partly a result of the fact that Deaver was asked to give many talks to many groups. More than that, however, it also reflects Deaver's desire to emphasize that medical care is something that goes on in an individual, person-to-person fashion. Looking at laboratory tests not only physically distances the patient from the physician, but it also emphasizes abstract numerical values over personal characteristics. This, too, may have been part of Deaver's concern.

Those who held with Da Costa believed that counts were a new, necessary part of patient care. But using blood counts for patients with suspected appendicitis was only relevant if you were ready and willing to go in after the pus—which clinicians were increasingly willing and ready to do, thanks to the skills of surgeons such as Deaver. Deaver never changed his opinion, but eventually the surgical world came to use blood counts as part of the routine of patient care.

At both the New York Hospital and the Pennsylvania Hospital the number of cases of appendicitis, and the number of appendectomies, steadily rose, consistent with the increasing importance of surgery and the surgical treatment of appendicitis in the early-twentieth-century U.S. hospital (see table 7.3). The percentage of patients who died was somewhat lower than the norm, reflecting, perhaps, better care provided at these two well-regarded hospitals.[121] At the New York Hospital the mortality rate, as would be expected, was higher in cases in which the appendix was removed later rather than earlier and in cases in which a drain was not properly employed.[122] The use of blood counts rose gradually at the Pennsylvania Hospital, from no blood counts in patients with appendicitis in 1900 to 33 percent in 1909, 40 percent in 1920, and 68 percent in 1925. At the New York Hospital approximately 50 percent of patients with appendicitis had a blood count done by 1910.

Physicians at the New York Hospital appear to have used blood counts much as the literature would suggest. For example, a nine-year-old Italian boy was admitted on Saturday, February 12, 1910, and on that same day had his appendix removed.[123] One of the ways in which his physicians monitored his progress after the operation was with a white blood count, which was done on March 2. They noted, perhaps with relief, that the "leucocytosis [was] down." The fact that the white cell count was not elevated was evidence that there was no residual pus left behind, and, indeed, the young man was discharged, cured, on March 14.

Sometimes the blood count led physicians away from an

Table 7.3 *Appendicitis and Blood Counts at Pennsylvania and New York Hospitals, 1900–1925*

Year	No. of Cases	Patients with Appendicitis Who Had at Least One Blood Count (%)	Patients Who Had a Differential Count* (%)	Patients Who Died (%)	Patients with Appendicits Who Had Operation (%)
			PENNSYLVANIA HOSPITAL		
1900	6	0	0	0	83
1909	30	33	0	3	80
1920	15	40	0	7	87
1925	32	68	20	9	91
			NEW YORK HOSPITAL		
1900	9	33	0	0	89
1910	30	50	100	3	87
1920	37	45	100	3	95

*When a blood count was done.

operation. On July 28, 1920, a thirty-six-year-old German clerk came to the New York Hospital complaining of "cramp-like pains" in his right lower abdomen.[124] Although a case of acute appendicitis was suspected, a blood count done on the day of admission showed "no leucocytosis," and he was discharged, without an operation, a few days later on August 3. This case *might* have represented the foolish use of blood counts which Deaver feared. It is possible that the surgeon was unduly influenced by the blood count report and that the man, having an acute attack of appendicitis, was denied the chance for an early operative cure. Perhaps his appendicitis went on to rupture, with morbid sequalae. Perhaps. There is no indication that the patient was readmitted to the New York Hospital, although he could easily have gone elsewhere or could have suffered, or perhaps died, at home, without hospitalization. On the other hand, he may have been suffering only from indigestion, and the blood count saved him unnecessary surgery. This is obviously the scenario that his physicians thought most likely. We shall never know. There were other instances in which the blood count served to indicate the absence of serious disease, in which the notes next to the count included phrases such as "no leucocytosis" and "negative" and in which the patient was sent home within a day or two, with the diagnosis changed from "chronic appendicitis" on admission to "constipation" on discharge.[125]

Blood counts did not serve only to inhibit surgery. The blood count was at times used to indicate the need for an operation. Take, for example, the case of a twenty-three-year-old Swedish woman admitted on August 27, 1920, with complaints referable to the tonsils.[126] She developed a set of confusing symptoms soon after she entered the hospital, and a blood count done on August 29 showed a leucocytosis, with a white count of 16,000—a definite, but not striking elevation. The differential count revealed that 82 percent of the white cells were polymorphonuclear leucocytes, and its interpretation was "Suspect appendicitis." On the next day surgeons removed her appendix. Here, then, was an instance in which the blood count led the physicians caring for this woman to perform an operation. Deaver might not have approved of the blood count, but one suspects that he would have approved of the outcome.

A DIFFERENTIAL QUESTION

One striking finding in the examination of case records is that physicians at the New York Hospital did more differential counts for patients with appendicitis, and started to do them sooner, than did physicians at the Pennsylvania Hospital. At the New York Hospital 100 percent of all cases of appendicitis had a differential count done by 1910. In sharp contrast physicians at the Pennsylvania Hospital did a differential count much less often. No differential counts were done until 1925, and then only 20 percent of the cases had one done. In fact, for all three of the diseases discussed—pneumonia and typhoid fever as well as appendicitis—differential counts were done more frequently at the New York Hospital. If we choose to look at all patients, with all diagnoses, we see a similarly dramatic difference in the use of these counts: 13 percent of patients at the Pennsylvania Hospital who had a blood count done also had a differential count done, as compared with 90 percent of such patients at the New York Hospital.[127] The two institutions were both well-respected hospitals with academic affiliations, located within a few hours of each other and acquainted with the same literature.[128] Why was there this difference in practice?

There was a solid clinical rationale for doing a differential count for patients with appendicitis or suspected appendicitis. Even if the white count were normal, a high percentage of polymorphonuclear leucocytes would lead the clinician to suspect a purulent infection, as Gibson's charts were designed to show. There was a somewhat less compelling clinical rationale for doing a differential count in patients with pneumonia or patients with typhoid fever. Although the differential count in these disorders had been described in the literature, and such a count might be useful for prognosis, in most instances no action needed to follow the findings. The fact that a similar difference in doing a differential count is seen between the New York and the Pennsylvania hospitals with all three diseases, including two diseases usually cared for by internists and one cared for by surgeons, suggests an explanation: physicians at the two institutions behaved differently as a matter of local style. It also undercuts the simplistic idea that the variation merely reflected a difference between specialties, as the same variation is seen for both surgical and medical cases.

The low number of differential counts performed at the Pennsylvania Hospital cannot be ascribed to lack of either facilities or expertise. The Ayer Clinical Laboratory had been founded with a fifty-thousand dollar donation in 1898, with the distinguished pathologist Simon Flexner soon placed as its head.[129] From the laboratory's first reports pathologists gave detailed hematological findings, including multiple differential counts.[130] But, upon closer examination of the reports and the purpose of the Ayer laboratory, it is not surprising that attention to the morphology of the various white cells did not find its way into the care of ordinary patients with pneumonia, typhoid fever, or appendicitis. The first article to come from the Ayer laboratory was about Hodgkin's disease, a disease known to involve the blood and the blood-forming tissue. In another study, of the bone marrow in typhoid fever, the bone marrow was treated as a blood-forming site, with the focus on that tissue rather than on the infectious agent. More important, Flexner made it clear at the outset that the *Ayer Bulletin* would not be a means for discussing the "routine examinations" of either pathology or the clinical departments; the Ayer laboratory was intended to remain quite distinct from routine clinical service.[131]

Flexner's dreams for a major research endeavor at the Ayer laboratory remained unfulfilled. He eventually left for the Rockefeller Institute, at which a far larger endowment permitted a more active research enterprise.[132] For a few years after he left the annual reports of the Pennsylvania Hospital continued to refer to the Ayer laboratory in terms of its contributions to the scientific literature: in 1905 the report points with pride to the fact that research from the lab was being referred to in German and U.S. medical journals; in 1906 the report states that the lab "has successfully utilized the valuable material which our hospital affords for scientific work, and the publication of these researches has reflected much credit on the institution." Only later does the report note that the Ayer work has contributed to "caring for the sick."

The balance between scientific investigation and clinical service gradually shifted. A decade after its founding the Ayer laboratory started to be "swamped with routine work."[133] By 1909 allusions in the *Ayer Bulletin* are made to the increase in routine work, and in 1911 the emphasis is reversed: the laboratory is now said to be "aiding greatly in the treatment of patients and adding to the general knowledge of disease." By 1924 the transition was complete, and the director of the Ayer laboratory expressed his wish to try to recover from being swamped with clinical work and to focus once again on the original mission of the unit, scientific research. Thus, at first the Ayer laboratory was focused on research, not patient care. It clearly had the facilities to support differential blood counts, but routine clinical care was not central to its mission, at least not at first.

The situation at the New York Hospital was quite different. The pathology laboratory hired additional staff starting in 1897, about the same time as the Ayer laboratory was being founded in Philadelphia, but the mission was explicitly clinical, not aimed at research.[134] Only in 1907 did the unit claim that it was starting to do some investigative work, but this was clearly not its primary focus. Although many of the tests on blood, sputum, and the like were done by house staff on the wards, the pathological laboratory at the New York Hospital, unlike the Ayer laboratory at the Pennsylvania Hospital, was intimately involved with the day-to-day testing on clinical units. The hospital's annual reports include detailed information on clinical services. In addition, starting in 1915 the pathologist held weekly conferences with some of the surgical divisions.[135]

The use of differential counts was no doubt encouraged by the presence of Charles L. Gibson, who served as a deputy attending surgeon at the New York Hospital House of Relief starting in 1907 and who in 1913 was named attending surgeon at the hospital.[136] As discussed in chapter 6, Gibson was an enthusiast for the value of the differential count. His graph, as previously noted, could easily inform the physician if the percentage of polymorphonuclear leucocytes was what one would expect for the given level of leucocytosis. "Gibson's chart," as it came to be known, was not only used routinely in the New York Hospital but also received wide notice in the medical literature, the scientific and the *vade mecum*, the allopathic and the sectarian.

Gibson's graph was important on its own terms, but it also marked a general emphasis on the scientific efficiency movement. Gibson later established a rational "follow-up" system for his surgical division, which he used to study the outcomes of patients who had been under his care.[137] The other surgical division at the New York Hospital did not escape the excitement of the Progressive era.

On that service a systematic program of efficiency was instituted, complete with charts of people's movements during operations, hand signals to communicate during operations, a careful end result system, and particular attention to making sure that appropriate laboratory examinations were made without delay.[138]

Even the annual reports of the two institutions show a clear difference in their interest in presenting a neat, systematic summary of the work that had been done. The New York Hospital reports are consistent in their use of terms and present the number of exams done in a wide range of consistent categories. The Pennsylvania Hospital reports are much more variable, with tests such as Widals and blood counts being included in different categories from year to year. Since both laboratories came under new leadership at about the same time—1904 for the Ayer laboratory and 1906 for the New York Hospital—the differences in record keeping do not reflect turmoil at the leadership positions so much as a different style of operation and a different definition of what the laboratory should be doing. At the New York Hospital the Progressive ideology of consistent, standardized information gathering and retrieval seems to have been taken to heart. At the Pennsylvania Hospital there was less effort made to be consistent and efficient. Recall that there were similar differences between the two hospitals, discussed in chapter 2, with regards to financial record keeping.

The pathology department at the New York Hospital took an active role in patient care. Not content with merely doing the laboratory examinations that clinicians requested, pathologists evaluated the appropriateness of the requests. Moreover, they did so from a perspective explicitly focused on the clinical needs of patients, rather than the research desires of investigators.[139] The research they did was focused on ideas of efficiency and management.

A major reason to count blood cells derived from a general faith in record keeping. Part of the Progressive era ideology about record keeping held that careful, detailed observations of information, often recorded in graphic form, could eventually provide useful insights. The blood count, it was claimed around the turn of the century, was becoming a part of the regular chart in many hospitals, often compared with temperature and pulse charts. Moreover, this information was valuable, or would soon become so, even if one did not know what the records of the blood counts signified. One physician

predicted: "I believe the near future will demonstrate the significance of changes which have as yet no interpretation."[140] He was
sure that the meaning of such records would be better understood
someday, soon. This attitude reveals a faith in science, in progress.
More than that, it gives a specific indication of precisely *how* progress will take place. Not by faith in God. Not by the clinicians'
carefully honed operative technique. Not through hard work and
perspiration and sitting at a patient's bedside all night long. But,
rather, by numbers and tests and science.

And science was increasing in status in U.S. society in general. Yet
another reason for a physician to do blood tests was "to hold the
confidence of the public and retain his standing in the profession."[141]
Lab tests need not mean a less complete or less skilled bedside
examination. They added something new, something better. The
public was becoming increasingly sophisticated and aware of the
latest scientific advances. Failure to be proficient in laboratory
medicine would, eventually, mean that a physician would lose his or
her patients to those who were able to use the new techniques, for
the lay world was fast coming to believe in the "superior ability of
those who have adopted these methods."[142] The physician, it was
said, would be proved legitimate through the use of science, not
through long experience.

The ideas of Deaver and Da Costa eventually came to be seen
as not opposing each other. After surgeons came to embrace laboratory science as one touchstone of clinical excellence the proper
interpretation of a blood count came to be part of what it meant to
be clinically excellent, and at that point having the blood count be
considered an element of the overall clinical picture was no longer in
doubt.

8

MACHINES AND MEDICINE
Lessons from the Early Twentieth Century

At the beginning of this book we met two people, people we called
Messrs. James Moran and Richard Scott. Each of these two gentlemen of Philadelphia broke his leg many years ago; each was admitted to the Pennsylvania Hospital. Both have long since departed that
hospital, as have the many other patients whose care, individually
and collectively, has become part of this study of medical practice in
the first few decades of the twentieth century. We have examined the
process of medical care for Mr. Moran, Mr. Scott, and others, to learn
something about how and why medical technology has become such
a routine part of U.S. medical practice. In so doing, we have also
explored the ways in which medical care was part of a larger system
of people and ideas. Beyond increasing our historical understanding
of U.S. medical care in the early years of the twentieth century, this
analysis may also be valuable for those interested in contemporary
health policy. For in the late twentieth century health care reform
has become a central issue for national discussion, and a major
part of the debate revolves around the appropriate use of medical
technology.

Historical analysis may enable us better to understand the relationship between technology and health care by demonstrating the importance of studying how technologies are used and defined within
a specific social context. This finding undermines the misleading
assumption that technology is some kind of autonomous, self-
defining force. People living in the late twentieth-century United

States (as well as in much of the industrialized world) are bombarded daily with messages about the ways in which technology is changing their lives, changing how they travel, changing how they communicate with other people, changing the ways they go about the most personal of their everyday activities. The dominance of technology appears to be even more obvious for the case of medical care. Today medical machines can replace vital organs; they can sustain life from the moment of birth, as when a premature infant is whisked away to a neonatal intensive care unit, up until the end of human life, when turning off a respirator may be the event that defines the very moment of death. Technology not only sustains life; it may also improve the quality of life or even prolong a healthy life. Amazing imaging devices produce color-coded pictures of the inside of the human body. Sometimes, when used as a screening test for detecting disease, the images may save lives. Mammograms appear to prolong the lives of some women, though at present we are not certain precisely which ones. Other types of technology are being represented as holding great promise. Blood tests based on molecular biological techniques may soon be used to detect asymptomatic people at risk of disease, in order that they may be "cured" before their disease ever becomes manifest. Looking at all of these prominent features of contemporary clinical practice, it is not surprising that medical technology is often cited as the dominant feature and the driving force of the U.S. health care system.

Certainly, medical technology enables us to see, and to do, that which was previously unseeable and undoable. It is one thing, however, to describe technology as an easily identifiable, central feature of late-twentieth-century medical care. It is quite another to describe technology as a causal force leading to change, to say, as many have, that "the American health care system is driven by technology."[1] Such statements reflect a dominant model, perhaps *the* dominant model, about the relationship between technology and society: that technology is the driving force for change.

Yet is this the best model? Is it useful, or accurate, to conceptualize technology as an agent shaping U.S. health care? Perhaps not. As we have seen earlier in this book, when people in the early twentieth century debated whether to use the latest and most scientific technology, when they decided to do a urinalysis, take an x ray, or examine the blood, their decisions were taken within a specific social context. Although they were constrained by the physical artifacts at their disposal, those practitioners made choices; they determined the ways those artifacts would be used and how meaning would be derived from what they found. History can help identify what past choices have been made and what the effects of those choices have been, or, perhaps most important, to identify that there were in fact choices to be made. These insights may enlighten present analyses about what health care decisions are being made and who is making them, by pointing out that technology does not arrive at the bedside with its meanings already determined but, rather, ideas about how tests and tools can be used reflect a social context as well as a technical function.[2]

This imbedding of technology within a larger set of values is of more than merely theoretical interest. To conceptualize technology as autonomous is to deny the contingent and cultural nature of the choices that people made, and continue to make, about what technology means, what it does, and how it should fit into our larger systems of action and belief. Donald MacKenzie and Judy Wajcman, two historians of technology, point out that to ask the unilluminating question "How can society best adapt to changing technology?" assumes a set of passive responses to an external agent.[3] Thus formulating the question implies that change comes from somewhere "outside" of a society. Moreover, it also implies that members of society are limited in their role: they can only react to the new technology.

Another conceptualization is to say that technology is distinct from, and also derived from, science. This approach is no more useful. In addition to making an assumption that may or may not be true about the source of technology, it too often assumes that "science" somehow exists apart from social context, an assumption that has been effectively debunked by past decades of studies in the history and sociology of science.

Far better (and more useful) not to privilege technology but to look at it, instead, as being created within and inextricably defined as part of a specific social system. This book has explored how some examples of medical technology can best be understood as part of the context of a particular time and place.[4] We have thus seen how medical technology has been associated with changes in the nature of medical care in ways that say a great deal more about how we think of patient care than about the physical characteristics of the artifacts themselves. Consider how technology informs the doctor-patient relationship of the late twentieth century, a period in which trends begun in the early years of the century have intensified. Medical technology is increasingly relied upon to make diagnoses, as when, for example, a patient visits his or her physician complaining of a headache and concerned about the possibility of a brain tumor. Perhaps medical machines save time by providing information necessary to make diagnoses more efficiently. If the machine can save time, there is no reason implicit in the machine why physicians could not use that extra time to talk longer with their patients, getting to know them better. Yet that is not how medical technologies are depicted, nor, in fact, is it likely to be the case that using new imaging devices will cause physicians to spend more time talking with their patients. Doctors spend less time with their patients because, for whatever reasons, both groups have come to expect such behavior, and society rewards it. The shiny machines we used then and continue to use now do not create our social values. The surfaces are curved and the image that we see when we look at the machine may be distorted. But the machines do not create social assumptions about their use any more than they create our own appearance; rather, they reflect both of them back to us.[5]

Unlike some previous works on the history of medical technology, this study's primary goal has not been to assign priority for a particular invention nor to examine the uses of technology to further scientific research. Although they may be interesting, such histories tell us little about the social history of medicine, nor do they offer many useful insights for policymakers.[6] Instead, I have tried to understand how caregivers made choices about using clinical technology for individual hospitalized patients. Having asked a different set of questions, I have, not surprisingly, arrived at a different set of conclusions, which emphasize the introduction of technology as a process rather than as an event as well as a view of technology as contingent rather than autonomous.

Focusing on patient care enables one to examine how medical technology has been used at the level of the "shop floor." Historians of other types of technology have shown how factory workers do not simply import a new device: they shape it, mold it, and negotiate a position for any new tool within their specific environment.[7] This was also true for medical technologies in the early twentieth century. Physicians decided precisely what they wished to include when performing a given test—what parts of the test were to be done and what parts of the test, despite their being advocated by some, were to be omitted. Even after having decided that a test was to be done, the physician could decide how much accuracy was needed in a specific instance, how to balance the cost in time (and perhaps in money) with the gain in precision (and perhaps in the patient's outcome). Those decisions were made differently in different settings. Physicians working alone had considerable flexibility in their choices. They had no professional colleagues to answer to, at least not on a regular basis, and few patients were likely to have critiqued their decisions. On the other hand, physicians working in hospitals were part of a more clearly articulated system; they were subject to controls originating from above, from administrators and laboratory supervisors. Yet, even within the efficient systems that their administrators chose to impose, they still made individual decisions about whether to use a given test. Having decided to do a blood count, someone also made a choice about whether to include a white blood cell differential count. Someone made a decision about whether to measure the urinary sugar when doing a urinalysis and by what method. Like workers on the shop floor, physicians were finding ways to exist within a system that came to value scientific, laboratory tests. At some times, and in some places, they were able to exercise considerable flexibility in their decisions; in other settings, at other times, they were more constrained. I have chosen to emphasize the individual choices about how to care for patients which physicians made in specific clinical instances.

Physicians in the 1990s still have considerable control over the use of laboratory tests, but for at least two reasons they may have less flexibility as compared to physicians earlier in the century. First, increasing specialization and automation has meant that those who see a patient at the bedside rarely do the laboratory tests on that person. Most physicians have never done a blood count in a clinical setting; the blood is examined in the laboratory, and the results appear on a patient's chart or on a computer screen. The laboratory is supervised by a physician who rarely sees the patients on whose bodily fluids the tests are being done. The x-ray results are interpreted by radiologists. Unlike in 1925, most physicians, even those who specialize in radiology, have no idea how to operate an x-ray machine; the actual test is done by technicians.

Second, tests are often grouped in ways over which the person ordering the test has no control. Urine sent for analysis will automatically have a number of tests done on it, including those for color, specific gravity, and sugar (glucose), whether or not these tests are specifically requested. A complete blood count will report a number of indices in addition to the requested red and white blood cell count. The differential white count, interestingly, must still be requested as a separate test from the complete blood count in most institutions.

Rules and formalities notwithstanding, physicians still use diagnostic tests in ways that reflect individual, specific choices. Responding to laws that require formal permission from a patient in order to test their blood for the virus that causes AIDS, some physicians choose to stay within the letter (though not the spirit) of the law by testing instead the CD4 count, a surrogate marker that suggests infection with HIV, the virus that causes AIDS.

If technology use is defined by individual choices that are social and contextual, to understand the use of technologies one might best look at their introduction not as a single event but, rather, as a process of negotiation.[8] Within that process voices are raised in support of and in opposition to the use of a new tool. New technologies are not immediately adopted and used. There was, for example, a lag period, perhaps surprisingly long, between the introduction and eventual use of a new technology as dramatic as the x-ray machine. Similar lags existed for other types of technology during this period, such as incubators for premature infants.[9] It is not a new idea to suggest that there is a difference between theory and practice, between ideology and behavior. The existence of such delays suggests, however, that historians should not treat the eventual acceptance of a technology that we now consider to be useful as natural or inevitable; rather, they should seek explanations for its use at the same time and with the same level of intensity as they construct explanations for its invention.

One major theme of this book has been the importance of examining sources of resistance to the introduction of new technologies. I have tried to hear the arguments that were made against using the x ray to help diagnose fractures or against using the blood count to help diagnose appendicitis. If we are to understand how technologies are defined, how they are placed in the larger health care system, we need to attend to those who spoke (and acted) both for and against the new tools. This is as relevant at the end of the twentieth century as at the beginning. Any change, any introduction of a new technology, threatens the status quo; what one group gains in power and prestige, another group loses. As new technologies become accepted, people who once based their expertise on skill and experience obtained without the new technologies find their contributions devalued. As laboratory tests came to be seen as the touchstone of clinical decision making, carefully honed bedside diagnostic skills could not help but be seen as less important.

The introduction of new diagnostic systems in the 1900s rewarded those who had the technical skills to use them while diminishing the value of the clinical skills of those who had learned to get along without them. Perhaps one reason for the early widespread use of the urinalysis was the insidious nature of its proliferation as a monitoring device. Invisible in the background, the urinalysis attracted little attention, and thus little opposition. Because it could not be done inconspicuously, the blood count, at about the same time, stirred up a good deal more resistance.

A similar dynamic exists today when a new technology is introduced. For example, physicians once relied upon the stethoscope to identify diseases within the chest, particularly lesions on the valves of the heart. There are four such valves, each of which can either let through blood when it should not (i.e., be regurgitant) or not let through enough blood when it should (i.e., be stenotic). More than one valve may be impaired, or a single valve may be both incompetent and stenotic. Until fairly recently cardiac auscultation was the primary means of identifying those lesions, and physicians who were skilled at making the diagnosis were highly regarded. Yet, with the introduction of a quick, (relatively) inexpensive, safe, and painless method of obtaining the same information, the cardiac ultrasound, that has largely changed. The same physicians who once were skilled at making auscultatory diagnoses have access to the cardiac ultrasound, and, thus, their overall ability to correctly identify valvular lesions has increased. But, although their previously valued ability to make the same diagnoses with only a stethoscope has not become irrelevant, its perceived value has certainly diminished a great deal.

Perhaps this is what people who resisted some of the technologies we discussed had feared. Deaver certainly had access to blood counts for his hospitalized patients. But access is not the same as power. By allowing the meaning of blood counts to influence the clinical judgment of the bedside examiner, the power to decide whether a patient needed an operation shifted. If the blood count was seen as important, the value of the bedside exam would diminish, along with the clinical influence of those who were best skilled in that examination.

LOCAL CULTURE

Medicine is by its very nature an interactive process. First, patients must, perforce, interact with their caregivers. This interaction may be long and complex, as when patient and physician together negotiate a diagnostic and therapeutic plan, or brief and inadequate, as when a physician uses his or her power to deny a patient the opportunity to be treated as other than a pathological specimen. Nonetheless, medical practice cannot exist without a patient and a caregiver.[10]

At times more than one person may be involved in caring for a specific patient. This has probably been true more often for those who are sickest, who may require intensive treatment. It is probably also true for patients who are confined to bed or who are unable to move about and care for themselves. Whenever several people care for patients together, they need to communicate and interact with one another. One characteristic feature of medicine from the end of the nineteenth century to the end of the twentieth is a steady increase in the number of caregivers associated with each patient, perhaps nowhere so much as in the hospital.

During the early years of the twentieth century, as more units were formed within the hospital and more students—medical, nursing, and others—used the hospital as a training ground, more different types of people were thrown together on the hospital wards. There they had to make decisions about how to interact with one another and with patients. They also needed to decide how to apply the fruits of the new revolution in scientific medicine to patient care. Together they formed a local culture and arrived at a set of decisions at each institution about how things were to be done. Despite the best efforts at standardizing clinical care, this local culture informed, and continues to inform, the practice of medicine at a micro level.[11]

This book has not explicated the precise manner in which the interaction between people at a specific site led to a particular way of doing things nor who the most important leaders were and how and when they exerted their influence over others at the institution. Such an explanation may simply be unknowable for the early twentieth century, given the passage of years and the dearth of sources. Nonetheless, contemporary research may be able to guide our understanding of human behavior in the first few decades of the twentieth century. It suggests that local culture shapes medical care through personal, informal contacts among caregivers in a specific institution. For example, practitioners in the late twentieth century, when prescribing drugs to patients, often need to choose between several that have similar indications, efficacies, and toxicities. They could make that decision based on a number of different parameters. They might choose on the basis of cost to their patients. Or they might decide based on the likelihood that their patients would correctly follow instructions about how to take the medication, the likelihood of their "compliance." Or the choice of which drugs they prescribe might be random. Instead, people tend to be influenced by how others around them behave. The most common reason for physicians' choice of a specific drug is simply because it is commonly used at their institution.[12]

We do not know, of course, if a similar pattern of influences occurred at the New York and the Pennsylvania hospitals between 1900 and 1925, but it is clear that local factors were important in determining medical care. People at the two hospitals behaved differently in some areas, ranging from the decision to do a differential blood count to whether to take x rays of men and women with the same diseases. The process of defining the role of a new technology is, to a large extent, contingent, social, and local.

Obviously, the hospitals I studied determined the specific results of this study. These two hospitals were chosen in part because they have preserved much of the necessary historical documentation, including patient records. This fact alone should make the reader wonder about how typical these two institutions were.[13] But the findings, I hope, transcend any claims that might be made about how generalizable the specific events at the New York Hospital and the Pennsylvania Hospital were to other institutions. They exemplify the general relationship between ideas, artifacts, and the care of patients. Perhaps as well, the history of what went on at these two institutions can tell us something about the ways in which we should think about the history of medical technology.[14] The fact that the New York Hospital and the Pennsylvania Hospital were in some ways similar and yet had some very different practice patterns demonstrates the importance of local culture.

It would be extremely useful to know about other hospitals and about other types of hospitals, such as rural hospitals and womens' hospitals. Or one might wonder to what extent hospital practice was like or unlike practices outside of the hospital. It seems unlikely that patterns were totally different, but it is also unlikely that they were the same. Hospitals were moving to center stage at the start of the twentieth century; they may be moving more to the periphery at the end of the century. It is hard to predict the implications of this decentralization of care for the shared beliefs that I have called local culture.

DIFFERENT TECHNOLOGIES, DIFFERENT STORIES

Just as it is dangerous to generalize too far based on a few hospitals, so, too, it is dangerous to generalize based on a few technologies. Many other technologies from 1900 to 1925 could have been discussed in this book. Some technologies were included in the book's data set (such as blood pressure and smears to detect tuberculosis), and some were not (such as cystoscopy and endoscopy). The technologies considered in this book were similar in some ways but also different in other important ways. The urinalysis, a very old test (at least in name), was part of a nineteenth-century meaning of medicine which was shared by patients and their physicians.[15] Its very familiarity made it, perhaps paradoxically, well suited to serve as the leading edge of a transition to laboratory-based medicine. As compared to blood tests, obtaining the sample for a urinalysis was less painful or frightening for the patient, analyzing the sample was simpler for the physician (at least for the color and specific gravity), and the test in general was far easier for both. There was an intense chemical literature on urinalysis. Although perhaps important in broad strokes, this literature of complex analytic technique, born in elite scientific laboratories, appears to have had little impact on actual clinical practice. Thus, although some medical technologies may have started as research tools, the roots of the urinalysis appear not to lie in that domain.

The urinalysis seems at first glance too insignificant, too mundane, to be an important element in any transition to a technology-based medicine. But the historical importance of "little-ticket" technologies, such as the urinalysis, was, in part, as a model for how others would be applied.[16] Having become familiar with using urinalysis to monitor clinical status, health care providers could more easily imagine blood tests in that role. Eventually, blood tests became more familiar and supplanted urine tests. Today, many blood tests are also little-ticket technologies, almost seen as "nontechnologies." Although their cost (in both money and pain) may be small in each instance, in aggregate the cost may be quite large.[17]

New technologies also provided an opportunity for hospital administrators and physicians to work out systems for applying those technologies within the hospital.[18] Having established a system for one, the pattern could then be easily applied to another. Once a system was developed for having separate departments, with a person supervising that department who did tests and charged for them, as for the x ray, that system could be easily extended, as the x-ray system was extended for the electrocardiogram. Once a system was developed for reporting results of a few laboratory tests, that system could report all manner of results. All of these systems eventually became part of the fabric of the institution, appearing to be natural and inevitable. They blended into the background so that we are today only rarely aware of their existence or of the way in which they define the process of health care.

All technologies did not follow the same trajectory. Technologies went through different patterns of development. Some that were initially used to diagnose specific diseases later changed to permit a more general application. Blood counts, for example, were used first for patients with diseases of the blood and later for patients with a more general set of diseases. Conversely, some technologies changed from a more general to a more specific application. The urinalysis was at first a general test done on everyone who came into the hospital; it later became a specific test done as a monitoring device on people who were sick and needed to be closely observed. In the process the technology itself changed. What it meant to "do a urinalysis" or "take an x ray" was not the same in 1925 as it had been in 1900. Nor is it the same today. That change reflects more than a difference in tools and techniques; it reflects a change in the overall social and intellectual structure of medical care.

Different technologies produced different products and entered the public debate in different ways. The fact that the x-ray image was at first accessible to the public led to debates over its ownership which were not a feature of debates over the results of other types of technologies. Radiologists started at a fairly low level of status—certainly lower than pathologists, who at first studied things such as blood counts—and thus devoted some time and effort to establishing the standing of radiology within medicine. Now radiologists have enhanced their position considerably, and questions about whether patients should be allowed to see the images of their bodies are no longer seen as particularly important or threatening. Images from within the bodies of pregnant women have become, in some social circles, something to be expected as a routine part of pregnancy.[19] Easy public accessibility of the images has become an advantage rather than a disadvantage. People today expect to see, and cherish, images of their unborn fetuses, just as people in the 1890s and 1900s cherished x-ray images of themselves or their beloved. But by the 1910s and the 1920s physicians were threatened by public access to the pictures, and ownership of the x-ray image was an important battleground for radiologists. How did this episode in the early history of the specialty shape its future course? We cannot say. But it seems reasonable to speculate that technologies that produce pictures will have an inherently different history than technologies that do not.

As we have seen, these pictures' meanings are socially constructed and contingent on specific historical circumstances, as is the case for every technology. To say, however, that the meaning of a technology is socially constructed is not to say that it is infinitely variable. There were constraints on the ways that different technologies could be applied. That the blood count could be done with small, simple equipment made it an ideal tool to identify people in rural areas who urgently needed invasive surgical care, a need particularly relevant when situated in a world of changing means of transportation and rapidly expanding surgical interventions, particularly when surgeons were primarily located in urban areas and worked in urban hospitals. The x ray—a tool that required space, people, and money—could not as effectively serve that need. The urinalysis would have made an excellent tool for the rural physician, perhaps even better than the blood count, if the requisite information for distinguishing between a patient with appendicitis, who thus required surgery, and an essentially healthy one with gas pains could have been obtained from an examination of, say, the urine's color and odor.

The historian of technology Thomas Hughes points out that technology is not infinitely malleable and calls for an interactive model, what he calls a "systems approach."[20] This approach is similar to the one developed in this book, in which medical technology is seen as only making sense when viewed as part of a larger system. Hughes also warns against the dangers of widespread systematization, the possibility that as the health care system changes it may become "another set of extremely large systems, systems that will become virtually impervious to social control." Perhaps. But probably not. The intensely personal nature of the relationship between patient and caregiver is likely to resist attempts at systematization and standardization in the future, just as it has in the past.

TECHNOLOGY AND PEOPLE

Medical technologies are used on people, for people, and by people. For many of the examples considered in this book, physicians made the decision about whether to use technology. Clinical practice in the Pennsylvania and New York hospitals from 1900 to 1925 reflected the care of hundreds of physicians. Little attempt was made in this book to explore the personal nature of specific physicians' practices. One fruitful source for further historical study would be to examine the relationship between the characteristics of individual physicians and the use of technology. Some of the transitions that were observed may reflect changes with succeeding generations of physicians, trained in different ways. The extent to which generational transitions explain changes in clinical practice could, perhaps, be studied in hospitals or other training institutions, such as the Pennsylvania Hospital or the New York Hospital. But such a study would be difficult because of the inherently diffuse nature of the decision-making process in a teaching institution. That is, it would be difficult to establish precisely who was responsible for any specific decision—the attending physician? the house staff? which one? Nonetheless, learning more about the people who made the decisions is likely to prove fruitful.

Most of those people were men; a few were women. The relationship of medical technology to gender also deserves more attention. Much contemporary study of the relations of gender and medical technology focuses on technology use during pregnancy and childbirth.[21] While useful, such studies miss the most widespread applications of technology to women, most of which involve women who are not pregnant. And, of course, a full understanding of the relations between gender and technology should include men as well. This book attempted to do so while exploring how the patient's gender may have informed x-ray use, in chapter 5.

Another way to study the relationship between gender and clinical practice could be to look at the physician's gender, and to examine differences between how male and female physicians have used medical technology. At about the same time as technologies such as the x-ray machine were starting to become widely used in the United States, there was a higher percentage of female physicians than there would be again for a very long time. The percentage of female physicians peaked in Boston at 18.2 percent in 1900 and at 6 percent in the country as a whole in 1910.[22] Did the introduction and widespread use of machines after 1900 play a role in discouraging women from entering medicine? Did the fact that medicine became even more male dominated in the ensuing decades make it more likely that those (male) physicians would want to use machines? Did women use technology differently? Because there were extremely few female physicians at the New York Hospital and the Pennsylvania Hospital from 1900 to 1925, this study could not address these questions. If sources for such studies could be located, perhaps in hospitals associated with women's medical schools, it would be interesting to compare and contrast how female and male physicians in hospitals treated female and male patients.[23]

Sources constrain all historical research. The part of this analysis that is based on patient records is limited to what was written down. It is certainly possible that tests were done and not recorded in a patient's chart. Those tests have probably disappeared forever from the historical record. Yet, because systematic recording of hospital activities was one of the most striking features of the period under study, when someone used a technology it was probably noted in the chart. Even when a test was recorded it is not always possible to discern why. One can note patterns among patients and patterns in the time course of the application of a technology and, when possible, by using narrative notations that were made in the chart, along with other written material.

These inferences can sometimes be extended to a patient's experience. Nonetheless, the analysis from the medicine-centered written record is necessarily indirect; it remains difficult to know precisely how patients experienced a given technology. Yet, since we are unlikely ever to be able to do for the early twentieth century the kind of ethnographic, anthropological study that would now seem to be ideal, this type of analysis may have to suffice.

By focusing at the level of individual patient care, we can ask questions about how medical technology changed patient care and in that way address some of the concerns of social historians about the relationships between health care and day-to-day life. There is little doubt that technology use was a major feature of patients' experiences by a decade or two into the twentieth century.

This book, however, does not attempt to establish the appropriateness of technology use, to decide if physicians who used technology helped their patients or hurt them. I cannot assess what was the "right" way to use a technology, to say, for example, that people at the New York Hospital were doing too many differential counts in 1920 or people at the Pennsylvania Hospital too few. Such a task would be ahistorical if we attempted to use contemporary standards and definitions, and it would be quite difficult to unpack adequately the values and goals of the patients upon whom the new technology was applied. Even when evaluating present-day care, it is often difficult to identify when techniques or technologies are being used in ways that help patients.

CONTEMPORARY ECHOES

Historians are intrinsically dubious about "routine proclamations of a new departure in policy."[24] Historical analysis may be useful for contemporary health policy if it can show that apparently new ideas and innovations have their historical roots in much older concepts. Several of the themes that we have explored for the early years of the twentieth century have now reappeared near the end of that century, sometimes with a new name, sometimes not. Perhaps the most striking parallel is that, as was the case for the early twentieth century, some of the most important medical technologies are organizational systems rather than mechanical artifacts, and some of these technologies have been imported to medicine from the world of business.

Machines that we would now think of as medical, such as the x-ray machine, did not drive the early-twentieth-century transformation of the U.S. hospital. The technology that played a key role in changing the hospital was introduced from the world of business, sometimes in the form of physical artifacts, such as the adding machine, and sometimes in the form of systems, changes in the internal organization of the hospital, both in the formal sense of cost accounting and in the more general (and probably more important) sense of a desire for efficient, quantitative analysis. The tendency to import methods and ideas from business into hospitals has continued and perhaps intensified as the twentieth century draws to a close.

As this book is being written, U.S. health care is being besieged on (it seems) all sides by advocates of a managerial philosophy (or, as it often referred to, a paradigm) known as Total Quality Management, or TQM.[25] Although often treated as something new, the similarities between TQM and the efficiency movement of the early twentieth century are inescapable. Both have been promoted as systems that can lead to continuous improvement in the quality of health care. (Both movements, in fact, are advocated as improving virtually all aspects of organized activity.) Both movements appeared to achieve remarkable success in the world of nonmedical business before being imported into the world of the hospital. Both are based on incorporating not only tools and systems but also a proper "attitude" toward work.[26] Both also result in an increased role for management, particularly those administrators who are most active in promoting the new management style. Just as was the case for the efficiency movement, those who preach TQM talk about desire to incorporate all physicians into TQM organizational improvement.[27] Also similar to the efficiency movement, as TQM becomes a wide-spread part of health care administration, health care providers find themselves pressured to adopt at least the language of TQM. The effort to recruit physicians to the cause has, so far, met with relatively little success, perhaps because of a consistent disquiet among health care providers about seeing medicine treated so overtly as a business.

The terms of TQM usually allude to improving quality as a primary goal. It is clear, however, that another primary goal of this new managerial system is to reduce the cost of health care, which, unlike in the early twentieth century, has become a central topic of national concern. Critics have blamed medical technology for much of the increase in the cost of health care over the past few decades.[28] Confronted with the assertion that technology is "the culprit behind rising health care costs," proponents of technology research have countered by claiming that better technologies lead to better treatments and that better treatments need not lead to higher expenditures. Instead, they claim that improving the quality of health care saves money, by allowing better and cheaper treatment of common conditions.[29] Whatever the outcome of the debate, the discussion has focused attention on the process by which technologies are invented and, more important, the process by which their use is encouraged or discouraged.[30]

Concerns about rising health care costs have led academics and politicians to question whether the United States is making optimum use of health care resources, particularly in light of considerable regional variation in health care delivery. If we wish to understand why regional variation now exists, it may help us to know something about its history. This book has demonstrated significant variation between how physicians at the New York and the Pennsylvania hospitals provided health care between 1900 and 1925, perhaps most dramatically in the ways that they used a little-ticket technology, the differential white blood cell count. The variation between the two hospitals existed in the context of significant national variation in the purchase of medical care during this time period.[31] Thus, the regional variation we see at the end of the twentieth century is not a new phenomenon. A full explanation for regional variation ought to explain both its existence from the early twentieth century and its persistence for almost one hundred years.

It is important to realize, however, that "regional variation" as a concept, as something to be considered and explained, did not exist in the 1910s and 1920s. Before this concept could be created, ideas about disease had to move away from a localistic, particularist philosophy of medical care. Around the turn of the twentieth century many caregivers and their patients believed that diseases in different climates and different environments would naturally take separate clinical courses and require different treatments. Moreover, as each patient's set of unique personal characteristics defined how disease would affect him or her, a health care provider could not possibly know how to treat someone without knowing about that person's temperament, upbringing, and personal life story. Thus, many observers did not believe that the inherent nature of disease would permit someone, even in theory, to devise a diagnostic and therapeutic schema that would apply to different patients in different places. If the concept had been explained to them, many of these caregivers would probably have seen regional variation as an appropriate reflection of the natural world, rather than as a topic to be labeled and studied.

Today clinical ideas about disease have shifted by almost 180 degrees. Medical writers have little difficulty combining clinical studies from different societies, even for diseases as loosely defined as "dyspepsia" or "irritable bowel syndrome," lumping together data from Asia, North America, and Europe as though disease is a purely biological construction, not affected by social and cultural context. The active work by historians and sociologists on the social construction of diseases appears to be having little impact on clinical studies.[32]

Within a medical world in which disease has come to be seen as susceptible to precise scientific analysis, regional variation has gone from being an appropriate reflection of the natural world to an aberration that should be studied and dealt with. If one chooses to believe that criteria for health care can be clearly defined, unexplained variation in health care delivery becomes a thing to be challenged. The existence of variation between otherwise comparable groups of people implies that someone must be receiving too much care or too little, thus, that someone must be receiving inferior health care. Variation among useful or expensive technology implies either that some area is getting too little care or that some area is spending too much money on care. To address such issues the federal Agency for Health Care Policy and Research has taken the leading role in a federal initiative to write clinical practice guidelines that are intended to synthesize the current state of knowledge and insure a uniform standard of medical practice.[33] Those guidelines themselves, along with the means of implementing them, constitute a form of technology, albeit a form very much in dispute.[34]

We have, of course, seen something akin to clinical practice guidelines before. The debates in the 1900s over whether all patients with potential fractures needed to have an x-ray examination done or whether all patients who might have appendicitis did (or did not) need a blood count made were based on a view about medical care which eventually led to the formal creation of clinical practice guidelines. Asking general questions about the appropriateness of a given technology contrasted sharply with the usual nineteenth-century model of medical care, based on the care of each individual patient within his or her specific, personal context. The tension between seeing medical decisions as fundamentally personal and individual and seeing medical decisions as fundamentally based on universal scientific principles has existed throughout the twentieth century. Despite intensive scientific research, concerns persist about the ill effects of attempting to reduce medical practice to a set of formal guidelines, guidelines that may threaten to undermine the value of clinical expertise and its basis in personal medical care. Although many physicians perceive clinical practice guidelines as providing useful advice, a sizable group see them as "oversimplified" and "too rigid to apply to individual patients"[35]

Current attempts to promote practice guidelines are not oblivious to these concerns. Their authors attempt to incorporate what are seen as the relevant variables for each patient.[36] How to define those variables has not been obvious. Until recently, studies of patient care have tended to exclude women, at times because of a fear that they might be pregnant, and clinical studies could put the fetus at risk. A more general reason for the absence of women from clinical studies is a tendency to conceptualize men as representing a universal clinical model and women as a separate, special case. Perhaps as a result, women (as well as African Americans) are less likely to receive the latest treatments when they suffer illnesses such as heart disease.[37] Of course, without knowing whether those treatments are helpful (as is often the case), one does not know if failure to be treated with them is a harm or a benefit.

During the early 1990s investigators have started to incorporate more women into the clinical studies upon which practice guidelines will be based. However, the previous exclusion illustrates a problem inherent in any attempt to promote universal guidelines for medical care. Those people who do the studies used to create the guidelines cannot help but do so within a specific social context, and that context is very likely to be one that privileges certain types of patients as the exemplar for the type of medical care to be studied.

Clinical trials have been used by physicians to identify certain clinical actions as appropriate for a given set of circumstances. Nonetheless, these results are frequently not used in clinical care. Many contemporary observers regularly bemoan the disparity between "optimum" care, as described in published literature, and "actual" care, as provided to patients. Present-day anomalies in physician behavior can sometimes be understood better by shifting the level of analysis from published ideas to individual decisions. For example, 1980s and 1990s studies suggested that clinical decisions can be made better with sets of formal, quantitative rules and that the decision analysis can be operationalized with small, hand-held computers. Using standard, validated scales that many at the end of twentieth century define as superior to an individual clinician's judgment, investigators claim that the decisions made using hand-held computers are superior to decisions made without such tools.[38] Nonetheless, these tools are rarely used to make patient care decisions, perhaps because they are perceived as compromising a physician's autonomy to make clinical judgments and subordinating his or her personal experience to a set of abstract guidelines. Similar sentiments were also true for earlier medical technologies. There may have been a distrust of artifacts, a desire not to have to rely on machines, a deep-seated cultural bias in favor of an individual clinician's clinical judgment, or a fundamental belief that individual clinicians make decisions using information and modes of analysis which simply cannot be captured by any set of formal rules or procedures. Deaver feared that laboratory-based guidelines, such as a white blood cell count, would undercut his clinical skills and impede his ability to effect a cure. This concern overwhelmed his ability to hear that some cell counts could, and did, often lead to more abdominal operations, an outcome that would have pleased Deaver. He wanted not to calculate but, rather, to cut. His message—that the individual clinician's clinical judgment cannot and should not be reduced to a set of formally articulated decision points—continues to be heard in the present day.

Yet some things have changed. Perhaps the single most important technological change, one that has already had widespread effects for health care in its broadest sense, is the availability of new types of machines for dealing with information.[39] There simply did not exist the computing technology in the early twentieth century to study medical practice involving more than a handful of physicians. As insightful as they were, E. A. Codman's outcomes charts would have quickly become unusable for analyzing any significant number of practice patterns.[40] Even in the early 1980s data analyses of the modest scale required for this book could be done only on a mainframe computer that sat in a single location. Today, in the mid-1990s, huge data sets can be analyzed using portable notebook computers that are no larger (or heavier) than the computer magazines one can purchase at a newsstand. This technology is a straightforward extension of the typewriters, adding machines, and punch cards that were discussed in chapter 2.[41] Just as was the case then, these technologies were originally adopted for use by hospital business departments, which used them to create large administrative data sets. Originally intended to be used to track the flow of money, the data sets have been used by health services researchers to analyze the delivery of medical care.[42] The computing technology may soon be used to track compliance with practice guidelines and to encourage (though precisely what this means is unclear) compliance with those guidelines.

It is hard to predict what changes the new health care system being discussed in the mid-1990s will bring. But it seems clear that, just as earlier in the twentieth century, money and accounting will again be central. Hospitals will probably need to become part of larger, integrated systems and, to compete effectively, will need to do a better job of analyzing costs and charges. These pressures are very similar to the push for cost accounting in the early years of the century. Hospitals will need to devise better systems for tracking both clinical and financial data, using computerized techniques that are both reminiscent of and directly derived from the Hollerith cards. These administrative changes are likely to have dramatic, though unpredictable, effects on the ways that patients are cared for.

Clinical information is important for patient care. We have seen how creating accurate means for circulating health care information throughout the system was a major concern of those who wished to make early twentieth-century health care more efficient. The issue of timely access to health care records persists. The United States does not yet have a single, centralized mechanism for keeping track of a person's medical records, although one is now being discussed as part of President Clinton's health care reform initiative.[43] Even though diagnostic technology may have been used to make a diagnosis, patients may suffer because information about their care is not easily transferred from one unit to another. A recent study reported on ten children who were taken to a pediatric emergency department for care of a previously undiagnosed disease. In each of these cases a screening test had already detected the disease, yet the information had not been properly transmitted and thus was not available to health care providers attempting to aid the children.[44] People are considering various forms of electronic patient records. Using technology to keep track of medical information may be as important to patient care as using technology used to create that medical information. Keeping efficient patient records was a concern in the 1900s and 1910s and still is today.

The precise determinants of change in medical technology use between 1900 and 1925 are not known and may never be, but at least this study should lay to rest some persistent myths about the relationship between science, medicine, technology, hospitals, and U.S. society which have long guided our historical perspective on the process by which the practice of medicine in the United States has come to depend so much on the use of machines. Technology was not quickly adopted because it was shown to be useful for the care of the ill: the change to a science- and technology-based model for medical care took several decades and was implemented in a nonhomogeneous way, certainly as reflected in the way medicine was practiced day to day for most Americans. Nor did medical technology in the form of the x ray, or other devices usually thought of as medical technology, drive the formation of the U.S. hospital. The most important technologies were, instead, those derived from the efficiency movement, and these changed the hospital and made it a more open environment for a host of more directly clinical devices. Still today, the technologies that we use, the machines that we choose to make a part of patient care, are used in ways that reflect the underlying social concerns and beliefs of a society.

APPENDIX

Sampling Techniques and Coding Forms

Choice of Sampling Method

Ideally, given infinite time, the researcher's historical conclusions about the events at a particular hospital would be based on an examination of the case records of each and every patient who was admitted. Yet in the case of hospitals such as the New York Hospital and the Pennsylvania Hospital between 1900 and 1925, when there were over four thousand admissions per year for each hospital, such a comprehensive survey is impossible, and it is necessary to reduce the total number of records looked at. The selection of records is crucial. Simply looking at the patients who experience an intervention of choice, such as the x ray, is not enough; to understand patients who were examined by x rays in the overall context of the hospital requires knowing about similar patients who, for whatever reason, did *not* have an x ray taken. Similarly, a researcher leafing through the records might be drawn to longer records or those written in a more legible hand or those covered with less dust or those that simply happen to be nearer to where he or she is standing in the archive.

In order to avoid the inevitable bias that comes with any arbitrary selection of case records, researchers need to use some form of probability sampling, a sampling method for which every patient record in the total population has a known, nonzero chance of being included in the sample. With a probability method one can use standard statistical techniques to derive estimates, such as the mean, from the total population from which the sample is drawn. One can also make estimates, such as confidence intervals, about the likelihood that the true, population mean (i.e., the mean that would have been found by looking at every available record rather than a sample of the total) will lie within a specified range.

Selecting a proper sample size is critical. Using too small a sample will make it difficult to arrive at a meaningful conclusion; collecting too large a sample will become prohibitively expensive and time-consuming. Based on a pilot study, I estimated the percentage of patients who would receive most of the interventions that I wished to study at between 1 and 25 percent.[1] To detect a difference of 10 percent with a power of 80 percent, one needs a sample size of approximately four hundred. There are several ways of obtaining a probability sample; I chose to use systematic sampling.[2] Other sampling methods would perhaps have worked as well, but they would have been less practical. With systematic sampling one starts with a record randomly selected between 0 and k and then simply takes every kth record throughout the series of casebooks. Each casebook—usually big, heavy, bulky volumes—thus needs to be taken off the shelf only once.[3] Although there are some rare situations in which systematic sampling is theoretically problematic, most notably when the records are placed in a pattern with a cycle length equal to k, this situation is usually obvious by simple inspection. The patient records used for this book appear to have been bound in simple chronological order, and thus systematic sampling is a valid method.

Availability of Records

Each hospital presented practical sampling problems. The patient records for the New York Hospital were stored by diagnosis rather than by year starting in 1914. Thus, the sampling from the New York Hospital was more difficult after that time. As each diagnosis volume was located, a sample was selected in the usual fashion. The difficulty of finding those volumes is reflected in the lower number of cases from 1920 and the absence of any cases from 1925. The more common diagnoses occupied more space, however, so they were more likely to have been located for the sample.

At the Pennsylvania Hospital the selection of records for 1910 was incomplete, so 1909 was sampled instead. Not all of the patient records were saved for 1920 and 1925. For purposes of this study, samples were systematically taken from the remaining volumes. The sample size, for the New York Hospital, was: 384 in 1900, 391 in 1910, and 165 in 1920; and, for the Pennsylvania Hospital, 383 in 1900, 402 in 1909, 441 in 1920, and 396 in 1925. The variance from four hundred records, when adequate numbers of records were available, is due to small inconsistencies between the published number of cases (which was used to derive k) and the actual number of cases located.

Forms Used to Collect Data

For each record a series of computer readable forms was filled out, either by me or by one of two outstanding research assistants, Chris Bass and Grace Brill. For each patient a basic patient data sheet was filled out which included data such as age, sex, and marital status. The information recorded on that sheet is listed in table A.1. By the year 1900 hospital patient records had become quite detailed, and most of the demographic information was available for most of the cases sampled.

Then, for each patient record, a form was completed for each of eight types of diagnostic technology if that technology was used. A separate form was completed for each instance in which that technology was used, with the exception of urinalysis. Because so many urinalyses were performed, only the first three tests were recorded in detail, and for those remaining (up to a maximum of fifteen tests) only the date of the test was recorded. The basic items included are listed in table A.2.

Obviously, not all of the information needed to understand a given interaction can be captured in code. Thus, each form had space to include any other information that was thought to be of value for understanding the particular case record. In addition, some information requested on the form (such as comments in the chart) was not coded but was simply recorded verbatim.

Table A.1 *Basic Data Recorded and Coded for Each Patient*

Column	Data
1–5	ID number (sequential)
6	Deck number
7–8	Hospital
9–10	Type of service to which patient was admitted
11–12	Location of admission service
13–15	Name of attending physician (on admission)
16–18	Name of house staff (on admission, who signed admission note)
19	Sex
20–21	Age
22	Marital status
23	Race
24–26	Nationality/place of birth
27–29	State or province of birth
30–32	Country of residence
33–35	State or province of residence
36	Religion
37–39	Occupation
40	Vertical level of occupation
41–44	Volume number of patient record
45–48	Page number (or case number)
49–51	Year of volume
52–54	Year of admission
55–56	Month of admission
57–58	Day of admission
59–61	Year of discharge
62–63	Month of discharge
64–65	Day of discharge
66	Duration of primary illness prior to hospitalization
67	Had the patient been hospitalized at this hospital before?
68	How many times had the patient been hospitalized here before?
69	Condition on discharge
70–76	Admission diagnosis
77–83	Discharge diagnosis
84–90	Reason for entering the hospital (chief complaint)
91	Was there an operation performed?
92–98	What was the operation?
99	Was anesthesia used?
100–101	What type?
102	Was the anesthesia record a separate printed form?
103–5	Who administered the anesthesia?

Table A.1   *Continued*

Column	Data
106–8	Length of the record (in pages)
109–10	Number of graphs in the record[a]
111-13	Number of separate forms in the record[b]
114	Are there drawings in the record?
115	Are there photographs in the record?
116	Did the MD use a stamp to indicate physical findings?
117–19	Year of operation
120–21	Month of operation
122–23	Day of operation
124–33	Columns for additional demographic data of interest

[a]A graph is defined here as any representation of data which uses points or a line defined by two orthogonal axes.
[b]A form is any separate piece of paper designed to be used in a patient record, such as an x-ray form, a laboratory form, a form for recording operative procedures, etc. A form will often, but need not, entail a graph.

Codebook

The codebook was initially developed based on a version used during the pilot study. As records were collected, the codebook was modified as needed. I coded the initial series of records for each hospital, and all of the admission and discharge diagnoses, using a disease classification system from the period.[4] I also coded the type of operation (if one was performed) and the type of anesthesia. The codebook contains codes for missing data and for illegible writing.

Data Entry and Analysis

After the code sheets were completed, data was entered into a microcomputer database program. At the start of this project the amount of data generated could not be analyzed statistically on a microcomputer, so it was uploaded to the University of Michigan mainframe system, and initial analyses were done using a statistical program known as MIDAS. Changes in computer hardware and software, however, now make data sets of this size easily manageable on a microcomputer system, and all of the later analyses were done on a DOS-based system using the statistical package STATA.[5]

Table A.2   *Data Recorded for Technology Use*

X ray Use

1–5	ID number
6	Deck number
7	Number (in order) of this x-ray examination
8	Was this use reported on a separate form?
9	Is that form printed?
10	Does the form indicate standard items to be evaluated?
11	Was there comment in the chart about the x ray? What was the comment?
12	Did the x ray result in a change in the patient's diagnosis? What were the first and second diagnoses?
13–15	Year of the exam
16–17	Month of the exam
18–19	Day of the exam
20–21	Type (location) of x-ray diagnostic study or therapy
22	Was the x ray used for therapy?
23–24	Area irradiated
25	Was there comment about technical inadequacies of this or previous exams or studies?

Electrocardiogram (ECG) Use

1–5	ID number
6	Deck number
7	Number of this ECG
8	Was this use reported on a form?
9	Is that form printed?
10	Does the form indicate standard items to be evaluated?
11	Was a copy (or the original) ECG in the chart?
12	How many leads are recorded?
13	Was there comment in the chart about the ECG? If yes, what was the comment?
14	Did the ECG change the patient's diagnosis? If yes, what were the first and second diagnoses?
15–17	Year of the exam
18–19	Month ECG use
20–21	Day ECG use

Urinalysis (UA) (First Three Exams)

1–5	ID number
6–7	Deck number
8	Number of this UA (1–3)
9	Were results reported on a separate form?
10	Was that form printed?

Table A.2   *Continued*

11	Was that form a general form for laboratory tests?
12	Did that form list specific items in the UA to be performed?

For each of the following, indicate whether:

1	Recorded
2	Indicated but not recorded
3	Neither indicated nor recorded

13	Specific gravity
14	Color
15	Albumin
16	Sugar
17	Rxn (acid or alkali)
18	Acetone (ketone) bodies
19	Microscopic examination (undifferentiated)
20	Bacteria
21	Casts
22	Crystals (all types)
23	Blood (red)
24	Blood (white; pus)
25	Urea
26	Indican
27	Bile
28	Other (list)
29	Was there comment in the chart about the UA? If yes, what was the comment?
30	Did the UA change the patient's diagnosis? If yes, from what to what?
31–33	Year of exam
34–35	Month of UA
36–37	Day of UA

Urinalysis (Fourth Exam and Subsequent)

1–5	ID number
6–7	Deck number
8–10	Year of fourth exam
11–12	Month of fourth exam
13–14	Day of fourth exam
15–17	Year of fifth exam
18–19	Month of fifth exam
20–21	Day of fifth exam

(etc., through column 90 for fifteenth exam)

Table A.2 *Continued*

Blood Counts

1–5	ID number
6	Deck number
7	Number of this blood count
8	Was the blood count reported on a separate form?
9	Was that form printed?
10	Was that form part of a general form for laboratory tests? What other tests were on that form?
11	Did the form indicate specific items to be evaluated? If so, list these items.
12	Was a differential blood count performed?
13	Was there comment in the chart about the blood count? If yes, what was the comment?
14	Did the blood count change the patient's diagnosis? If yes, what were the first and second diagnoses?
15–17	Year of exam
18–19	Month of blood count
20–21	Day of blood count

Tuberculosis (TB) Exam (Microbiological)

1–5	ID number
6	Deck number
7	Number of this TB exam
8	Was this reported on a separate form?
9	Was that form printed?
10	Was that form part of a general laboratory form? If yes, what other tests were included on the form?
11	Was there comment about the results in the chart? What was the comment?
12	Did the exam for TB change the patient's diagnosis? If yes, from what to what?
13–15	Year of the exam
16–17	Month of exam for TB bacilli
18–19	Day of exam
20	Was there a drawing of the findings?
21	Was there a photograph of the findings?

Widal Reaction (Rxn)

1–5	ID number
6	Deck number
7	Number of this Widal Rxn
8	Were results presented on a separate form?
9	Was that form printed?

Table A.2   *Continued*

10	Was that form part of a general laboratory form? If yes, what other tests were included?
11	Was there comment about the results in the chart? What were they?
12	Did the Widal exam change the patient's diagnosis? From what to what?
13–15	Year of exam
16–17	Month of exam
18–19	Day of exam

Blood Pressure (BP)

1–5	ID number
6	Deck number
7	Number of this BP exam
8–10	Value of systolic pressure
11–13	Diastolic pressure
14–16	Pressure when only one number given
17	Did the BP change the patient's diagnosis? From what to what?
18	Was there a form that specified taking the BP?
19–21	Year of exam
22–23	Month of exam
24–25	Day of exam

Pulse

1–5	ID number
6	Deck number
7	Number of this exam
8–10	Value of pulse rate
11	Was there comment on the pulse value? What was it?
12	Was there a qualitative comment on the pulse?
13	Who took the pulse?
14–16	Year of exam
17–18	Month of exam
19–20	Day of exam

Data-Checking Protocol

After the data was entered into the computer, standard error checking was done to find out-of-range values (i.e., sex coded as "5" when that is not a valid code) and illogical conclusions (i.e., a patient who was discharged from the hospital before he or she had entered it).

These errors were often due to obvious mistakes, such as column shifting during data entry, and were easily corrected. More difficult to identify are errors such as entering the age as "17" rather than "71." To obtain an estimate of the overall error rate, after entry was completed I recoded one hundred records directly from each hospital and found an overall accuracy rate of over 99 percent.

Deposit of Data for Public Use

At the conclusion of this study the electronic data will be deposited at the Inter-University Consortium for Political and Social Research, in Ann Arbor, Michigan, along with codebooks and explanatory material. At that time researchers who wish to use the data for other purposes can do so. A great deal of the material that was collected was not used, and there is much more to be done with the data than can be accomplished in a single book.

NOTES

CHAPTER I: PHYSICIANS, PATIENTS, AND MEDICAL TECHNOLOGY

1. "Mr. Moran" probably died long ago. His relatives, however, may still be alive. In order to protect his confidentiality, as well as that of all other patients mentioned in this book, I shall use pseudonyms throughout. Those wishing to examine the case record will find it in volume 84 (1900): 215, of the Pennsylvania Hospital Case Records (henceforth PHCR).

2. PHCR 956 (1925): 5639.

3. None of this discussion should be taken to imply that physicians, patients, and administrators were the only people in the hospital. Nurses played an important role; the best place to start for a discussion of nursing in the early-twentieth century hospital is Susan Reverby, *Ordered to Care: The Dilemma of American Nursing, 1850–1945* (Cambridge: Cambridge University Press, 1987). Most of the explicit decision making, however, was thought to lie in the hands of physicians, and it is on the relationships of physicians and patients that we shall focus our attention. See also Barbara Melosh, *"The Physician's Hand": Work Culture and Conflict in American Nursing* (Philadelphia: Temple University Press, 1982).

4. On the general changes that took place within the American hospital, see Charles E. Rosenberg, *The Care of Strangers: The Rise of America's Hospital System* (New York: Basic Books, 1987).

5. Stanley Joel Reiser, *Medicine and the Reign of Technology* (New York: Cambridge University Press, 1978); Edward Shorter, *Bedside Manners: The Troubled History of Doctors and Patients* (New York: Simon and Schuster, 1985).

6. Mark Weiser, "The Computer for the Twenty-first Century," *Scientific American* 265, no. 3 (September 1991): 94–194.

7. PET scans (positron emission tomography scans), for example, are usually examined in black and white for diagnostic purposes and only given color when distributed for the popular press.

8. Norbert Gleicher, "Expansion of Health Care to the Uninsured and Underinsured Has to Be Cost Neutral," *Journal of the American Medical Association (JAMA)* 205 (1991): 2388–90.

9. On this in childbirth, see Judith Walzer Leavitt, *Brought to Bed: Childbearing in America, 1750–1950* (New York: Oxford University Press, 1986).

10. Kathryn Montgomery Hunter, *Doctor's Stories: The Narrative Structure of Medical Knowledge* (Princeton: Princeton University Press, 1991).

11. Many hospitals were, in fact, buildings originally constructed as houses, which had later been converted to use as hospitals.

12. For examples, see the annual reports from the period for almost any voluntary hospital.

13. See, for example, "The New York Hospital," *New York Times*, November 22, 1891, 20; "The New York Hospitals," *New York Times*, January 31, 1901, 12.

14. There has been relatively little attention paid to the history of medical technology. The standard works in the field are Audrey B. Davis, *Medicine and Its Technology: An Introduction to the History of Medical Instrumentation* (Westport, Conn.: Greenwood Press, 1981); and Reiser, *Medicine*. See also Stuart Blume, *Insight and Industry: On the Dynamics of Technological Change in Medicine* (Cambridge, Mass.: MIT Press, 1992); and Jonathan Liebenau, "Medicine and Technology," *Perspectives in Biology and Medicine* 27 (1983): 76–92

15. It is perhaps worthy of note that near the end of the twentieth century, perhaps as a result of increased competition, perhaps as a result of changing public perceptions of medical care, some hospitals are once again becoming more attuned to the importance of amenities such as food and style as well as medical technology.

16. For a cogent analysis, see Ellen Breckenridge Koch, "The Process of Innovation in Medical Technology: American Research on Ultrasound, 1947 to 1962" (Ph.D. diss., University of Pennsylvania, 1990), 296–313; and Thomas J. Misa, "Theories of Technological Change: Parameters and Purposes," *Science, Technology, and Human Values* 17 (1992): 3–12. See also Joel D. Howell, "Machines' Meanings: British and American Use of Medical Technology, 1880–1930," (Ph.D. diss., University of Pennsylvania, 1987).

17. Thomas Hughes, *American Genesis: A Century of Invention and Technological Enthusiasm* (New York: Viking, 1989), 5–6.

18. Such as that given by Renaldo N. Battista, "Innovation and Diffusion of Health-Related Technologies: A Conceptual Framework," *International Journal of Technology Assessment in Health Care* 5 (1989): 227–48; and the United States Congress Office of Technology Assessment (OTA), *Development of Medical Technology* (Washington, D.C.: Government Printing Office, 1976), 4.

19. "General Introduction" to Wiebe E. Bijker, Thomas P. Hughes, and Trevor J. Pinch, *The Social Construction of Technological Systems: New Directions in the Social History of Technology* (Cambridge, Mass.: MIT Press, 1989), 4.

20. For discussion of the relationship between power and the use of medical technology, see Sandra Harding, "Knowledge, Power, Technology, and Social Relations," *Journal of Medicine and Philosophy* 3 (1978):

346–58; and, emphasizing the importance of profits for some technology use, Howard Waitzkin, "A Marxian Interpretation of the Growth and Development of Coronary Care Technology," *American Journal of Public Health* 69 (1979): 1260–68.

21. For an introduction to the field, see Bijker, Hughes, and Pinch, *Social Construction*; Ruth Schwartz Cowan, *More Work for Mother: The Ironies of Household Technology from the Open Hearth to the Microwave* (New York: Basic Books, 1983); and Donald Mackenzie and Judy Wajcman, eds., *The Social Shaping of Technology: How the Refrigerator Got Its Hum* (Philadelphia: Milton Keynes, 1985).

22. Bryan Pfaffenberger provides an outline of a similar perspective from the sociological literature, which he calls the "Standard View of Technology," along with a plea for the relevance of anthropology, in "Social Anthropology of Technology," *Annual Review of Anthropology* 21 (1992): 491–516. Examples of this "standard view" may be implicitly found in most clinical accounts of new medical machines published in medical journals.

23. Charles E. Rosenberg, one of the historians most responsible for interest in the social history of medicine, recently commented on the general consensus among both historians and physicians about the "fundamental place" of technology in medical care. "Technology and Modern Medicine," *Newsletter: American Association for the History of Medicine* 42 (1993): 1–2. Similarly, Stuart Blume notes how medical technology is seen as different because it is seen as potentially lifesaving. *Insight and Industry*, 3.

24. Rosenberg, *Care of Strangers*; Rosemary Stevens, *In Sickness and in Wealth: The American Hospital in the Twentieth Century* (New York: Basic Books, 1989).

25. Eric H. Monkkonen, *America Becomes Urban: The Development of U.S. Cities and Towns, 1780–1980* (Berkeley: University of California Press, 1988).

26. Although the precise definition of a "failed" technology becomes less and less clear the more precisely one attempts to locate it. All technologies must succeed, if only at some very local level, or else historians would never know about that technology. On the other hand, given enough time, all technologies are likely to become failed technologies.

27. A 1991 symposium at the University of Southern California Law School considered how technology was shaping the way in which we view the world. One could also consider the reverse: how technologies were shaped by, as well as helped to shape, the ideological content of their times. Joel D. Howell, "Diagnostic Technologies: X-Rays, Electrocardiograms, and CAT Scans," *Southern California Law Review* 65 (1991): 529–64, as well as the entire issue. For another discussion of how the way that a technology is used in medicine reflects broader ideas about the role of that technology, see Bonnie Kaplan, "The Medical Computing 'Lag': Perceptions of Barriers to the Application of Computers to

Medicine," *International Journal of Technology Assessment* 3 (1987):
123–36.

28. For an introduction to this aspect of the social history of medicine, see
Susan Reverby and David Rosner, "Beyond the Great Doctors," in
Health Care in America: Essays in Social History, edited by Susan
Reverby and David Rosner, 3–16 (Philadelphia: Temple University
Press, 1979).

29. "A Plea for a 'Behaviorist Approach' in Writing the History of Medicine," *Journal of the History of Medicine and Allied Sciences* 22 (1967):
211–14.

30. For example, see Ellen Dwyer, *Homes for the Mad: Life inside Two
Nineteenth Century Asylums* (New Brunswick, N.J.: Rutgers University Press, 1987); Dorothy Porter and Roy Porter, *Patient's Progress:
Doctors and Doctoring in Eighteenth-Century England* (Stanford: Stanford University Press, 1989); and Roy Porter, *A Social History of Madness: The World through the Eyes of the Insane* (New York: Weidenfeld
and Nicholson, 1988). For an overview of attempts to capture patients'
experiences of more recent times, particularly people depending on
chronic renal dialysis, see Harry M. Marks, "Medical Technologies:
Social Contexts and Consequences," in *Companion Encyclopedia to
the History of Medicine,* edited by W. F. Bynum and Roy Porter, 2:
1592–1618 (London: Routledge, 1993). An innovative account is given
by Sheila M. Rothman, *Living in the Shadow of Death: Tuberculosis
and the Social Experience of Illness in American History* (New York:
Basic Books, 1994).

31. For a general discussion of such fiction, see John G. Cawelti, *Adventure,
Mystery, and Romance: Formula Stories as Art and Popular Culture*
(Chicago: University of Chicago Press, 1976). Much of the book is an
analysis of the various formulas that were used. Cawelti does not
attempt to identify a specific audience for the stories. For another inter-
pretation of the role of fiction, here about a specific group, see Barbara
Melosh, " 'A Special Relationship': Nurses and Patients in Twentieth-
Century Short Stories," in *Images of Nurses: Perspectives from History,
Art, and Literature,* edited by Anne Hudson Jones, 128–49 (Philadelphia: University of Pennsylvania Press, 1988).

32. Caroline W. Latimer, "The Treatment of Medicine in Fiction," *New
Science Review* 2 (1896): 253–62.

33. For a review of some recent work in this area, see Guenter B. Risse and
John Harley Warner, "Reconstructing Clinical Activities: Patient Records in Medical History," *Social History of Medicine* 5 (1992): 183–205.
For examples of work using case records, see Michael MacDonald, *Mys-
tical Bedlam: Madness, Anxiety, and Healing in Seventeenth-Century
England* (Cambridge: Cambridge University Press, 1981); Martin S. Pernick, *A Calculus of Suffering: Pain, Professionalism, and Anesthesia in
Nineteenth-Century America* (New York: Columbia University Press,
1985); Guenter B. Risse, *Hospital Life in Enlightenment Scotland: Care*

and Teaching at the Royal Infirmary of Edinburgh (Cambridge: Cambridge University Press, 1986); and Nancy Tomes, *A Generous Confidence: Thomas Story Kirkbride and the Art of Asylum-Keeping, 1840–1883* (Cambridge: Cambridge University Press, 1983). Using these records to reconstruct the lives of large numbers of people is an approach similar to that used by some practitioners of urban history, who have used sources such as city directories and parish registers. Theodore Hershberg, ed., *Philadelphia: Work, Space, Family and Group Experience in the Nineteenth Century: Essays towards an Interdisciplinary History of the City* (New York: Oxford University Press, 1991), intro., xii–xiii. This volume contains several essays from the Philadelphia Social History Project, an example of what was termed at the time "the new urban history."

34. Barbara Duden, *The Women beneath the Skin: A Doctor's Patients in Eighteenth-Century Germany,* translated by Thomas Dunlap (Cambridge, Mass.: Harvard University Press, 1991).

35. The heart station was a place designated in early-twentieth-century hospitals as a repository for various types of machines to study the heart as well as, perhaps even more important for the history of the medical profession, those people who devoted themselves to the study of heart disease. The cystoscopy suite was a place where physicians used tubes to look into the patient's urinary bladder.

36. In order to record an electric signal, early versions of the electrocardiogram machine had the patient immerse his or her arms and legs into buckets of water to which salt had been added in order to facilitate the flow of electric signals.

37. For a magnificent example, see Jacalyn Duffin, *Langstaff: A Nineteenth-Century Medical Life* (Toronto: University of Toronto Press, 1993). Christopher Crenner has also used case records of a single practitioner to good effect in "Professional Measurement: Quantification of Health and Disease in American Medical Practice, 1880–1920," (Ph.D. diss., Harvard University, 1993).

38. There has been a productive literature on this topic over the past several decades. Charles E. Rosenberg, whose incisive essay "Inward Vision and Outward Glance: The Shaping of the American Hospital, 1880–1914" (*Bulletin of the History of Medicine* 53 [1979]: 346–91) was one of the seminal events of the reworking of this history, has provided in *The Care of Strangers* perhaps the best place to start reading about the history of the American hospital. In that book he places the beginnings of the changes before 1890; undoubtedly in smaller, more rural hospitals (about which we still know very little) the changes probably came after 1925. Nonetheless, the decade or so around the turn of the twentieth century still seems a reasonable place to start to look at the creation of the new institution that we now call a hospital. For other sources on the history of the hospital at the turn of the twentieth century, see David Rosner, *A Once Charitable Enterprise: Hospitals and Health Care in*

Brooklyn and New York, 1885–1915 (Cambridge: Cambridge University Press, 1982); and Morris Vogel, *The Invention of the Modern Hospital: Boston, 1870–1930* (Chicago: University of Chicago Press, 1980). On city hospitals, see Harry F. Dowling, *City Hospitals: The Undercare of the Underprivileged* (Cambridge, Mass.: Harvard University Press, 1982).

39. A. J. Ochsner, *Modern Hospital* 1 (1913): 1–13.
40. Kenneth M. Ludmerer, *Learning to Heal: The Development of American Medical Education* (New York: Basic Books, 1985).
41. Or at least the clinical training necessary to obtain a medical degree. It has long been obvious that hospital training may not be the best way to train physicians to deliver care outside of the hospital. In the 1990s there is a new, apparently strong movement to encourage medical training in ambulatory primary-care settings, away from the hospital-dominated medical center.
42. George Rosen, *The Structure of American Medical Practice, 1875–1941* (Philadelphia: University of Pennsylvania Press, 1983).
43. Stevens, *In Sickness and in Wealth.*
44. John Harley Warner, *The Therapeutic Perspective: Medical Practice, Knowledge, and Identity in America, 1820–1885* (Cambridge, Mass.: Harvard University Press, 1986).
45. Thomas Misa has written insightfully about the history of U.S. business, a topic that will be dealt with at greater length in chapter 2. See "How Machines Make History, and How Historians (and Others) Help Them to Do So," *Science, Technology, and Human Values* 13 (1988): 308–31; and "Theories of Technological Change: Parameters and Purposes," *Science, Technology, and Human Values* 17 (1992): 3–12.
46. The presence of variations in medical practice has been of interest in the Anglo-American medical literature for much of the twentieth century. For general discussion, see J. Alison Glover, "The Incidence of Tonsillectomy in School Children," *Proceedings of the Royal Society of Medicine* 31 (1938): 1219–36; Paul A. Lembcke, "Measuring the Quality of Medical Care through Vital Statistics Based on Hospital Service Areas. 1. Comparative Study of Appendectomy Rates," *American Journal of Public Health* 42 (1952): 276–86; Mark R. Chassin, Jacqueline Kosecoff, R. E. Park, Constance M. Winslow, Katherine L. Kahn, Nancy J. Merrick, Joan Keesex, Arline Fink, David H. Solomon, and Robert H. Brook, "Does Inappropriate Use Explain Geographic Variations in the Use of Health Services? A Study of Three Procedures," *JAMA* 258 (1987): 2533–37; and J. Wennberg and A. Gittelsohn, "Variations in Medical Care in Small Areas," *Scientific American* 24 (1982): 120–34.
47. Two recently released examples include guidelines for the management of acute pain and of urinary incontinence. Agency for Health Care Policy and Research, *Clinical Practice Guideline: Acute Pain Manage-*

ment—*Operative or Medical Procedures and Trauma*, AHCPR Publication 92-0032 (Washington, D.C.: U.S. Department of Health and Human Services, 1992); *Clinical Practice Guideline: Urinary Incontinence in Adults*, AHCPR Publication 92-0038 (Washington, D.C.: U.S. Department of Health and Human Services, 1992).

48. William H. Williams, *America's First Hospital: The Pennsylvania Hospital, 1751–1841* (Wayne, Pa: Haverford House, 1976); Francis R. Packard, *Some Account of the Pennsylvania Hospital from 1751 to 1938* (Philadelphia: Engle Press, 1938).

49. The first hospital building burned down; the next was used for a variety of war purposes during the Revolutionary War. For background, see Eric Larrabee, *The Benevolent and Necessary Institution: The New York Hospital, 1771–1971* (New York: Doubleday, 1971); Eugene H. Pool and Frank J. McGowan, *Surgery at the New York Hospital One Hundred Years Ago* (New York: Paul B. Hoeber, 1929). On the hospital's case records, see Helen B. Lincoln, "Records Then and Now," *Modern Hospital* 56 (1937): 56–59.

50. Rosenberg, *Care of Strangers*, 109.

51. John Shrady, "Two Hundred Years of Medicine," in *The Memorial History of the City of New-York [sic]*, edited by James Grant Wilson, 4:408. (New York: New York History Company, 1892–93).

52. *Sesqui-Centennial 150th Annual Report of the Board of Managers of the Pennsylvania Hospital; The Society of the New York Hospital Annual Report for the Year 1900.*

53. Using a chi-square test.

54. Vogel, *Invention of the Modern Hospital.*

CHAPTER 2: SCIENCE, SCIENTIFIC SYSTEMS, AND SURGERY

1. Quotation from David A. Hollinger, "Science and Anarchy: Walter Lippmann's *Drift and Mastery*," *American Quarterly* 29 (1977): 463–75.

2. For more on the general ideas and ideals, see Samuel Haber, *Efficiency and Uplift: Scientific Management in the Progressive Era, 1890–1920* (Chicago: University of Chicago Press, 1964); Walter Lippmann, *Draft and Mastery: An Attempt to Diagnose the Current Unrest* (New York: Mitchell Kennerly, 1914); Daniel Nelson, ed., *A Mental Revolution: Scientific Management since Taylor* (Columbus: Ohio State University Press, 1992); and Robert H. Wiebe, *The Search for Order, 1877–1920* (New York: Hill and Wang, 1977). The term *efficiency craze* is used by Haber.

3. Edward T. Morman, ed., *Efficiency, Scientific Management, and Hospital Standardization: An Anthology of Sources* (New York: Garland Publishing, 1989). There was even published an article entitled "The Bible:

Textbook of Efficiency." Jesus was portrayed as the founder of modern business in the popular novel by Bruce Barton, *The Man Nobody Knows: A Discovery of the Real Jesus* (Indianapolis: Bobbs-Merrill, 1925).

4. Charles S. Maier, "Between Taylorism and Technocracy: European Ideologies and the Vision of Industrial Productivity in the 1920s," *Journal of Contemporary History* 5 (1970): 27–61. Maier examines how the ideology of Taylorism was transferred and adopted in France, Germany, and Italy.

5. It was not, so the Taylorites held, an invention of a person or people but, rather, the elucidation of fundamental laws of nature, which could not be ignored. See Edwin T. Layton, *The Revolt of the Engineers: Social Responsibility and the American Engineering Profession* (Baltimore: Johns Hopkins University Press, 1986), chap. 6: "Measuring the Unmeasurable: Scientific Management and Reform," esp. 143–44.

6. For the best discussion of changing organizations in American business, see Alfred Chandler, *The Visible Hand: The Managerial Revolution in American Business* (Cambridge, Mass.: Harvard University Press, 1977).

7. David Rosner, *A Once Charitable Enterprise: Hospitals and Health Care in Brooklyn and New York, 1885–1915* (Cambridge: Cambridge University Press, 1982).

8. "Introduction," *On the Administrative Frontier: The First Ten Years of the American Hospital Association, 1899–1908*, edited by Morris J. Vogel (New York: Garland, 1989), v.

9. Anthony G. Hopwood, "The Archaeology of Accounting Systems," *Accounting, Organizations, and Society* 12 (1989): 207–34.

10. Although the most widespread use of cost accounting came with the nineteenth-century railroad, the English Wedgewood china manufacturer used a similar system much earlier. See Hopwood, "Archaeology of Accounting Systems."

11. Robert S. Kaplan, "The Evolution of Management Accounting," *Accounting Review* 59 (1984): 390–418; H. Thomas Johnson and Robert S. Kaplan, *Relevance Lost: The Rise and Fall of Management Accounting* (Boston: Harvard Business School Press, 1987). See also Gary John Previts and Barbara Dubis Merino, *A History of Accounting in America: An Historical Interpretation of the Cultural Significance of Accounting* (New York: John Wiley and Sons, 1979); and Robert S. Kaplan, "Management Accounting for Advanced Technological Environments," *Science* 245 (1989): 819–23.

The concept of cost accounting is not itself immutable. Cost accounting can be carried out at the level of the department, as it was in the period under discussion. It can also, with more powerful computational devices, be carried out at the level of the individual patient, as it is today in some hospitals.

12. Aaron Waldheim, "Increasing the Efficiency of Hospital Administrators," *Modern Hospital* 14 (April 1920): 298–99.

13. F. C. Townsend, "Hospital Cost Accounting," *Modern Hospital* 3 (1914): 233. Of course, cost accounting, like any other innovation of the period, did not always mean the same thing to different people or even to the same person at different times.

14. Rosner, *Once Charitable Enterprise*, 50–61.

15. Final Report of a 1905 New York City Committee on Hospital Needs and Hospital Finances, chair John E. Parsons; quoted in William H. Allen, "Hospital Efficiency," *American Journal of Sociology* 12 (1906): 298.

16. For many years the Michigan State Legislature provided care for all poor patients at the "State Hospital in Ann Arbor." During the 1910s and 1920s they were quite concerned that funds designated for patient care should not go toward medical education.

17. J. R. Coddington, "Hospital Records," Fourth Annual Conference of the American Hospital Association (AHA), 1902, 102; and C. Irving Fisher, "Private Patients in General Hospitals," with discussion, Sixth Annual Conference of the AHA, 1904, 93–104, in Vogel, *On the Administrative Frontier*.

18. Henry M. Hurd, "Discussion," of "Hospital Records and Reports," Fourth Annual Conference of the AHA, 1902, 94–98, in Vogel, *On the Administrative Frontier*.

19. William H. Allen, "Hospital Efficiency," *American Journal of Sociology* 12 (1906): 308; reprinted in Morman, *Efficiency*. The actual forms, including those used in the New York Hospital, may be found in *The Forms of Hospital Financial Reports and Statistics* (Boston: Thompson-Brown, 1908).

20. Edward Martin, George E. Deschweinitz, Robert G. Leconte, Charles B. Penrose, Wilmer Krusen, John D. McLean, Joseph S. Neff, and Richard Waterman, "Philadelphia Investigates Its Hospitals," *Modern Hospital* 3 (1914): 388–90.

21. See Allen, "Hospital Efficiency," 305–7, for examples. One cannot be sure that more detailed records were not being kept somewhere else and that these more detailed itemizations were simply not preserved. Yet given the widespread concern about the state of records, this seems unlikely.

22. The astute reader will also note the "omitted" expenses of heat, water, and fuel, which remain unaccounted for in this chart. One wonders if this was covered, perhaps, by the state. The point about the need for more careful bookkeeping remains the same.

23. The letterpress was an effective, though laborious, way of keeping copies of written material. For discussion of its use and importance, see JoAnne Yates, *Control through Communication: The Rise of System in American Management* (Baltimore: Johns Hopkins University Press, 1988).

24. Townsend, "Hospital Cost Accounting."

25. Allen, "Hospital Efficiency." In *On the Administrative Frontier* Vogel astutely points out that the move to a management science that was

distinctly masculine in style may have been, in part, a reflection of the desires of the new, "professional," male hospital superintendents to differentiate themselves from the previous, largely female generation. See also Morris Vogel, "Managing Medicine: Creating a Profession of Hospital Administration in the United States," in *The Hospital in History,* edited by Lindsay Granshaw and Roy Porter, 234–60 (London: Routledge, 1989); and Stephen J. Kunitz, "Efficiency and Reform in the Financing and Organization of American Medicine in the Progressive Era," *Bulletin of the History of Medicine* 55 (1981): 497–515.

26. For discussion of adding machines, see Derek de Solla Price, "A History of Calculating Machines," *IEEE Micro* 4 (1984): 23–52; Michael R. Williams, *A History of Computing Technology* (Englewood Cliffs, N.J.: Prentice Hall, 1985); and "Early Calculation," in *Computing before Computers,* edited by William Aspray, 3–58 (Ames: Iowa State University Press, 1990); and, particularly on the trajectories of the various companies that made the machines, James W. Cortada, *Before the Computer: IBM, NCR, Burroughs, and Remington Rand and the Industry They Created, 1865–1956* (Princeton: Princeton University Press, 1993). See also J. A. V. Turk, *Origin of Modern Calculating Machines: A Chronicle of the Evolution of the Principles That Form the Generic Make-up of the Modern Calculating Machine* (Chicago: Western Society of Engineers, 1921).

27. E. St. Elmo Lewis, *Efficient Cost Keeping,* 3d ed. (Detroit: Burroughs Adding Machine Company, 1914). This volume is filled with examples of the time saved in doing specific calculations as well as photographs of hard-working people being productive in a variety of business settings, but always using a Burroughs product.

28. Hollerith worked on the card in large part at the suggestion of the physician John Shaw Billings, who founded the library that later became the National Library of Medicine. See Keith S. Reid-Green, "The History of Census Tabulation," *Scientific American* (February 1989): 98–103; and Geoffrey D. Austrian, *Herman Hollerith: Forgotten Giant of Information Processing* (New York: Columbia University Press, 1982). For an insightful essay on the cultural meaning of the card, see Steven Lubar, " 'Do not fold, spindle, or mutilate': A Cultural History of the Punch Card," *Journal of American Culture* 15, no. 4 (1992): 43–55.

29. James R. Beniger, *The Control Revolution: Technological and Economic Origins of the Information Society* (Cambridge, Mass.: Harvard University Press, 1986), 413; Herbert Arkin, "Development and Principles of the Punched Card Method (Hollerith), in *Practical Applications of the Punched Card Method in Colleges and Universities,* edited by G. W. Baehne, 1–8 (New York: Columbia University Press, 1935). The New York City trial revealed a major flaw in the original design: punching too many holes in heavy paper led to a marked loss of strength in the operator's hands. This led to the invention of a new machine with which to make the punches in the cards.

30. Raymond Pearl, "Modern Methods in Handling Hospital Statistics" *Johns Hopkins Hospital Bulletin* 32 (1921): 184–94 (emphasis on the word *accurate* in original). That the author was the statistician to the Johns Hopkins Hospital may, certainly, have bearing on how one reads his remarks. On the other hand, the fact that the administrators of the Johns Hopkins Hospital chose to employ a statistician is also an indication of the seriousness with which they viewed the acquisition of quantitative data.

31. See Cortada, *Before the Computer,* 51; and Halbert L. Dunn, "Application in Medical Research and Hospitals, chapter 1: Hospital and Clinical Statistics in General," in Baehne, *Practical Applications,* 241–70, esp. 266–69.

32. Yates, *Control through Communication.* This work is a masterful description of the importance of various genres of internal communication for U.S. business.

33. For a general overview of records, primarily in Canada and the United Kingdom, see Barbara L. Craig, "Hospital Records and Record-Keeping, Part 1: The Development of Records in Hospitals," *Archivaria* 29 (1989–90): 57–60; "Hospital Records and Record-Keeping, Part 2: The Development of Record-Keeping in Hospitals," *Archivaria* 30 (1990): 21–38; "The Role of Records and of Record-Keeping in the Development of the Modern Hospital in London, England, and Ontario, Canada, c. 1890–1940," *Bulletin of the History of Medicine* 65 (1991): 376–97.

34. For describing a body of data, such as the length of the patient record, which has extreme values in one direction, the median often provides a better description than the mean.

35. The value went from 0.167 pages per day in 1900 to 1 page per day in 1925. The increase is even greater if one eliminates from consideration charts of people admitted for removal of their tonsils, who typically stayed for only one day. Similar findings are noted by David Juchau in his 1993 University of Michigan Ph.D. dissertation, "Transitions in American Medical Therapy and the Older Patient, 1820–1920."

    The values for the New York Hospital are slightly higher than those from the Pennsylvania Hospital. This is due to the fact that the sampling procedure for the New York Hospital included a large number of charts with a zero length of stay—that is, patients went home the same day that they were seen. It is not clear whether these people were ever "admitted" to the hospital, although they were included in the bound volumes of hospitalized patients. For the purposes of this calculation I excluded them from the analysis. The general point does not depend upon this decision; the trend is the same with them included as with them excluded. When the data is deposited for public use, scholars will be able to make any decisions they like about which data to include and to exclude.

36. For example, at the Pennsylvania Hospital in the early twentieth century the Radiology Department, Dietetics Department, Anesthesiology

Department, Clinical laboratories, and Social Work Department all created their own forms. See also Stanley Joel Reiser, "Creating Form Out
of Mass: The Development of the Medical Record," in *Transformation
and Tradition in the Sciences*, edited by Everett Mendelssohn (Cambridge: Cambridge University Press, 1985), 26.

37. By 1925 a book devoted entirely to the use and design of forms had been
published: Wallace Clarke, *Shop and Office Forms: Their Design and
Use* (New York: McGraw-Hill, 1925).

38. The concept is taken from Yates, *Control through Communication*.

39. For some of many examples of such a system, see John A. Kolmer, "A
System of Laboratory Examinations and Records," *Journal of Laboratory and Clinical Medicine* 6 (1920): 505–19; or Howard T. Child, "A
Plea for Simplified Laboratory Reports for Hospitals," *Modern Hospital*
5 (1915): 19–20.

40. Rosemary Stevens, *American Medicine in the Public Interest* (New
Haven: Yale University Press, 1971). See also Franklin Martin, *Fifty
Years of Medicine and Surgery* (Chicago: Surgical Publishing Company
of Chicago, 1934); and "Conference on Hospital Standardization," *Bulletin of the American College of Surgeons* 3 (1917): 1–53.

41. Russell D. Carman and Albert Miller, *The Roentgen Diagnosis of Diseases of the Alimentary Canal* (Philadelphia: W. B. Saunders, 1917),
facing p. 30. For additional examples of forms, see I. Seth Hirsch, "The
Hospital X-ray Laboratory: Its Scope and Limitations," *Modern Hospital*
4 (1915): 254–57.

42. On a general tendency to portray the advantages of a machine age in
cleaner images than might be usual for the machine in question, see
Marianne Doezema, "The Clean Machine: Technology in American
Magazine Illustration," *Journal of American Culture* 11 (1978): 73–92.

43. Reiser, *Medicine*, 209.

44. In 1900 the mean number of forms per day at the Pennsylvania Hospital
was 0.0013; by 1925 there were 0.57 forms for each day of admission.

45. This history and interpretation of the use of the typewriter follows
closely Yates's analysis for business applications. See also M. H. Adler,
The Writing Machine—A History of the Typewriter (London: George
Allen and Unwin, 1973); W. A. Beeching, *Century of the Typewriter*
(New York: St. Martin's Press, 1974); Cortada, *Before the Computer*;
Carroll W. Pursell, Jr., "Machines and Machine Tools, 1830–1880," in
Technology in Western Civilization, vol. 1, edited by Melvin Kranzberg
and Carroll W. Pursell, Jr., 392–408 (New York: Oxford University Press,
1967); and Trevor I. Williams, *A Short History of Twentieth-Century
Technology, c. 1900–c. 1950* (New York: Oxford University Press, 1982),
292–95.

46. Joseph B. Howland, "Hospital Records," *Modern Hospital* 3 (1914):
288–91.

47. Using a typewriter also promoted safety, by rendering notes and pre-
scriptions legible. "Safety First: It Demands the Use of the Silent Seven

Oliver" (advertisement), *The Modern Hospital* 1 (1913): advertisements section, 33.

48. Or put it there in the first place, although the point remains the same whether one sees this specific typewriter as there "naturally" or not.

49. For locating this vignette I am indebted to Joshua Newman and his unpublished manuscript, "The Use and Usefulness of X-ray Machines for Routine Patient Care at the University of Michigan Hospital: 1925 through 1934."

50. "The Graphic Method," *Nation* 29 (October 9, 1879): 238–39. Prior to the 1870s graphs in the United States were generally confined to uses in vital statistics. Howard Grey Funkhauser, "Historical Development of the Graphical Representation of Statistical Data," *Osiris* 3 (November 1937): 269–404. On the role of Etienne-Jules Marey, who pioneered use of the graphic method (and later the motion picture) as a means of capturing motion, see Marta Braun, *Picturing Time: The Work of Etienne-Jules Marey (1830–1904)* (Chicago: University of Chicago Press, 1992); and on the use of graphs and photography as a means of making visible the previously invisible parts of the human body, analogous to the x ray, see Lisa Cartwright, " 'Experiments of Destruction': Cinematic Inscriptions of Physiology," *Representations* 40 (1992): 129–52. My choice to present some information in this book in graphic form reflects many of the same social and cultural ideas about graphs which were important in the early twentieth century.

51. Kenneth M. Ludmerer, *Learning to Heal: The Development of American Medical Education* (New York: Basic Books, 1985).

52. For an excellent discussion of the long-term implications of this educational change, see Merriley Borell, "Training the Senses, Training the Mind," in *Medicine and the Five Senses*, edited by W. F. Bynum and Roy Porter, 244–61 (Cambridge: Cambridge University Press, 1993).

53. On the changing world of physiology, see W. Bruce Fye, *The Development of American Physiology: Scientific Medicine in the Nineteenth Century* (Baltimore: Johns Hopkins University Press, 1987).

54. For an idiosyncratic but illuminating look at uses of the graphic method, see Siegfried Giedon, *Mechanization Takes Command: A Contribution to Anonymous History* (Oxford: Oxford University Press, 1948).

55. Such records appear as early as 1870 at the Massachusetts General Hospital. Reiser, *Medicine*, 207.

56. Karl G. Karsten, *Charts and Graphs: An Introduction to Graphic Methods in the Control and Analysis of Statistics* (New York: Prentice Hall, 1925).

57. Lester Adams, "A Rubber Stamp for Hospital Charts," *Modern Hospital* 3 (1914): 131–32.

58. From 0.05 per day in 1900 to 0.51 per day in 1925. After 1900 the number of graphs per day was higher for surgical than for nonsurgical patients,

showing that, at least in the use of graphs, the practice of surgery, as well as its ideology, was strongly influenced by the ideas of science.

59. John R. Williams, "A Simple Method of Plotting Charts," *Journal of Laboratory and Clinical Medicine* 2 (1916–17): 247–51.

60. For this section of the chapter I am indebted to Barbara Marie Stafford for starting me thinking about the visual, artistic nature of how information is presented in patient charts and for an engaging and provocative session of slide viewing in March 1992. For more on the uses of visual evidence in medicine, see her book *Body Criticism: Imaging the Unseen in Enlightenment Art and Medicine* (Cambridge, Mass.: MIT Press, 1991).

61. Of course, it is difficult to know exactly what emotions were present in the minds of those who created these marks, and these readings must be treated as inferential.

62. For a review of sociological approaches to the use of visual imagery in science, generally, see Jan Golinski, "The Theory of Practice and the Practice of Theory: Sociological Approaches to the History of Science," *Isis* 81 (1990): 492–505.

63. Charles E. Rosenberg, *The Cholera Years: The United States in 1832, 1849, and 1866* (Chicago: University of Chicago Press, 1962), 157.

64. For a sensitive discussion of the process, see Christopher Lawrence, "Democratic, Divine, and Heroic: The History and Historiography of Surgery," in *Medical Theory, Surgical Practice: Studies in the History of Surgery*, edited by Christopher Lawrence, 1–47 (London and New York: Routledge, 1992).

65. Lawrence, "Democratic, Divine, and Heroic."

66. As they in fact were, well into the twentieth century. For detailed descriptions of the travails of operating in homes throughout Vermont, see Johns Brooks Wheeler, *Memoirs of a Small-Town Surgeon* (Garden City, N.Y.: Garden City Publishing, 1935). The matter of operations in private houses is discussed in Hunter Robb, *Aseptic Surgical Technique: With Especial Reference to Gynaecological Operations, Together with Notes on the Technique Employed in Certain Supplementary Procedures* (Philadelphia: J. B. Lippincott, 1894).

Once the decision was made to move surgery into the hospital, U.S. hospitals required many more rooms than did hospitals in Europe, as U.S. hospitals allowed more surgeons to operate within. Edward F. Stevens, "The Surgical Unit: European and American Architecture Compared—Descriptions of Equipment," *Modern Hospital* 1 (1913): 18–21.

67. Pennsylvania Hospital Annual Report (1896–97), 17–23. On electric light, see Wolfgang Schivelbusch, *Disenchanted Night: The Industrialization of Light in the Nineteenth Century*, trans. Angela Davies (New York: Oxford University Press, 1988). For discussions and advertisements about hospital lighting, see almost any volume of the *Modern Hospital* for the first several years after the initial issue of 1913.

68. Van Buren, "Address Delivered on the Occasion of the Inauguration of the New Building," *Report of the Building Committee, Society of the New York Hospital* (1877), 22.
69. New Operating Theater of the New York Hospital: Finished and Opened for Service, May 1907. (Apparently) printed for the hospital, 1907.
70. Although the operating theater as used for teaching was becoming smaller, perhaps due to a desire to minimize the potential for infection in light of ideas about asepsis. Brent V. Stromberg, "The Operating Room: An Historical Perspective," *Journal of the South Carolina Medical Association* 81 (1985): 31–33.
71. See the introduction by James M. Edmonson, "Introduction on Truax, and the Development of the American Surgical Industry," to Charles Truax, *The Mechanics of Surgery* (1899; reprint, San Francisco: Norman Publishing, 1988).
72. "General Introduction," in *The Social Construction of Technological Systems,* edited by Wiebe E. Bijker, Thomas P. Hughes, and Trevor Pinch, 1–6 (Cambridge, Mass.: MIT Press, 1989).
73. The 1925 *Annual Report of the Pennsylvania Hospital* does not list the numbers of operations by type, only the total number. The yearly breakdown is based on a handwritten, manuscript book listing the numbers of the most common operations, located in the archives of the Pennsylvania Hospital. The handwriting is similar throughout the book, suggesting that the same person did all the tabulations. This makes it likely that the person used the same criteria for deciding how to categorize the operations, and I have thus chosen to compare the types of operations from that single source. The manuscript book does not, however, give grand totals for admissions to the hospital, and for that tally I have used the annual reports.
74. The general pattern was similar at many other institutions. At the University of Michigan, for example, in 1898 the most frequent operation was appendectomy—done 22 times. Second was repair of urethral stricture (19), removal of varicocele (15), and excision of hemorrhoids (13). Contrast this pattern with that for 1919, during which there were 1,285 tonsillectomies and/or adenoidectomies, 202 appendectomies, 124 inguinal hernia repairs, and 42 thyroidectomies. The pattern was thus almost identical with that at the Pennsylvania Hospital.
75. This theory—by 1924 an "established fact"—was based at least partially on information provided by the x ray. Thomas Horder, "The Influence of Radiology upon Our Conception of Disease," *British Medical Journal* 2 (1924): 89–94.
76. Seth Scott Bishop, *Diseases of the Ear, Nose, and Throat* (Philadelphia: F. A. Davis, 1897), 382.
77. This catalog of the library of the United States Surgeon General's office was a standard reference source for many years. The first series listed everything held by the library up to the time that the index catalog began.

78. Chevalier Jackson, *The Life of Chevalier Jackson: An Autobiography* (New York: Macmillan, 1938), 89–90.
79. Harold Wilson, "The Tonsils," *Grace Hospital Bulletin* 2, no. 4 (April 1918): 7–8. For an overview of techniques, see Neil Weir, *Otolaryngology: An Illustrated History* (London: Butterworths, 1990), 239–40.
80. Draft report, "The Tonsil and Adenoid Situation in New York City," in file "Tonsil and Adenoid Cases, 1913–1921," New York Academy of Medicine.
81. Jackson, *Life of Chevalier Jackson*, 89–90, 124.
82. Cf. Thomas Henry Manley, *Hernia: Its Palliative and Radical Treatment in Adults, Children and Infants* (Philadelphia: Medical Press, 1893), with a leading advocate of mechano-therapy, George Herbert Taylor, *Pelvic and Hernial Therapeutics* (New York: J. B. Alden, 1885).
83. Sir J. Burdon-Sanderson, "An Address on the Relation of Science to Experience in Medicine," *British Medical Journal* 2 (1899): 1333–35. Burdon-Sanderson had resigned his hospital appointments in 1870 to devote himself to scientific research. He became Regius Professor of Medicine at Oxford in 1895. See Gerald L. Geison, "John Scott Burdon-Sanderson," in *Dictionary of Scientific Biography*, edited by Charles Gillispie, 2:598–99 (New York: Charles Scribner's Sons, 1970).
84. Both the total number of operations and the percentage of patients who had an operation are important measures. But they measure different things. To the people who ran the operating rooms, who bought the supplies and hired the help, the number of times an operating room was used was the important feature. To the patient, whether or not he or she was operated on was probably of central concern. Certainly, an increased number of operations would also have been a matter to be noted by each patient. But the data and clinical reasoning suggests that a small number of patients would have had more than one procedure.

    In 1925, 52 percent of patients had an operation. Of the 6,668 admissions, that would include 3,467 operations. Yet the annual report lists 3,606 operations as having been done in the hospital. The difference between those two numbers is 139 operations. (The difference would be greater if some of the patients reported in the *Annual Report* as having been operated on outside of the hospital did not have that fact clearly noted on their charts and thus were included in the 52 percent of the samples that was operated on.) We do not know whether that reflects 139 patients who had two operations or some smaller number of patients who had two or more operations. It is likely that some patients, particularly those with chronically infected conditions, would have had several operations to debride dead tissue or to drain an abscess repeatedly.
85. As is discussed in the appendix to this book, sampling for New York Hospital records after 1914 presents technical difficulties. The annual reports do not give this value. Thus, the exact percentage of patients who underwent surgery is difficult to establish with precision. It should

be noted, however, that, as the primary criteria for sampling 1920 records at the New York Hospital was (unavoidably) the ability to locate volumes bound for a specific diagnosis, one may assume that records of patients admitted with the more common diagnoses would be more likely to be included in the sample, simply because their records occupy more space. It does not appear that any records were discarded.

Problems with locating patient records notwithstanding, the evidence seems to consistently point to a dramatic increase in the percentage of patients in U.S. hospitals undergoing an operation between 1900 and 1925.

86. Stevens, *In Sickness and in Wealth*, 33–34.

87. For an excellent historiographic discussion of the creation of these myths, see Lawrence, "Democratic, Divine, and Heroic."

88. Martin Pernick, *A Calculus of Suffering* (New York: Columbia University Press, 1985), 82–83. Pernick explores the use of anesthesia, primarily in the mid-nineteenth century.

89. Among the sample used for this book. While there may have been a few who did not, the percentage would have to be very small.

90. On the "creation" of Listerism as a revolutionary change in surgical practice by small changes in the surgical community as a whole rather than as the specific suggestions of a single person (or small group of people) at a single moment, see Christopher Lawrence and Richard Dixey, "Practising on Principle: Joseph Lister and the Germ Theories of Disease," in Lawrence, *Medical Theory*, 153–215. See also Thomas P. Gariepy, "The Introduction and Acceptance of Listerian Antisepsis in the United States," *Journal of the History of Medicine and Allied Sciences* 49 (1994): 167–206; and Lindsay Granshaw, " 'Upon This Principle I Have Based a Practice': The Development and Reception of Antisepsis in Britain, 1867–90," in *Medical Innovations in Historical Perspective*, edited by John V. Pickstone, 17–46 (New York: St. Martin's Press, 1992).

91. William Stewart Halsted, "The Training of the Surgeon," *Bulletin of the Johns Hopkins Hospital* 15 (1904): 267–75, esp. n. 19.

92. Robert T. Morris, *Fifty Years a Surgeon* (New York: E. P. Dutton, 1938). Morris's text, *How We Treat Wounds Today: A Treatise on the Subject of Antiseptic Surgery Which Can Be Understood by Beginners* (New York: G. P. Putnam's Sons, 1886), went through three editions. Also, Arpad Geyza Gerster, another New York City surgeon, claimed to have sold over eleven thousand copies of his book *The Rules of Aseptic and Antiseptic Surgery* (New York: D. Appleton, 1888), in his *Recollections of a New York Surgeon* (New York: Paul B. Hoeber, 1917), 236–38. The subject reached prominence in the canon of surgical textbooks with William Williams Keen and James William White's enormously popular *An American Text-Book of Surgery* (Philadelphia: W. B. Saunders, 1892), in which the very first section of book 1, on general surgery, is "Surgical Bacteriology," and the very first word in the book is *bacteria*. Also for

general discussion, see Frederick W. Cartwright, *The Development of Modern Surgery* (London: Arthur Barker, 1967).

93. Morris J. Vogel, *The Invention of the Modern Hospital: Boston, 1870–1930* (Chicago: University of Chicago Press, 1980), 60–61, 66.

94. By 1895 Charles Milton Buchanan could devote four chapters on the history of antisepsis in his *Antisepsis and Antiseptics* (Newark: Terhune, 1895), and near the end of the century students at the University of Michigan received regular instruction in the field, as indicated in Charles Beylard Guerard Nancrede, *Lectures upon the Principles of Surgery* (Philadelphia: W. B. Saunders, 1899). See also Charles E. Rosenberg, *The Care of Strangers: The Rise of America's Hospital System* (New York: Basic Books, 1987), 147–50. Of course, none of the printed sources can be relied on, in fact, to accurately reflect what transpired in the operating rooms of the period. If sources could be found, the history of surgical practice in this period would make a fascinating topic. Nonetheless, there appears to have been no radical shift in the ideology of aseptic or antiseptic surgery in the period 1900–1925, the period during which hospital patient records reveal such a drastic change in practice.

95. Paul Starr, in *The Social Transformation of American Medicine* (New York: Basic Books, 1982), 156, notes this transformation and suggests that it was due in part to "creative excitement" and notes further that "improvements in diagnostic tools, particularly the development of X-rays in 1895, spurred the advance." Creative excitement is hard to measure, but at the Pennsylvania Hospital, as well as the New York Hospital, use of the x-ray machine was not associated with operations. In fact, fewer people who underwent an operation had an x-ray image taken than did not. The x ray was infrequently used in 1900 and 1909. In 1920, however, only 8 percent of those people who underwent an operation had an x ray taken as compared to 24 percent of those who did not. In 1925 the figures were 14 percent and 38 percent. With only 14 percent of patients undergoing an operation having an image taken, it is difficult to sustain the argument that x-ray use was the dominant force.

96. Clarke, *Shop and Office Forms*, 128–29.

97. Perhaps the best source on Codman is Codman himself, in the autobiographical preface and prologue to *The Shoulder* (Boston: Thomas Todd, 1924). See also Susan Reverby, "Stealing the Golden Eggs: Ernest Amory Codman and the Science and Management of Medicine," *Bulletin of the History of Medicine* 55 (1981): 156–71; and George Rosen, "The Efficiency Criterion in Medical Care, 1900–1920: An Early Approach to the Evaluation of Health Service," *Bulletin of the History of Medicine* 50 (1976): 28–44.

98. Stevens, *American Medicine*; and *In Sickness and in Wealth: American Hospitals in the Twentieth Century* (New York: Basic Books, 1989), 75–79. See also Loyal Davis, *Fellowship of Surgeons: A History of the American College of Surgeons* (Chicago: American College of Surgeons,

1973); "Conference on Hospital Standardization," *Bulletin of the American College of Surgeons* 3, no. 1 (1917): 1–53; and Franklin Martin, *Fifty Years of Medicine and Surgery* (Chicago: Surgical Publishing Company of Chicago, 1934).

99. "Hospital Standardization Series: General Hospitals of 100 or More Beds," *Bulletin of the American College of Surgeons* 4, no. 4 (1919): 5.

100. "Editorial," *Hospital Management* (May 1919).

101. On Gilbreth, see Brian Price, "Frank and Lillian Gilbreth and the Motion Study Controversy, 1907–1930," in Nelson, *Mental Revolution*, 58–76; and Albert Jay Nock, "Efficiency and the High-Brow," *American Magazine* (1913): 48–50.

102. Frank B. Gilbreth, "Motion Study in Surgery," *Canadian Journal of Medicine and Surgery* 40 (1916): 23; "Scientific Management in the Hospital," *Modern Hospital* 3 (1914): 321–24.

103. Robert L. Dickinson, "Standardization of Surgery: An Attack on the Problem," *Journal of the American Medical Association* 63 (1914): 763–65; "'Efficiency Engineering' in Pelvic Operations: One- and Two-Suture operations," *Surgery, Gynecology, and Obstetrics* 18 (1914): 559–71. The article is far broader than its title would suggest.

104. Gilbreth, "Motion Study," 30.

105. John Allen Hornsby, "The Items in Hospital Efficiency," *Modern Hospital* 2 (1914): 173–75.

CHAPTER 3: THE CHANGING MEANING OF URINALYSIS

1. Theodore Wm. Schaefer, "A Brief Historical Retrospect of the Examination of the Urine in Ancient and Modern Times," *Boston Medical and Surgical Journal* 136 (1897): 623–26; American Medical Association (AMA), *The Evolution of Urine Analysis: An Historical Sketch of the Clinical Examination of Urine* (London: Burroughs Wellcome, 1911); Ronnie Beth Bush, "Urine Is a Harlot, or a Lier," *JAMA* 208 (1969): 131–34. For a list of examples of uroscopy found in various arts, see Joseph H. Kiefer, "Uroscopy: The Clinical Laboratory of the Past," *Transactions of the American Association of Genito-Urinary Surgeons* 50 (1958): 161–72. Another overview is provided by Meryl H. Huber, "Pisse Prophecy: A Brief History of Urinalysis," *Clinics in Laboratory Medicine* 8, no. 3 (September 1988): 415–47 (the entire issue is devoted to urinalysis).

2. AMA, *Evolution of Urine Analysis*, 61–73.

3. The situations arise in the second scene of *Henry IV, pt. 2*, and in act 3, scene 4, of *Twelfth Night*. I am indebted to Leonard Barkan for pointing out these two references.

4. Charles E. Rosenberg, "The Therapeutic Revolution," in *The Therapeutic Revolution: Essays in the Social History of American Medicine,*

edited by Morris J. Vogel and Charles E. Rosenberg (Philadelphia: University of Pennsylvania Press), 2–25.

5. Such as the Massachusetts General Hospital. By the 1880s analyses were reported on standardized forms. At Commercial Hospital of Cincinnati urinalysis was common in the 1860s and 1870s, although chemical analysis was not used so frequently at the Commercial Hospital of Cincinnati as at the Massachusetts General Hospital. John Harley Warner, *The Therapeutic Perspective: Medical Practice, Knowledge, and Identity in America, 1820–1885* (Cambridge, Mass.: Harvard University Press, 1986), 156–57. Also see Christopher Crenner, "Professional Measurement: Quantification of Health and Disease in American Medical Practice, 1880–1920" (Ph.D. diss., Harvard University, 1993), 69–70, in which he indicates that at Massachusetts General Hospital urinalysis was expected to be done on every patient by 1899.

6. Andrew Cunningham and Perry Williams, "Introduction," in *The Laboratory Revolution in Medicine*, edited by Andrew Cunningham and Perry Williams, 1–13 (Cambridge: Cambridge University Press, 1992).

7. For a general overview, see Stanley Joel Reiser, *Medicine and the Reign of Technology* (Cambridge: Cambridge University Press, 1978).

8. Here, as elsewhere, it is impossible to know about tests that were done and not recorded. Nor, unfortunately, can we ascertain with any consistency who was actually doing the test—that is, whether it was the medical student or the house officer who actually went to the laboratory bench and examined the urine.

9. Pennsylvania Hospital Case Records (henceforth PHCR) 81 (1900): 3116; PHCR 82 (1900): 3426; 85 (1900): 848.

10. One concern might be that at least some of the injuries involved the pelvis or abdomen, for which physicians might logically (at least in the late twentieth century) suspect traumatic injury to some part of the urogenital system. Such was not the case, however, as the vast majority of the trauma involved fractures of the extremities or lacerations.

11. The median value is the middle value. It is a better estimation of the central value than the mean, because it is not so influenced by a few extreme values. For example, take the hypothetical instance that there were five patients and that the number of days before a urine analysis was done was 1, 1, 1, 1, and 100 days. The mean value would be 20.8 days. The median would be 1 day. One could make a reasonable argument that the mean of 20.8 days misrepresents the best summary of the central tendency, as the vast majority of patients (80 percent) had the test within one day. The 75th percentile is the value that one would find if one divided all of the values into four equal parts and took the value that comes at the dividing line between the third and the fourth quartile.

12. The term *ritual* is used here to indicate a repetitive process, not a ritual in a precise anthropological sense. For a rich discussion of the concept of occupational rituals in medical care, see Charles L. Bosk,

"Occupational Rituals in Patient Management," *New England Journal of Medicine* 303 (1980): 71–76. Barbara A. Koenig has described how rituals associated with machine use change as people gain experience using a plasmapheresis machine in "The Technological Imperative in Medical Practice: The Social Creation of a 'Routine' Treatment," in *Biomedicine Examined*, edited by M. Lock and D. R. Gordon, 465–96 (Dordrecht: Kluwer Academic Publishers, 1988). Also useful for medical rituals is Zane Robinson Wolf, *Nurses' Work: The Sacred and the Profane* (Philadelphia: University of Pennsylvania Press, 1988).

13. This conclusion also illustrates the value of not drawing conclusions from aggregate statistics alone. Hospital annual reports are often fruitful sources of data that were compiled at the aggregate level of all of the patients admitted to a particular hospital. If one wishes to understand the nature of patient care at the level of an individual patient, however, it helps to look at data at that level.

14. For 1900 the sample taken for this book included thirteen patients with kidney disease. Of that group seven had their urine examined once and the remainder between two and five times.

15. For 1925 the sample included six patients. One had his urine examined once, two had their urine examined more than five times, and the remainder between two and five times.

16. In the context of this chapter one cannot, obviously, do a fractional urine analysis. For example, when there was a mean of 0.25 urine analysis done per day, that means that, on average, each patient had one urine analysis done for each four days in the hospital.

17. AMA, *Evolution of Urine Analysis*, 12–14.

18. Reiser, *Medicine*, 122–24.

19. This method has been replicated by a late-twentieth-century nephrologist and medical historian, with reasonable results. See Steven J. Peitzman, "Richard Bright and Mercury as the Cause and Cure of Nephritis," *Bulletin of the History of Medicine* 52 (1978): 427 n. 31; "Bright's Disease and Bright's Generation—Toward Exact Medicine at Guy's Hospital," *Bulletin of the History of Medicine* 55 (1981): 307–21.

20. For discussion of the role of albumin in the diagnosis of Bright's disease, see Reiser, *Medicine*; and especially the works of Steven Peitzman, "Nephrology in America from Thomas Addis to the Artificial Kidney," in *Grand Rounds: One Hundred Years of Internal Medicine*, edited by Russell C. Maulitz and Diane E. Long, 211-41 (Philadelphia: University of Pennsylvania Press, 1988); "From Bright's Disease to End-Stage Renal Disease," in *Framing Disease: Studies in Cultural Disease*, edited by Charles E. Rosenberg and Janet Golden, 3–19 (New Brunswick, New Jersey: Rutgers University Press, 1992).

21. Peitzman, "Richard Bright," 419.

22. William Coleman, "Experimental Physiology and Statistical Inference: The Therapeutic Trial in Nineteenth-Century Germany," in *The Probabilistic Revolution*, vol. 2: *Ideas in the Sciences*, edited by Lorenz

Krüger, Gerd Gigerenzer, and Mary S. Morgan, 201–26 (Cambridge, Massachusetts: MIT Press, 1987).

23. Robert E. Kohler, *From Medical Chemistry to Biochemistry: The Making of a Biomedical Discipline* (Cambridge: Cambridge University Press, 1982), esp. 227–31. A brief chronology is provided by Wendell T. Caraway, "The Scientific Development of Clinical Chemistry to 1948," *Clinical Chemistry* 19 (1973): 373–83.

24. Kohler, *From Medical Chemistry*, 219, 228.

25. A. McGehee Harvey, *Science at the Bedside: Clinical Research in American Medicine, 1905–1945* (Baltimore: Johns Hopkins University Press, 1981), 50. See also Russell H. Chittenden, *Development of Physiological Chemistry in the United States* (New York: Chemical Catalog Company, 1930); Samuel Meites, *Otto Folin: America's First Clinical Biochemist* (American Association for Clinical Chemistry, 1989); and P. A. Shaffer, "Otto Folin," in *Biographical Memoirs of the National Academy of Science* 27 (1952): 47. For a fuller discussion of these two individuals in the context of U.S. biomedical research, see Kohler, *From Medical Chemistry*.

26. K. B. Hoffman and R. Ultzmann, *Guide to the Examination of Urine, with Special Reference to Diseases of the Urinary Apparatus* (Cincinnati: Peter G. Thompson, 1879); also translated and published the same year as *Analysis of the Urine: With Special Reference to the Diseases of the Genito-Urinary Organs* (New York: D. Appleton, 1879).

27. R. B. H. Gradwohl and A. J. Blaivas, *The Newer Methods of Blood and Urine Chemistry* (St. Louis: C. V. Mosby, 1917), 20.

28. Charles E. Simon, *A Manual of Clinical Diagnosis by Means of Microscopic and Chemical Methods*, 3d ed. (Philadelphia: Lea Brothers, 1900), 284.

29. Alfred L. Loomis, *Lessons in Physical Diagnosis* (New York: William Wood, 1896), 180; Ralph W. Webster, *Diagnostic Methods: Chemical, Bacteriological, and Microscopical: A Textbook for Students and Practitioners*, 6th ed. (Philadelphia: P. Blakiston's Son, 1920), 194.

30. "A New Urinometer," *Modern Hospital* 2 (1914): 319.

31. Jacalyn Duffin, *Langstaff: A Medical Life* (Toronto: University of Toronto Press, 1993), 66.

32. Richard C. Cabot, "Clinical Examination of the Urine: A Critical Study of the Commoner Methods," *JAMA* 44 (1905): 837–42, 943–50.

33. Some devices were described for more accurately determining the color of a urine specimen, but these color scales were thought by some observers to be no more accurate than simple description. I have found no evidence that they were ever used. See Webster, *Diagnostic Methods*, 185.

34. Reiser, *Medicine*, 126, 135–36. For a description of the various tests, as well as an account of early attempts to do home tests, see Joseph Litwins, "Sugar in Urine: Determination by Reduction of Copper—Methods from 1841 to 1941," *New York State Medical Journal* 77 (1977):

1001–2. For more discussion of the details of the pitfalls of tests for sugar in urine, and a brief precis of the changes in sugar measurement, see J. M. Davison and G. A. Cheyne, "History of the Measurement of Glucose in Urine: A Cautionary Tale," *Medical History* 18 (1974): 194–97. Although the debate was quite heated, it appears that most of the protagonists were addressing the investigative use of the methods more than their clinical application. A slightly different selection for a chronology may be found in Diana W. Guthrie and Selby S. Humphreys, "Diabetes Urine Testing: An Historical Perspective," *Diabetes Educator* 14 (1988): 521–25. For detailed discussion of various tests in the primary literature, see Webster, *Diagnostic Methods*, 298–322; and Simon, *Manual of Clinical Diagnoses*, 402–22.

35. Duffin, *Langstaff*, 66.
36. Loomis, *Lessons in Physical Diagnosis*, 189–92. A. H. Sanford, in "Clinical Laboratories: Their Place in Hospital Functions," *Hospital Progress* 1 (1920): 302–4, describes the measurement of specific gravity and states that albumin and sugar are the two most important pathological substances found in urine. Sanford was at that time at the Mayo Clinic.
37. Henry A. Christian, "A Critical Estimation of the Fermentation Specific Gravity Method of Quantitating Sugar in Diabetic Urine," *Boston Medical and Surgical Journal* 157 (1907): 178–81.
38. Michael Bliss, *The Discovery of Insulin* (Chicago: University of Chicago Press, 1982).
39. PHCR 566 (1920): page 2891.
40. One of the most influential texts was Frederick M. Allen, Edgar Stillman, and Reginald Fitz, *Total Dietary Regulation in the Treatment of Diabetes* (New York: Rockefeller Institute for Medical Research, 1919). Allen advocated an extremely low-calorie diet. Others advised a high-fat diet, such as Louis Harry Newburgh; see Steven Peitzman, "Louis Harry Newburgh and Metabolism at Michigan," in *Medical Lives and Scientific Medicine at Michigan, 1891–1969*, edited by Joel D. Howell, 129–51 (Ann Arbor: University of Michigan Press, 1993). When insulin became available the debate over which of these two approaches became moot, and a whole new set of dietary questions arose.
41. The condition is technically known as hypoglycemia, and it continues in the 1990s to be a complication of insulin therapy.
42. For example, see PHCR 926 (the cases starting on page 2891 and 2900).
43. Peitzman, "Bright's Disease."
44. Loomis, *Lessons in Physical Diagnosis*, 181–83.
45. Cabot, "Clinical Examination of Urine."
46. Webster, *Diagnostic Methods*, 230 and the section from 229–37; see also Simon, *Manual of Clinical Diagnosis*, 322–45.
47. Thomas Dixon Saville, *A System of Clinical Medicine*, 3d ed. (New York: William Wood, 1912), 385.
48. PHCR 86 (1900): 1398.

49. PHCR 606 (1920): 4503; 956 (1925): 5662; and 556 (1920): 5195.
50. This appears to have been Charles Franklin Mitchell (1875–1962), who received an M.D. degree from the University of Pennsylvania in 1898, was a member of the American Surgical Association, and was on the faculty and staff of several Philadelphia institutions, including the Pennsylvania Hospital. For an obituary, see *JAMA* 182 (1962): 1131.
51. Cabot, "Clinical Examination of Urine," 947, 950.
52. Miles J. Breuer, "The Construction of Clinical Laboratory Equipment," *Journal of Laboratory and Clinical Medicine* 2 (1916–17): 427–36.
53. See Charles W. Purdy, *Practical Uranalysis* [sic] *and Urinary Diagnosis: A Manual for the Use of Physicians, Surgeons, and Students*, 3d ed. (Philadelphia: F. A. Davis, 1897). This book appears to have been quite popular, going through six editions between 1894 and 1901, and receiving favorable notice in the *Boston Medical and Surgical Journal* by Schaefer, "Brief Historical Retrospect."
54. Breuer, "Construction of Clinical Laboratory Equipment," 427.
55. O. Hensel, "Progress in Clinical Pathology," in *Festschrift zur Vierzigjährigen Stiftungsfeir des Deutschen Hospitals* (New York: Lemcke and Buechner, 1909), 576–89; Stuart Hart, "The Collection, Preservation, and Transportation of Clinical Material for Laboratory Examination," *New York Medical Journal* 71 (1900): 907–10.
56. In a 1990s medical analysis we might speak of multiple tests for this purpose as increasing the sensitivity (i.e., increasing the likelihood that someone with a particular disease would be identified by testing) at the risk of decreasing the specificity (i.e., decreasing the likelihood that someone who has a positive test result will actually have the disease).
57. Purdy, *Practical Uranalysis* [sic], 1.
58. See, for example, Webster, *Diagnostic Methods*, 179. One could also suppose that multiple analyses would diminish the likelihood of a single technical error in the means used to measure the urine, although this possibility is not generally discussed in the literature of the time. For a general historical discussion of such problems with diagnostic tests, see Reiser, *Medicine*.
59. With the exception of patients admitted to diabetic hospitals. John Christopher Feudtner is preparing a Ph.D. dissertation at the University of Pennsylvania which uses patient records to address the twentieth-century treatment of patients with diabetes by specialists who worked in hospitals for diabetic patients.
60. Kenneth M. Ludmerer, *Learning to Heal: The Development of American Medical Education* (New York: Basic Books, 1985).
61. Cabot, "Clinical Examination of the Urine."
62. Charles Sherrington describing a 1907 tour of U.S. medical schools; quoted in Kohler, *From Medical Chemistry to Biochemistry*, 56–57.
63. Kohler, *From Medical Chemistry to Biochemistry*, 115. On the tension between the U.S. laboratories as elitist or egalitarian (they were both), see John Harley Warner, "The Rise and Fall of Professional Mystery:

Epistemology, Authority, and the Emergence of Laboratory Medicine in Nineteenth Century America," in Cunningham and Williams, *Laboratory Revolution in Medicine*, 110–41. See also Ludmerer, *Learning to Heal*.

64. Walter C. Allen, "The Role of the Intern in the Standardization of Hospitals," *Modern Hospital* 12 (1919): 318–19.

65. C. N. B. Camac, "Hospital and Ward Clinical Laboratories," *JAMA* 35 (1900): 219–27; Henry M. Hurd, "Laboratories and Hospital Work," *Bulletin of the American Academy of Medicine* 2 (1896): 483–95. The excitement over hospital laboratories in some places should not obscure the fact that such facilities were distributed unevenly. For example, for much of the first decade of the twentieth century the Reading Hospital pathology laboratory was located either in the pharmacy, where the few test tubes and microscope that were available were used on the pharmacy table, or in space shared with the morgue. *History of Reading Hospital, 1867–1942* (n.p.: Reading Hospital, 1942), 80.

66. This is a common theme. This example comes from a prominent address by a prominent clinician: James B. Herrick's "Oration on Medicine," delivered to the annual meeting of the American Medical Association, "The Relation of the Clinical Laboratory to the Practitioner of Medicine," *Boston Medical and Surgical Journal* 156 (1907): 763–68. For a similar discussion, see Paul G. Wooley, "Relation of the Clinical Laboratory to the General Practitioner," *Journal of Laboratory and Clinical Medicine* 9 (1923–24): 130–37.

67. Charles P. Emerson, "Some Clinical Aspects of Chemistry," *JAMA* (1902): 1359–62.

68. Stanley Joel Reiser, "Technology and the Eclipse of Individualism in Medicine," *Pharos* (Winter 1982): 10–15.

69. The choice to define fever purely on the basis of the temperature was one that was only made late in the nineteenth century. It was also a choice that served to define a condition purely on the basis of a finding by a laboratory instrument.

70. These categories represent the most common ways of reporting the test results. Obviously, one could count the numbers of casts or, more simply, report them as "numerous" or "rare." Similarly, one could report only the presence or absence of sugar.

71. Literally. The coding system I used listed only the first fifteen urine examinations. Given the overall pattern of use, it seems unlikely that much additional information would have been gathered in obtaining information on more than fifteen tests, and the cost in computing resources would have been considerable. This case is to be found in PHCR 596: 3566.

72. If one divides the patients into groups along two dimensions—whether or not they had a urine analysis done and whether or note they were noted to be "worse" or "dead" at the time of discharge—one can do a chi-square test, a simple statistical measure of association, to see if one

group is more likely to have a urine analysis done. It shows that in 1900 there was no statistically significant difference between the two groups, but at the end of the study period there was a statistically significant difference, with the people who were sicker being more likely to have had a urine analysis done.

73. Such charts are found in the 1868 New York Hospital records.

74. See, for example, Edward S. Wood, "Urinary Diagnosis," *Boston Medical and Surgical Diagnosis* 130 (1894): 484–87, 505–8. This article does little to differentiate between the essential and the optional among a long list of possible tests and diagnoses.

75. Joanne Yates, *Control through Communication: The Rise of System in American Management* (Baltimore: Johns Hopkins University Press, 1989), 80.

76. Purdy, *Practical Uranalysis*, includes a form that lists the physical examination: transparency, color, specific gravity, chemical reaction, solids, and quantity. Later Clyde Lottridge Cummer, in *A Manual of Clinical Laboratory Methods* (2d ed. [Philadelphia: Lea and Febiger, 1926]), asserts that a routine exam includes color, appearance, reaction, specific gravity, quantitative tests for albumin and sugar, and microscopic examination of sediment.

77. These came from the Cornell Division; it should be noted that Cornell was not, at this time, affiliated with the New York Hospital. C. N. B. Camac, "Hospital and Ward Clinical Laboratories," *Journal of the American Medical Association* 35 (1900): 219–27. This is but one example; there are many others in the medical literature of the period.

78. See, for example, Cummer, *Manual of Clinical Laboratory Methods.*

79. Wooley, "Relation of the Clinical Laboratory."

80. Kohler, *Medical Chemistry*, 228. Kohler's conclusions follow naturally from the object of his book. He writes about the development of biochemistry. He makes it clear that he is not writing about the use of tests for patient care, and his attention does not extend to the nonchemical study of urine. This chapter suggests that the urine analysis may have played an important role in the institutional development of biochemistry in the United States. The increased use of the "old" urinalysis may have led to a "new" urinalysis, which may then have made the utility of the biochemist more apparent.

81. Simon, *Manual of Clinical Diagnosis*, 335; see also Herbert Thomas Brooks, *Diagnostic Methods* (St. Louis: C. V. Mosby, 1916), 33–34.

82. One could also point out that there are many, many tests listed in the hospital pathology books today, most of which are not done on a regular basis. This would simply emphasize the difference between medicine as described in books and medicine as practiced on people.

83. The highest public profile for the urinalysis is probably as a screen for the use of illicit drugs. The urine analysis was done 36.7 million times in 1988; the most common test was the complete blood count. See Dixie

Farley, "Urinalysis: Looking into the Void," *FDA Consumer* 23 (1989): 16–21.

84. William N. Berkeley, "Some Practical Remarks on Clinical Examination of the Blood," *New York Medical Journal* 71 (1900): 599–601.

85. See, for example, H. Miller Galt, "On the Value of the Blood Count as an Aid to Diagnosis in Obscure Bacterial and Other Infections," *British Medical Journal* 2 (1913): 1367–69; George Dock, "Correlation of Laboratory and Clinical Teaching," *Southern Medical Journal* 10 (1917): 187–91; Lucien Achard, "The Place of the Modern Medical Laboratory in the Diagnosis of Disease," *Medical Record* 101 (1922): 418–19; Harry Gauss, "The Evolution of Clinical Pathology," *Journal of Laboratory and Clinical Medicine* 8 (1923): 703–16.

86. Achard, "Place of the Modern Medical Laboratory," 419.

CHAPTER 4: CLINICAL USE OF THE X-RAY MACHINE

Portions of this chapter have been previously published as Joel D. Howell, "Early Use of X-ray Machines and Electrocardiographs at the Pennsylvania Hospital: 1897–1927," *Journal of the American Medical Association (JAMA)* 255 (1986): 2320–23; "Machines and Medicine: Technology Transforms the American Hospital," in *The American General Hospital: Communities and Social Contexts*, edited by Diana Elizabeth Long and Janet Golden, 109–34 (Ithaca: Cornell University Press, 1989); "Diagnostic Technologies: X-rays, Electrocardiograms, and CAT Scans," *Southern California Law Review* 65 (1991): 529–64. When no reference is explicitly given, information specific to the Pennsylvania Hospital and the New York Hospital is derived from the minutes of their governing bodies and from the hospital annual reports.

1. George Sarton, "The Discovery of X-rays," *Isis* 26 (1937): 349–64.

2. *Ueber eine neue Art von Strahlen* [*Vorläufige Mittheilung*] (On a New Kind of Rays [preliminary communication]), *Sitzsber. Physik.-med Ges. Würzburg.*, 137 (1895): 132–41. An excellent translation and discussion is to be found in Otto Glasser, *Dr. W. C. Röntgen* (Springfield, Ill.: Charles C Thomas, 1945).

3. The secondary literature on Röntgen's discovery is vast. See particularly Ruth Brecher and Edward Brecher, *The Rays: A History of Radiology in the United States and Canada* (Baltimore: Williams and Wilkins, 1969).

4. In this discussion I do not consider the use of x rays for therapeutic purposes nor the (related) use of radium for treatment. These two issues, particularly the use of radium, often were addressed by a different community of practitioners than addressed diagnostic radiology. On this, see Lawrence Badash, *Radioactivity in America: Growth and Decay of a Science* (Baltimore: Johns Hopkins University Press, 1979). I look instead at the use of the machines as a tool for diagnostic purposes. I also

focus primarily on the production of radiographs rather than the use of fluoroscopy. During the early years of the x-ray technology U.S. manufacturers were unable to produce screens for amplifying the image which were as effective as those that could be obtained in Germany. "Report Relative to the Meeting of the Röntgen Ray Society, held at Chicago December 10–11, 1902," W. C. Borden to Surgeon General, U.S. Army, January 3, 1903. MS.B.127, History of Medicine Division, National Library of Medicine, Bethesda, Md.

5. Unless otherwise noted, all information specific to these two hospitals comes from either the Pennsylvania Hospital patient records, minutes of the Board of Managers, and annual reports, located at the Pennsylvania Hospital Archives, 9th and Spruce streets, Philadelphia, or the New York Hospital patient records, minutes of the Medical Board, and annual reports, all of which are located in the hospital archives.

6. Henry W. Cattell, "Roentgen's Discovery—Its Application in Medicine," *Medical News* (N.Y.) 68 (1896): 169–70. The cost estimates soon escalated, however, until by the middle of the second decade of the century an x-ray facility was held to be quite expensive—"far more costly than . . . a pathological laboratory." I. Seth Hirsch, "The Hospital X-ray Laboratory," *Modern Hospital* 4 (1915): 11–14, 92–97, 254–57.

7. Stanley Joel Reiser, "The Science of Diagnosis: Diagnostic Technology," edited by W. F. Bynum and Roy Porter, 2:826–51, *Companion Encyclopedia of the History of Medicine* (London: Routledge, 1993).

8. For example, the Hospital of the University of Pennsylvania purchased a machine in 1896; it is not surprising that this elite university hospital should be in the forefront of U.S. hospitals purchasing such equipment. In fact, there is a controversy—unrelated to the medical application of x rays which we consider in this chapter—about the possibility that the first discovery of x rays was made at the University of Pennsylvania in 1890. See Lynne Allen Leopold, *Radiology at the University of Pennsylvania, 1890–1975* (Philadelphia: University of Pennsylvania Press for the Department of Radiology, 1981). Another elite institution, Jefferson Hospital, also acquired a machine in 1896. The 1896 annual report for that institution noted that a "fully equipped Roentgen Ray apparatus was donated." See also Simon Kramer and Robert M. Steiner, "Department of Radiology, Radiation Oncology, and Nuclear Medicine," in *Thomas Jefferson University: Tradition and Heritage,* edited by Frederick B. Wagner, 737–51 (Philadelphia: Lea and Febiger, 1989). The Philadelphia General Hospital purchased an x-ray machine somewhat later, in 1899. See George E. Pfahler, "Fifty Years of Trials and Tribulations in Radiology," in *The American Roentgen Ray Society, 1900–1950: Commemorating the Golden Anniversary of the Society* (Springfield, Ill.: Charles C Thomas, 1950), 15–24. A survey of "a large number of prominent hospitals in six of the leading hospitals of America" found that by about a year after Röntgen's discovery, one-third had x-ray equipment. D. W. Hering, "A Year of the X Rays," *Popular Science Monthly* 50 (1896–97): 654–62. By

1898 "almost every first-class hospital in the country" had the necessary equipment. *New York Times,* May 9, 1898, 14.

9. James H. Kenyon, who was in charge of the x-ray machine until 1903, claimed that the hospital had purchased some equipment in "1895 or 6." As the invention was barely published in 1895, it seems rather unlikely that the New York Hospital had managed to purchase it in that year, and 1896 seems more likely. James H. Kenyon to chairman of Visiting Committee of the New York Hospital, June 8, 1903. Also in file of the secretary-treasurer, box 35, folder 4.

10. Otto Glasser, *William Conrad Röntgen and the Early History of the Roentgen Rays* (Springfield, Ill.: Charles C Thomas, 1934). Other types of investigations were going on as well. For an outstanding discussion of early use of the x ray for gastrointestinal research, see Saul Benison, A. Clifford Barger, and Elin L. Wolfe, *Walter B. Cannon: The Life and Times of a Young Scientist* (Cambridge, Mass.: Belknap Press, 1987).

11. Eugene R. Corson, "Some Observations on Colles' Fracture by Aid of the X-ray," *Medical Record* (N.Y.) 51 (1897): 649–53. See also A. V. L. Brokaw, "An Exhibition of Radiographs with Remarks," *Transactions of the Southern Surgical and Gynecological Association* 10 (1898): 80.

12. Ross and Wilbert, "Five Hundred Cases of Fractures of Extremities Verified by Radiographs," *Philadelphia Monthly Medical Journal* (June 1899); cited in Francis H. Williams, *The Roentgen Rays in Medicine and Surgery* (New York: Macmillan, 1901), 467. Williams was considered by his contemporaries to be one of the most important early users of the x ray. See P. M. Hickey, "The First Decade of American Roentgenology," *American Journal of Roentgenology* 20 (1928): 150–57; Juan A. del Regato, "Francis Henry Williams," *International Journal of Radiation Oncology, Biology, and Physics* 9 (1983): 739–49. Williams cited the title of the article slightly incorrectly; the actual reference is G. G. Ross and M. I. Wilbert, "Fractures of the Extremities. A Report of 500 Consecutive Cases, Verified by Radiographs," *Philadelphia Monthly Medical Journal* 1 (1899): 330–36. Demonstrations of x-ray apparatus were widespread, and reports of such activities can easily be found. For example, to take early demonstrations from widespread geographical areas of the United States, see F. C. Robinson and C. C. Hutchins, "Demonstration of the Use of Röengten Rays," *Transactions of the Maine Medical Association* 12 (1896): 408–14; C. F. Lacombe, "The Roentgen Ray," *Colorado State Medical Society Proceedings* (1896): 261–78; Cuthbert Thompson, "The Uses of the Roentgen Ray in Surgery," *American Practitioner and News* (Louisville) 21 (1896): 164–66; Laurence Turnbull, "The Significance of the New Rays," *Georgia Journal of Medicine and Surgery* 2 (1898): 157–63. For world's fairs, see Edwin K. Hart and John C. Grady, *Pennsylvania Public Institutions at the World's Fair* (St. Louis, 1904).

13. Of course, not all fractures are alike. A fractured fifth finger of the hand and a fractured cervical vertebra (part of the spinal column in the neck)

carry very different implications. Even then there are many different ways to break both a finger and a vertebra. The question of how broadly (or how narrowly) to construct groupings of diagnostic categories is best resolved in reference to the specific question for which ones wishes an answer. In this case, the idea of detecting a broken bone with x rays was a widespread general revelation in the early days of the instrument. Also, this grouping is broad enough so that a meaningful collection of patient records can be assembled.

14. Much of this chapter is about decisions to take an x ray. In the absence of definitive evidence one way or the other, I shall assume that the decisions were being made by physicians. This is not to deny that patients could have had significant input; late in the twentieth century most ethicists would argue that they should. In a few instances, such as patients who were rather well-to-do, patients in the early twentieth century may have played a role in the decision-making process. But it seems safe to assume that the vast majority did not.

15. Lewis A. Stimson, *A Practical Treatise on Fractures and Dislocations,* 3d ed. (New York: Lea Brothers, 1900), 51.

16. Charles Lester Leonard, "Recent Progress in the Roentgen-Ray Methods of Diagnosis," *JAMA* 35 (1900): 147–52; Frank Leech, "The Röntgen Rays: Illustrated by Sixteen Photographs," *Maryland Medical Journal* 25 (1896): 345–48.

17. Leonard, "Recent Progress"; Williams, *Roentgen Rays,* 467.

18. "The Value of the New Photography in Military Surgery," *British Medical Journal* 1 (1896): 1059; Francis C. Abbott, "Surgery in the Graeco-Turkish War (1897)," *Lancet* 1 (1899): 80–83, 152–56.

19. W. C. Borden, *The Use of the Röntgen Ray by the Medical Department of the U.S. Army in the War with Spain (1898)* (Washington, D.C.: Government Printing Office, 1900).

20. Sanford Withers, "The Story of the First Roentgen Evidence," *Radiology* 17 (1931): 99–103. See also "Roentgen Rays in Court," *Medical Record* (N.Y.) 49 (April 4, 1896): 491; "The New Photography in Court," *Literary Digest* 12 (April 11, 1896), 707; "About X-ray Photography," *New York Times Magazine,* September 6, 1896, p 12; "The Roentgen Rays in the Witness-Box," *JAMA* 27 (1896): 168, in which the x ray is used to disprove rather than prove the diagnosis of a fracture (the patient was shown to have a dislocation with the x ray); "X-ray Photographs as Evidence," *JAMA* 29 (1897): 870; Samuel Donaldson, "Medical Facts That Can or Cannot be Proved by Roentgen-Ray: Historical Review and Present Possibilities," *Annals of Internal Medicine* 18 (1943): 535–50; R. Harvey Reed, "The X-ray from a Medico-Legal Standpoint," *JAMA* 30 (1898): 1013–19. A glance at the early issues of the *American Journal of Roentgenology* confirms that the legal implications of x-ray images were a major concern for those who wished to make their career using the new machines.

21. "X-rays," *Boston Medical and Surgical Journal* 134 (1896): 174–75.

22. James Burry, "Discussion," in Reed, "X-ray from a Medico-Legal Standpoint," 1018. This is a rather amazing claim and probably should not be taken entirely at face value, as it would imply—assuming that the person in question obtained a machine on January 1, 1896, and worked five days per week, fifty weeks per year until the day of the meeting, October 6, 1897—taking an average of eleven pictures per day. The fact, however, that Dr. Burry was willing to make the claim, and that none of those present decided to dispute it, suggests that such a level of use was not too far from believability. James Burry was the chief surgeon for the Illinois Steel Company and an early user of the x-ray machine in Chicago. E. R. N. Grigg, *The Trail of the Invisible Light: From X-Strahlen to Radio(bio)logy* (Springfield, Ill.: Charles C Thomas, 1965), 29.

23. Ross and Wilbert, "Fractures of the Extremities," 330. For a discussion of the use of x rays in fractures and other conditions during this period, see Barron H. Lerner, "The Perils of 'X-ray Vision': How Radiographic Images Have Historically Influenced Perception," *Perspectives in Biology and Medicine* 35 (1992): 382–97.

24. For example, Lewis A. Stimson's *A Treatise on Fractures and Dislocations*, originally published in 1883 (revised after the 3d ed. of 1900, at that time titled *A Practical Treatise on Fractures and Dislocations* [New York: Lea Brothers, 1900]), contained discussions of the use of x rays. For a general overview of medical literature on fractures, see Leonard F. Peltier, *Fractures: A History and Iconography of Their Treatment* (San Francisco: Norman Publishing, 1990).

25. Carl Beck, *Fractures: With an Appendix on the Practical Use of the Röntgen Rays* (Philadelphia: W. B. Saunders, 1900).

26. Charles Lester Leonard, "The Past, Present, and Future of the Röntgen Ray," *American Medicine* 10 (1905): 1082–85. This was the Presidential Address to the American Röntgen Ray Society, delivered at Johns Hopkins Hospital.

27. Frank E. Peckham, "The Importance of Röntgenology in Fracture Work," *Providence Medical Journal* 8 (1907): 122–24.

28. Owen Tully Stratton, *Medicine Man* (Norman: University of Oklahoma Press, 1989), 199.

29. This is generally true in medicine in the United States in the late twentieth century, with only a few exceptions, such as stress fractures or fractures in areas such as the wrist, where many bones overlap and make x-ray interpretation difficult.

30. Leo G. Rigler, "The Development of Roentgen Diagnosis," *Radiology* 45 (1945): 467–502; Peltier, *Fractures*, 228. Peltier nonetheless includes in his book ample evidence of skepticism about the usefulness of x rays, evidence that has generally not been accorded much attention in light of the fact that x-ray examination eventually did become routine.

31. "Death of President McKinley," *JAMA* 37 (1901): 779–86.

32. Richard W. Westbrook, book review, "A Practical Treatise on Fractures and Dislocations by Lewis A. Stimson, 3d ed.," *Annals of Surgery* 34 (1901): 719–22; "The Roentgen Rays in Surgical Work," *British Medical Journal* 2 (1899): 1026–27.

33. Ellsworth Eliot, "The Legal Responsibility to the Surgeon and Practitioner Which the Use of the X-ray Involves," *Annals of Surgery* 63 (1916): 483.

34. "Possibilities of the Roentgen Ray in Medicine," *Medical News* (N.Y.) 68 (1896): 210–11.

35. Stratton, *Medicine Man*, 131.

36. Ross and Wilbert, "Fractures of the Extremities," 330. For more on the debate over whether the sense of touch can equal instrumental aids for diagnosis, see Lawrence, "Incommunicable Knowledge"; and Howell, "Diagnostic Technologies."

37. The noted American physician George Dock critiqued the blind valuing of the x ray over physical diagnostic methods. At the same time, however, he argued for increased use of the x ray for some conditions, such as lung diseases. George Dock, "X-ray Work from the Viewpoint of an Internist," *American Journal of Roentgenology* 8 (1921): 321–27. See also Reiser, "Science of Diagnosis."

38. "Possibilities of the Roentgen Ray."

39. "Report of the Committee of the American Surgical Association on the Medico-Legal Relations of the X-rays," *Transactions of the American Surgical Association* 18 (1900): 429–61; also published in the *American Journal of the Medical Sciences* 120 (1900): 7–36.

40. Eliot, "Legal Responsibility," 479–85.

41. Exactly how many had x-ray machines is hard to say. Whereas the more prominent clearly did, as can be gleaned from annual reports, the next tier may have been somewhat slower. As late as 1916, it was claimed that "even in some large centres, some hospitals are conducted without the advantages of X-ray apparatus." Eliot, "Legal Responsibility," 484–85. This assertion was made in the context of an argument against the need for x rays and may be perhaps read as indicating that at least a few centers lacked x-ray equipment.

42. Charles E. Rosenberg, *The Care of Strangers: The Rise of America's Hospital System* (New York: Basic Books, 1987).

43. Ross and Wilbert, "Fracture of the Extremities," 330. The two authors worked at the German Hospital in Philadelphia.

44. Leon L. Solomon, "Modern Day Diagnosis: Clinical and Laboratory Diagnostic Methods as Practiced by the Staff of the Solomon Clinic," *Kentucky Medical Journal* 18 (1920): 15–22.

45. For a cogent discussion of accidents, fractures, and the development of orthopedics as a specialty in Britain, see Roger Cooter, *Surgery and Society in Peace and War: Orthopedics and the Organization of Modern Medicine, 1880–1948* (London: Macmillan Press, 1993).

46. Those five diagnoses were contusion of extremities, simple fracture of tibia and fibula, ankle sprain, and lacerated extremities. This conclusion is based on a review of six hundred consecutive admissions; for details on the sampling, see Howell, "Early Use of X-ray Machines." The x ray was also used rarely at the elite Johns Hopkins University Hospital. Frederick L. Hoffman, "The Statistical Experience of the Johns Hopkins Hospital, Baltimore, Maryland, 1892–1911," *Johns Hopkins Hospital Reports* 17 (1916): 344.

47. There is no single "right" way of presenting this type of analysis. I present the data with regards to x rays in two different ways—one might also stratify by age, sex, or any number of other variables, depending upon the question one wishes to answer.

48. Pennsylvania Hospital Case Records (henceforth PHCR) 96 (1902): 3300. Although we cannot know for certain, it seems likely that the finger abnormality was what we would now designate as "clubbing" of the fingers, often seen in patients with cyanosis due to heart disease.

49. The large confidence intervals reflect the low number of patients having the procedure done at each hospital.

50. On the New York Hospital's reputation, see John Shrady, "Two Hundred Years of Medicine," in *The Memorial History of the City of New-York, from Its First Settlement to the Year 1892,* edited by James Grant Wilson, (New York: New York History Company, 1893), 4:408.

51. See, for example, PHCR 196 (1912): 3161.

52. Pennsylvania Hospital, Minutes of the Board of Managers, November 24, 1914.

53. This analysis is not primarily concerned with the development of the specialty of radiology or the issue of how one might define a specialist in radiology. I shall use the term *radiologist* in a broad sense, to denote any physician who decided to focus his or her attention on using an x-ray machine. For more on the process of specialization, see Rosemary Stevens, *American Medicine and the Public Interest* (New Haven: Yale University Press, 1971).

54. Minutes of the Board of Managers, November 11, 1897.

55. Pennsylvania Hospital 1896–97 Annual Report, Description of the Walter Garrett Memorial Building, 17–23.

56. Herbert Reid Hawthorne, "Memoir of Walter Estell Lee," *Transactions and Studies of the College of Physicians* 20 (1952): 159; Minutes of the Board of Managers, April 25, 1911.

57. Ralph S. Bromer, "Memoir of David Ralph Bowen, M.D.," *Transactions and Studies of the College of Physicians* 8 (1940): 132–34; George E. Pfahler, "The Early History of Roentgenology in Philadelphia: The History of the Philadelphia Roentgen Ray Society, Part 1: 1899–1920 (1905–1920)," *American Journal of Roentgenology* 75 (1956): 14–22. For examples of Bowen's publications, see "Roentgen Examination of the Sphenoidal Sinus: Presenting a Vertical Technique, *American*

Journal of Roentgenology 1 (1914): 449–59; and "Acute Massive Collapse (Atelectasis) of the Lung," *American Journal of Roentgenology and Radium Therapy* 21 (1929): 101–41. The latter was presented in 1928 at the Second International Congress of Radiology in Stockholm, Sweden.

58. Manges had followed Bowen by almost a decade at Jefferson, graduating in 1903. Although initially appointed assistant demonstrator of Surgery in 1904, Manges also found himself head of the Department of Roentgenology in that same year, a position he held until his death in 1936. He was president of the American Roentgen Ray Society in 1918 and made a number of important contributions to radiology, including work on training of army officers during World War I and on biplane fluoroscopy to recover foreign bodies from the respiratory and gastrointestinal systems, the latter with Chevalier Jackson. See Kramer and Steiner, "Department of Radiology"; Ralph S. Bromer, "The History of Radiology in Philadelphia: The History of the Philadelphia Roentgen Ray Society, Part 2: 1920–1954," *American Journal of Roentgenology* 75 (1956): 23–29.

59. For a discussion of early attempts to professionalize radiology, see Julie Elisabeth Cohen, "Influences on American Radiological Thought, 1896–1913," (undergraduate) thesis, Harvard University, 1986, esp. chap. 3.

60. It appears to have been fairly typical for the period, close to the 60 percent–40 percent split advised by John M. Baldy, president of the Pennsylvania Board of Medical Education and Licensure, in "The Standards of Hospital Education for Interns," *Modern Hospital* 10 (1918): 397–403.

61. James H. Kenyon, to chairman of Visiting Committee of the New York Hospital, June 8, 1903. Also in file of the secretary-treasurer, box 35, folder 4. A document in the archives of the Mount Sinai Hospital of New York City claims that Mount Sinai was the first hospital in New York to purchase an x-ray machine, in 1900, providing inferential evidence that the New York Hospital probably did not advertise its ownership of an x-ray machine before that date. "Radiology," 9 p., unauthored, MS, in the Office of the Historian of Mount Sinai Hospital, box 2, file 19.

62. Kenyon, to chairman of the Visiting Committee, New York Hospital, June 8, 1903. Also in file of the secretary-treasurer, box 35, folder 4. (There are two letters in that file from Kenyon, which have the same date.)

63. A. H. Busby, to Executive Committee of the New York Hospital, Secretary-Treasurer's Papers, box 39, folder 3.

64. The annual report for 1907 documents that the most common diagnosis for which x-ray examinations were done, by far, was the 478 for fractures. Only 24 were done for foreign bodies, but Busby may have chosen to highlight this usage because it seemed more dramatic.

65. Minutes of the Medical Board, July 21, 1907.

66. Annual Report, 1910.
67. *The Medical Department of the U.S. Army in the World War, Volume 1: The Surgeon General's Office* (Washington, D.C.: Government Printing Office, 1923), 471.
68. U.S. Army, *History of the Pennsylvania Hospital Unit (Base Hospital No. 10, U.S.A.) in the Great War* (New York: Paul B. Hoeber, 1921); Edward H. Sheldon, "Historical Address," in "The Society of the New York Hospital, 1771–1921, A Commemoration of the One Hundred and Fiftieth Anniversary of the Granting of Its Charter, held in Trinity Church New York October 26, 1921," 11–44. For a description of the plan of the hospital, see "Red Cross Base Hospital Unit," *Society of the New York Hospital General Bulletin* 1, no. 6 (1916): 1–2. For discussion of the experiences of the unit, see Burton James Lee, "Experiences in Surgery with the Second Division of the American Expeditionary Force," *Society of the New York Hospital General Bulletin* 1, no. 12 (1919): 1–46.
69. Percy R. Turnure, "A Report at the Request of the Executive Committee of the New York Hospital," *Society of the New York Hospital General Bulletin* 1, no. 4 (1915): 1–15. This trip was made, obviously, before the United States entered the war, and before the establishment of Base Hospital Number 9.
70. Thomas Howell (superintendent of the New York Hospital), to L. A. Conner (secretary of the Medical Board), July 15, 1915; minutes of the Executive Committee, August 2, 1915. Hirsch, "Hospital X-ray Laboratory—Its Place," also comments on the need for attending staff to sign the requisition to check the "enthusiasm of an interested house staff for the Roentgen demonstration of conditions where no difficult problem exists in diagnosis."
71. The x ray was made an integral part of a portable operating room. Gelett Burgess, "French Surgical Automobiles," *Collier's* 54, no. 17 (January 9, 1915): 9–10.
72. Leonard S. Reich, *The Making of American Industrial Research: Science and Business at GE and Bell, 1876–1926* (Cambridge: Cambridge University Press, 1985), 89–91. For (much) detail on tubes, see Paul Rønne and Arnold B. W. Nielsen, *Development of the Ion X-ray Tube* (Copenhagen: C. A. Reitzel, 1986).
73. Arthur W. Fuchs, "Radiographic Recording Media and Screens," in *The Science of Radiology*, edited by Otto Glasser (Springfield, Ill.: Charles C. Thomas, 1933), 104–5. See also O. Gary Lauer, "Radiography in the United States Army during World War I," *Radiologic Technology* 56 (1985): 400–09.
74. *Medical Department of the U.S. Army*, 468–70.
75. Minutes of the Medical Board, 1917 and 1920.
76. Superintendent Howell, August 20, 1920, Minutes of the Medical Board.
77. PHCR 96 (1902): 3277.

78. One possibility for the late taking of an x ray would have been to ascertain if the fracture was properly set. If the rays could penetrate the cast, as was usually the case, the image could reveal any problems with bony union. Early observers of the rays noted this possibility; see, for example, "Possibilities of the Roentgen Ray." This use, however, does not appear to have been the case for the person described here, and it appears to have been rare for the cases described in this series.

79. In cases in which more than one x ray was taken, the figure indicates the length of time to the first one.

80. Consider a simple example: suppose that there were five cases and that the length of time to obtain an x ray in those five cases was 1, 2, 3, 4, and 100 days. What is the best measure of central tendency? The mean is the sum/the number, 110/5, which is 22 days. The median is the middle number, which is 3 days. As in this example, a single extreme value has a large effect on the mean but much less of an effect on the median. This is the case when examining the lag for patients with a fracture at the Pennsylvania Hospital in 1925. There is a single value of 12 days; all other values are 2 or fewer. The median is 0 days; that is, over half of the patients with a fracture had an x ray done on the day of admission. Whether this value or the mean value of 1.63 days is best for estimating the speed with which x rays were done is a matter of judgment.

81. New York Hospital Medical Board, February 25, 1916.

82. George E. Burch and Nicholas P. DePasquale, *A History of Electrocardiography* (1964; reprint, San Francisco: Norman Publishing, 1990); John Burnett, "The Origins of the Electrocardiograph as a Clinical Instrument," *Medical History*, supp. no. 5 (1985): 53–76.

83. The cost of installation was said to be about $215 and the annual cost of maintenance $60. No details are given about financial arrangements for the person who was to run the machine. Minutes of the Medical Board, September 25, 1914; October 30, 1914; and November 17, 1914.

84. The x ray was purchased with funds from a number of donors. See the 170th annual report, for 1921, 12.

85. The fees were $1.00 for ward patients, except for those taken for study, which should be marked "experimental." Private patient fees were to be $15–$25. Medical Board, to Cussler, September 15, 1924.

86. Brecher and Brecher, *The Rays*; see also Paul C. Hodges, "Development of Diagnostic X-ray Apparatus during the First Fifty Years," *Radiology* 45 (1945): 438–48. For an amusing contemplation about what were perceived as the major technical problems in 1916, see "A Radiologists Dream," *American Journal of Roentgenology* 3 (1916): 450–51.

87. Joel D. Howell, "Early Perceptions of the Electrocardiogram: From Arrhythmia to Infarction," *Bulletin of the History of Medicine* 83 (1984): 83–98.

88. On technical changes in the use of the electrocardiogram, see Joel D. Howell, "Frank Norman Wilson: Theory, Technology, and Electrocardiography," in *Medical Lives and Scientific Medicine at Michigan,*

1891–1969, edited by J. D. Howell, 101–27 (Ann Arbor: University of Michigan Press, 1993).

89. The increase in receipts is similar to that for the number of exams performed, although exact data on the totals for exams are not available.

90. Alfred D. Chandler, *The Visible Hand: The Managerial Revolution in American Business* (Cambridge, Mass.: Harvard University Press, 1977).

91. A. H. Busby, to Executive Committee of the New York Hospital, file of the secretary-treasurer, box 39, folder 3.

92. Busby noted in 1912 that inadequate facilities had caused the New York Hospital department to lose "over 200 valuable plates." Undated memo to the Medical Board, box for 1912.

93. See note from Underwood and Underwood, Inc., "Every Kind of Photographic Work," to the Committee of the Medical Board of the New York Hospital, offering to show a visitor how the company files its negatives. Undated letter, in group from 1916, box 48, folder 10.

94. On specialization in general in the U.S. context, see Stevens, *American Medicine.*

95. Hirsch, "Hospital X-ray Laboratory," 13.

96. The precise mechanism by which those who operated an x-ray machine in a hospital were to be paid was a long-standing concern. See, for examples from two different decades, "The Attitude of the Medical Profession towards Roentgenology" (editorial), *American Journal of Roentgenology* 2 (1915): 912–13; W. Edward Chamberlain, "Radiology as a Medical Specialty," *JAMA* 92 (1929): 1033–35.

97. Arthur V. Desjardins, "The Status of Radiology in America," *JAMA* 92 (1929): 1035–39—at a late enough date that one might have suspected the debate over status was over. This comment implies that it was not.

98. Hirsch, "Hospital X-ray Laboratory," 92–97.

99. By way of comparison, in 1896 you could have a half-gallon of milk delivered to the door for less than $0.14. The average industrial worker (excluding farm laborers) earned $462 per year, the average public school teacher $294, and the average minister $764. *Historical Statistics of the United States: Colonial Times to 1970, Part 1* (Washington, D.C.: Government Printing Office, 1975), 168, 213.

100. Morton (at no. 19, E. 28th St.), to Stieglitz, May 25, and June 10, 1896, New York Academy of Medicine Archives, MS 1048. It is interesting that some hospital annual reports, such as those for the New York Hospital, listed "negative cases" as a separate entry in their listing of uses of x rays. William James Morton received an M.D. degree from Harvard in 1872. He worked extensively with electricity as well as x rays and was the chair of Diseases of the Mind and Nervous System and Electro-therapeutics at the New York Post-Graduate Medical School. See James Joseph Walsh, *History of Medicine in New York: Three Centuries of Medical Progress* (New York: National Americana Society, 1919), 394–98; and Brecher and Brecher, *The Rays,* 61–62.

101. Stevens, *American Medicine and the Public Interest*.
102. Such stamps were found in other hospitals as well, and perhaps earlier at the Massachusetts General Hospital. Reiser, *Medicine*, 207; and "Creating Form out of Mass: The Development of the Medical Record," in Everett Mendelssohn, ed., *Transformation and Tradition in the Sciences: Essays in Honor of I. Bernard Cohen* (New York: Cambridge University Press, 1984), 303–16.
103. Henry E. Sigerist, "An Outline of the Development of the Hospital," *Bulletin of the History of Medicine* 4 (1936): 573–81.

CHAPTER 5: THE X-RAY IMAGE

This chapter is a direct result of being asked to give a talk on medical technology at the University of Michigan Institute for the Humanities, as part of the theme for 1991–92, "Histories of Sexuality." I am grateful for the invitation to the acting director for that year, Domna Stanton, and to the director, James Winn, as well as to the participants in that seminar, for their thoughtful comments, which have improved the chapter greatly.

1. Thomas Laqueur, "Orgasm, Generation, and the Politics of Reproductive Biology," *Representations* 14 (1986): 1–41.
2. Of course, we now choose to understand the "laws of physics" themselves in a specific social context. I do not wish to privilege that form of knowing called "physics" over other forms of knowing. Nor do I wish to explore the endless and, for purposes of this chapter, futile debate over how far one may consider knowledge to be socially constructed and when, or if, one comes across some basic, immutable physical reality. I may summarize my position briefly. I am, in general, quite sympathetic to a radical social construction view of knowledge. There are, however, limits to how far one can push such an analysis. One of those limits lies in the use of machines. An x-ray machine will not, try as one might, fly a person to the moon. Nor will it bring the dead to life. Which is my second point of ultimate reality, one that cannot be avoided in any discussion of matters medical. And that is, dead is dead. Our definitions at the margins may change (is "brain-dead" dead?), and we may debate the existence of a hereafter, but death, unlike disease, appears for the time being to be grounded firmly in a physical reality. For a cogent discussion of the limits of relativism and the finality of death, see Charles E. Rosenberg, "Disease and Social Order in America," in *AIDS: The Burdens of History*, edited by Elizabeth Fee and Daniel M. Fox, 12–32 (Berkeley: University of California Press, 1988).
3. For an introduction to much of the excellent work in this area, a good place to start is Charles E. Rosenberg and Janet Golden, eds., *Framing Disease: Studies in Cultural History* (New Brunswick: Rutgers University Press, 1992).

4. Recent scholarship has shown that this continues to be true in fields from clinical trials to court decisions. Gender clearly continues to be a central theme, even in such areas as science and law which might seem at first to be "objective" and thus independent of such influences.

5. For discussion of the ways in which visual evidence has unique properties, see Barbara Marie Stafford, *Body Criticism: Imaging the Unseen in Enlightenment Art and Medicine* (Cambridge, Mass.: MIT Press, 1991).

6. Nancy Knight, " 'The New Light': X Rays and Medical Futurism," in *Imagining Tomorrow: History, Technology, and the American Future*, edited by Joseph J. Corn, 10–34 (Cambridge, Mass.: MIT Press, 1986); C. F. Lacombe, "The Roentgen Ray," *Transactions of the Colorado Medical Society* (1896): 261–78.

7. The volume of works devoted to x rays is immense. For an excellent area study of coverage about the rays, see J. H. T. Connor, "The Adoption and Effects of X-rays in Ontario," *Ontario History* 74 (1987): 92–107.

8. This continues to be the case. As many generations of medical students can attest, seeing the illustrations of, say, the tissue planes for a hernia repair, no matter how clearly they may appear, is a far cry from actually differentiating those planes at the operating table.

9. Ludmilla Jordanova, Chapter 7, "Medical Images of the Female Body," *Sexual Visions: Images of Gender in Science and Medicine between the Eighteenth and Twentieth Centuries* (New York: Harvester Wheatsheaf, 1989), 135–59.

10. For one of many reproductions, see Herbert S. Klickstein, *Wilhelm Conrad Röntgen: On a New Kind of Rays*, vol. 1 (N.P.: Mallinckrodt Classics of Radiology, 1966).

11. Early work with the x-ray tube used a variety of devices to make the image accessible to human viewing. When recorded on a glass plate, the image was called a plate, a skiagram (from the Greek for *shadow*), and a roentgenogram, among other things.

Images were also observed on fluoroscopes. I shall not pay as much attention to these images, which were not transportable, as I shall to the forms of images that could be easily moved and reproduced. Moreover, it was the photographic images that attracted the most attention and were seen as the most interesting. See R. W. Wood, "Photographing the Unseen: A Symposium on the Roentgen Rays," *Century Magazine* 52 (n. ser. 30) (1896): 122–25.

12. James R. Beniger, *The Control Revolution: Technological and Economic Origins of the Information Society* (Cambridge, Mass.: Harvard University Press, 1986), 356–62; Martha Banta, *Imaging American Women: Idea and Ideals in Cultural History* (New York: Columbia University Press, 1987); Bram Dijkstra, *Idols of Perversity: Fantasies of Feminine Evil in Fin-de-Siècle Culture* (New York: Oxford University Press, 1986).

13. Stephen Fox, *The Mirror Makers: A History of American Advertising and Its Creators* (New York: Morrow, 1984), 34.

14. D. W. Hering, "A Year of the X-rays," *Popular Science Monthly* 50 (1896–97): 654–62.
15. *New York Times*, January 16, 1896, 9.
16. See Brecher and Brecher, *The Rays*, 24–25; and E. R. N. Grigg, *The Trail of the Invisible Light* (Springfield, Ill.: Charles C Thomas, 1965), 9–11.
17. Knight, "The New Light"; Frank R. Victor, "The Magic Eye: A Brief History of the Use of X-ray in Kansas," *Journal of the Kansas Medical Society* 68 (1967): 300–306.
18. *New York Times*, May 9, 1898, 14. This kind of reaction persists in the late twentieth century. Upon hearing this history one physician related the following story: while she was a second-year medical student, she had a chest x-ray image taken as part of an evaluation for what was eventually determined to be a benign, self-limiting condition. When shown the x ray she noted her ribs tapering toward her waist (which is quite small) and was quite surprised at how beautiful she found the image. She was also somewhat amazed at her reaction, quite troubled by the intensity of her feelings, and had never before felt comfortable telling anyone about her reaction. Anonymous communication to author, August 13, 1992.
19. Thomas Mann, *The Magic Mountain* (1924; reprint, New York: Vintage Books, 1969; translated in 1927), 348–49.
20. For an overview, see Ingrid D. Ebner and Glen P. Jenkins, *Skeletons in Our Closet: Skeletal Illustration as Represented in the Rare Book Collection of the Cleveland Health Sciences Library* (Cleveland: Cleveland Health Sciences Library, 1983.)
21. Mann, *Magic Mountain*, 218–19. The association of death and love is, of course, a common theme in art and literature, perhaps most beautifully expressed in Richard Wagner's opera *Tristan und Isolde*.
22. Lacombe, "Roentgen Ray." The ubiquity of hands as subjects was noted by Thomas Commerford Martin, the editor of the *Electrical Engineer*, who noted that, "while a large proportion of the inhabitants of the United States have had their hands 'taken,' only a single foot, so far as the writer is aware, has been made to reveal the secrets of its flesh-clad anatomy." In "Photographing the Unseen," 120–22.
23. *Electrical Engineer* 21 (June 3, 1896): 600.
24. C. H. T. Crosthwaite, "Röntgen's Curse," *Longman's Magazine* 28 (1896): 469–84.
25. The choice of surname is probably not accidental.
26. As Christopher Lawrence has pointed out, English physicians of the period were distinguished for their classical learning and their temperament and had little use for the new scientific paraphernalia. "Incommunicable Knowledge: Science, Technology, and the Clinical Act in Britain, 1850–1914," *Journal of Contemporary History* 20 (1985): 503–20.
27. Otto Glasser, ed., *The Science of Radiology* (Springfield, Ill.: Charles C Thomas, 1933), 8. Also noted as a humorous aside under "The Humour of It," *Photography* 8, no. 385 (March 26, 1896): 217.

28. Samuel D. Warren and Louis D. Brandeis, "The Right to Privacy," *Harvard Law Review* 4 (1890): 193–220.
29. "Scientific Inquisitors," *Littel's Living Age* 208 (March 21, 1896): 822–23.
30. *Wilson's Photo Magazine* 33 (1896); quoting the *Detroit Free Press.* Citation supplied by Nancy Knight.
31. From "The New Photography," *Punch* (London), January 25, 1896, 45. The poem is (mis)quoted in Glasser, *Science of Radiology,* 9, in which *off* in the second line of the excerpt is omitted.
32. Alice L. Callander, "A Debt to Science," *Argosy* 26 (1898): 105–15.
33. "The New Photographic Discovery," *Punch*, January 25, 1896, 45.
34. *Critic* 28 (January 18, 1896): 45–46; and 29 (August 22, 1896): 199–20.
35. Cited in Knight, "New Light."
36. *Punch* (January 25, 1896), 117.
37. "Reading the Contents of Envelopes," *Photography* 8, no. 381 (February 27, 1896): 145.
38. Julius F. Sachse, "The Roentgen (X) Rays," *American Journal of Photography* 17 (March 1896): 97–99. This article lists a number of amusing and erroneous claims made about the x ray but reports the bill being introduced as fact, suggesting that the bill may have actually been read. *Electrical Engineer* 21 (1896): 216. This citation, which indicates the laugh, was kindly supplied by Nancy Knight. Grigg also suggests that it was in jest. The event has been transmuted, in at least one article, into a claim that such a bill was actually passed. John L. Greenway, "Penetrating Surfaces: X-Rays, Strindlberg, and the *Ghost Sonata*," *Nineteenth Century Studies* 5 (1991): 31.
39. The newspapers of record for the New Jersey Legislature appear to have been the *Trenton Times* and the *Daily True American.* These newspapers listed the bills introduced in each chamber for each day the legislature was in session. A careful search of the listings from February 19 through February 28, 1896, failed to reveal any evidence of the alleged bill.
40. A quotation from the *Scarborough Post,* in "The New Horror," *Photography* 8, no. 381 (February 27, 1896): 146–47. For more examples of talk about the early x ray, presented so as to emphasize the foolish speculation, see Otto Glasser, *William Conrad Röntgen* (Springfield, Ill.: Charles C Thomas, 1934), esp. chap. 20, "Röntgen's Discovery in Contemporary Humor: Curious Suggestions on the Production of Röntgen Rays," 364–75.
41. "The Textile Wonder: 'Textile Buckskin,' in the *Toronto Globe,* February 27, 1896. Photocopy kindly supplied by Nancy Knight. See also "Commercial Application of X-rays," *Electrical World* 27 (March 28, 1896): 339, in which the "commercial application" of x rays by selling underclothing to women is noted to be making prey of ignorant women. See also Glasser, *Science of Radiology,* 8; Brecher and Brecher, *The Rays,* 25.

42. *Electrical Engineer* 21 (April 15, 1896): 377.

43. *Photography* (London), February 1896; quoted in Grigg, *Trail of the Invisible Light*, 33.

44. Linda Dalrymple Henderson, "X Rays and the Quest for Invisible Reality in the Art of Kupka, Duchamp, and the Cubists," *Art Journal* 47 (1988): 323–40; "Francis Picabia, Radiometers, and X-rays in 1913," *Art Bulletin* 71 (1989): 114–23.

45. *Life* 27, no. 687, February 27, 1896, 151.

46. S. G., in *The World*; quoted in *Photographic Times* 29 (July 1897): 347.

47. On Mann's use of the x ray to symbolize the "inner heart," see Peter Brooks, *Body Work: Objects of Desire in Modern Narrative* (Cambridge, Mass.: Harvard University Press, 1993), 263–65. This type of belief in the underlying importance of that part of a person's being which is hidden from view may have been related to the work being done at about the same time by Freud. The connection, however, is far from clear. Although Freud had already started his seminal writings on the unconscious when the x ray was first invented, his work was not particularly well-known in the United States at this time.

48. *The Complete Bachelor: Manners for Men* (New York: D. Appleton, 1897), 136. This book was a guide to etiquette. For another early example of the tube being perceived as rendering all things visible, see the cartoon of a tube saying "I see right through you" to a top-hatted image of a globe in a cartoon, in *Life* 27, no. 687, February 27, 1896, 153.

49. "Cathode Ray Criticism on 'Jude,'" *Life* 27, no. 687, February 27, 1896, 156.

50. "News Items," *Chicago Medical Recorder* 11 (1896): 295. *American Journal of Photography* (March 1896); citation supplied by Nancy Knight.

51. "Ordinary Photography and 'New Photography,'" *Life* 27, April 6, 1896; cited in Glasser, *William Conrad Röntgen*, 365.

52. A. Judson Quimby, "Laboratory Notes on Radiography," *Post-Graduate* 27 (1912): 174–89.

53. *Photographic Times*, September 1896; citation supplied by Nancy Knight. Also noted in "The Humour of It," *Photography* 8, no. 389, April 23, 1896, 279; and "The New Photography," *Electrical Engineer* 21, (March 13, 1896): 284.

54. *New York Times*, May 9, 1898, 14.

55. This discussion is based in large part on Ornella Moscucci, *The Science of Woman: Gynaecology and Gender in England, 1800–1929* (Cambridge: Cambridge University Press, 1990).

56. Elaine Showalter, *Sexual Anarchy: Gender and Culture at the Fin de Siècle* (New York: Viking, 1990).

57. The ways in which the ideas were expressed, particularly having to do with seeing into women, penetration, etc., are suggestive of other metaphors. It would be historically interesting to consider more closely if there were differences between the ways looking into men and

women were described, particularly around other "looking into" technologies, such as the ophthalmoscope or the cystoscope

58. Virginia G. Drachman, "The Loomis Trial: Social Mores and Obstetrics in the Mid-Nineteenth Century," in *Women and Health in America*, edited by Judith Walzer Leavitt, 166–74 (Madison: University of Wisconsin Press, 1984).

59. I am indebted to a seminar audience at the History Department of Indiana University in December 1992 for an insightful discussion of the nineteenth-century American gaze and its implications.

60. "Observations on Clinical Obstetrics," *New York Medical Gazette;* reprinted in *Medical News and Library* (October 9, 1850): 83–84; and quoted in Jane B. Donegan, " 'Safe Delivered, but by Whom?' Midwives and Man-Midwives in Early America," in Leavitt, *Women and Health,* 302–17.

61. Thomas Dixon Savill, *A System of Clinical Medicine,* 3d ed. (New York: William Wood, 1912), 436.

62. Mary Poovey, "Scenes of an Indelicate Character: The Medical 'Treatment' of Victorian Women," *Representations* 14 (1986): 137–68. The nineteenth-century American physician Samuel Gregory, quoting the French naturalist Count Buffon, *Man-Midwifery Exposed and Corrected* (1848); reprinted in *The Male Mid-wife and the Female Doctor: The Gynecology Controversy in Nineteenth Century America* (New York: Arno Press, 1974), 46.

63. For an overview of this subject I am indebted to Susan Lederer for allowing me to review her unpublished manuscript, "The New Photography: X-rays and Obstetrics in the Early Twentieth Century."

64. Edward P. Davis, "The Application of the Röntgen Rays, Part 3: The Study of the Infant's Body and of the Pregnant Womb by the Röntgen Rays," *American Journal of the Medical Sciences* 111 (1896): 263–70. On Davis, see James H. Lee, "Department of Obstetrics and Gynecology," in *Thomas Jefferson University: Tradition and Heritage,* edited by Frederick B. Wagner, 720–22 (Philadelphia: Lea and Febiger, 1989).

65. Sidney Lange, "The Present Status of the Roentgen Ray," *Lancet-Clinic* (Cincinnati) 58 (1907): 79–89.

66. At this early stage of work with the x ray there was not a great deal being said or written about potential dangers to the fetus or the mother from exposure to x rays. By shortly around the turn of the century some authors were expressing concern, based in part on experimental evidence. See William Rollins, "Notes on X-light," *Boston Medical and Surgical Journal* 146 (1902): 221; Ronald L. Kathren, "William H. Rollins (1852–1929): X-ray Protection Pioneer," *Journal of the History of Medicine and Allied Sciences* 19 (1964): 287–94. Long exposures were a consistent problem for work in obstetrics, due to the enlarged abdomen of pregnant women. Until the 1940s and the 1950s most obstetricians felt that x rays posed little threat to women or their fetuses. On this, see Anja Hiddinga, "X-ray Technology in Obstetrics: Measuring

Pelves at the Yale School of Medicine," in *Medical Innovations in Historical Perspective,* edited by John V. Pickstone, 124–45 (New York: St. Martin's Press, 1992).

67. I am indebted to Regina Markell Morantz-Sanchez for this observation.

68. Lacombe, "Roentgen Ray." See also Frank Leech, "The Roentgen Rays: Illustrated by Sixteen Photographs," *Maryland Medical Journal* 35 (1896): 345–48. Pregnant women were also used as markers for toxicity; it was noted that one was exposed to the beam for two hours without ill effect, though no mention was made of why. A series of three papers offering contrasting opinions about the efficacy of radiology for the diagnosis of pregnancy is useful: Dr. DeLee, "The Uses of the X-ray in Obstetrics," *Journal of the American Medical Association (JAMA)* 58 (1912): 750; Angus McLean and P. M. Hickey, "X-Ray Diagnosis of Pregnancy," ibid., 751; and Patrick S. O'Donnel, "X-ray Findings in the Differential Diagnosis of Early and Late Pregnancies," ibid., 748–49.

69. W. A. Newman Dorland and Maximilian John Hubeny, *The X-ray in Embryology and Obstetrics* (St. Paul, Minn.: Bruce Publishing, 1926), 259.

70. Norman Prince, *Roentgen Technic (Diagnostic)* (St. Louis: Mosby, 1917), 31. The pictures here are very interesting, in that the technician is a woman and the model patient is frequently an often unclad woman. Another explicit statement that the woman should wear a chemise is in H. Varnier, "Pelviography and Pelvimetry by Means of X-rays," Report to 12th International Medical Congress in Moscow in 1897, in André J. Bruwer, *Classic Descriptions in Diagnostic Roentgenology* (Springfield, Ill.: Charles C Thomas, 1964), 358–61.

71. *Electrical Engineer* 21 (June 3, 1896).

72. Crane, "X-Ray Clinic," 217–19.

73. Quimby, "Laboratory Notes," 182.

74. George E. Pfahler, "The Use of Roentgen Rays in the Treatment of Gynaecological Conditions," *American Journal of Roentgenology* 1(1913–14): 65–73.

75. *New York Times,* May 9, 1898, 14.

76. Davis, "The Study of the Infant's Body."

77. William Osler, *The Principles and Practice of Medicine* (New York: D. Appleton, 1892), 767. Similar descriptions may be found in most other standard textbooks.

78. Rosalind Pollack Petchesky, "Foetal Images: the Power of Visual Culture in the Politics of Reproduction," in *Reproductive Technologies: Gender, Motherhood, and Medicine,* edited by Michelle Stanworth, 59–80 (Cambridge: Polity Press, 1987).

79. The P value indicates that were the null hypothesis true—that is, were there no difference in the likelihood of x-ray use for men and women—one would expect to see differences of the magnitude noted in the sample less than once in one thousand samples. That is unlikely enough by standard criteria to assume that, in fact, there is a difference.

80. The difference in the incidence of broken limbs reflects differences in occupation between men and women. This, too, reflects differing perceptions of gender but in the area of appropriate employment rather than health care.

81. Some measure of class would have been useful. Such measures, however, are difficult to derive from patient charts. Occupation is one useful surrogate, but, as many women did not work, that value is missing more for women than for men, a difference that would skew the results. Correlating the patient's address with a knowledge of the city's geography would be another, extremely labor-intensive approach. Even using that approach, people who worked as household servants would lead to confusion, as their address would indicate a higher class than would be accurate.

82. As the outcome of interest is dichotomous (i.e., either a person did or did not have an x-ray image taken), it can be represented as either a 0 or a 1. This is then called the dependent variable. The technique is described in most standard statistical texts.

The independent variables used for the calculation were as follows:

XRAY: Dependent variable, 0 = no x ray, 1 = x-ray image taken.

SEX: Male = 1, Female = 2.

AGE: Continuous variable, from 0 to 85

YEAR2, YEAR3, YEAR4: Dummy variable for the years 1909, 1920, and 1925 (so that each is compared to the year 1900).

NATDUM: Dummy variable for nationality, U.S. vs. foreign.

XRAYPROB: A correction for the diagnosis. In order to estimate the equation, I aggregated the detailed diagnoses into larger groups (i.e., combining all cardiac valvular disease into a single category). All remaining diagnoses with fewer than ten patients were not included. This led to a fall in the total number of cases included in the analysis. For each remaining diagnosis I calculated the probability of having a x-ray image taken. That value was then included in the overall logistic regression as a case-mix adjustment.

RACED1, RACED2: White or "colored." The equation was run with RACED2 as the omitted variable.

See table N.1, p. 306.

83. Pennsylvania Board of Managers, meetings in the fall of 1920. The burns were as a result of treatment, not the diagnostic use of x rays, but the impact of local attitudes probably covered both types of use.

84. Pennsylvania Hospital, Board of Managers, September 24, 1923.

85. Owen Tully, *Medicine Man* (Norman: University of Oklahoma Press, 1989), 192.

86. Though somewhat less so. The P value indicates that one would see such a difference approximately 25 times in 1,000.

87. Values are defined as for the analysis of the Pennsylvania Hospital. See table N.2, p. 307.

Table N.1 *Logit Estimates*

Log Likelihood = −216.098

Number of obs = 1,041
Chi-square (8) = 270.19
Prob > chi-square = 0.0000

XRAY	Odds Ratio	Standard Error	t	P > |t|	[95% Confidence Interval]	
SEX	.535	.155	−2.158	0.031	.303	.944
AGE	1.014	.007	2.042	0.041	1.000	1.028
XRAYPROB	8308.075	6814.892	11.002	0.000	1661.356	41546.850
YEAR 2	6.864	4.387	3.014	0.003	1.958	24.058
YEAR 3	36.527	22.485	5.845	0.000	10.914	122.242
YEAR 4	70.778	44.200	6.821	0.000	20.783	241.039
NATDUM	.862	.255	−0.499	0.618	.481	1.543
RACED 1	.798	.273	−0.656	0.512	.407	1.563

XRAY	Coefficient	Standard Error	t	P > |t|	[95% Confidence Interval]	
SEX	−.625	.289	−2.158	0.031	−1.193	−.056
AGE	.014	.007	2.042	0.041	.000	.028
XRAYPROB	9.024	.820	11.002	0.000	7.415	10.634
YEAR 2	1.926	.639	3.014	0.003	.672	3.180
YEAR 3	3.598	.615	5.845	0.000	2.390	4.806
YEAR 4	4.259	.624	6.821	0.000	3.034	5.484
NATDUM	−.147	.296	−0.499	0.618	−.730	.434
RACED 1	−.224	.342	−0.656	0.512	−.896	.447
_cons	−6.090	.901	−6.759	0.000	−7.858	−4.322

Note: The analysis was run on a microcomputer using STATA, a statistical program written by Computing Resource Center, Santa Monica, Calif.

Table N.2 *Logit Estimates*

Log Likelihood = −66.28712

Number of obs = 501
Chi-square (6) = 83.36
Prob > chi-square = 0.0000

XRAY	Odds Ratio	Standard Error	t	P > |t|	[95% Confidence Interval]	
SEX	1.851	.896	1.272	0.204	.714	4.792
AGE	1.019	.014	1.427	0.154	.992	1.047
XRAYPROB	5311828.000	1.47e+07	5.580	0.000	22771.240	1.24e+09
YEAR 2	19.339	22.339	2.564	0.011	1.998	187.107
YEAR 3	86.960	103.055	3.768	0.000	8.474	892.368
NATDUM	.468	.230	−1.540	0.124	.177	1.232

XRAY	Coefficient	Standard Error	t	P > |t|	[95% Confidence Interval]	
SEX	.615	.4841	1.272	0.204	−.335	1.567
AGE	.019	.0137	1.427	0.154	−.007	.046
XRAYPROB	15.485	2.7749	5.580	0.000	10.033	20.937
YEAR 2	2.962	1.1551	2.564	0.011	.692	5.231
YEAR 3	4.465	1.1850	3.768	0.000	2.137	6.793
NATDUM 1	−.758	.4926	−1.540	0.124	−1.726	.209
_cons	−8.601	1.5239	−5.644	0.000	−11.595	−5.607

88. Thomas McKeown, *Role of Medicine: Dream, Mirage, or Nemesis?* (Princeton: Princeton University Press, 1979).

89. Lacombe, "Roentgen Ray."

90. Stephen Kern, *The Culture of Time and Space: 1880–1918* (Cambridge, Mass.: Harvard University Press, 1983).

91. Lange, "Present Status of the Roentgen Ray."

92. H. Kennon Dunham, quoted in Homer L. Sampson, "Diagnosis by X-rays," in *The Story of Clinical Tuberculosis*, edited by L. Brown, 212–32 (Baltimore: Williams and Wilkins, 1941), 226. Also *Archives of the Roentgen Ray* 17 (1913): 477–85. Some physicians at the time were not unaware of the dangers inherent in placing too much faith in x-ray images. See Barron H. Lerner, "The Perils of 'X-ray Vision': How Radiographic Images Have Historically Influenced Perception," *Perspectives in Biology and Medicine* 35 (1992): 382–97.

93. This use of technology often serves to strengthen the position of men, but women may also benefit. Patricia A. Cooper has nicely demonstrated such an event for women in the cigar industry. "What This Country Needs Is a Good Five Cent Cigar," *Technology and Culture* 29 (1988): 779–807.

94. On obstetrics, see Hiddinga, "X-ray Technology."

95. See, for example, H. J. W. Dam, "The New Marvel in Photography," *McClure's Magazine* 6, April 1896, 403–20.

96. James Burry, "A Preliminary Report on the Roentgen or X-rays," *JAMA* 26 (1896): 402–4.

97. Such as Walter J. Dodd at the Massachusetts General Hospital. He eventually obtained an M.D. degree. John A. Macy, *Walter James Dodd: A Biographical Sketch* (Boston: Houghton Mifflin, 1918); Frederick A. Washburn, *The Massachusetts General Hospital: Its Development, 1900–1935* (Boston: Houghton Mifflin, 1939).

98. "Editorial Department," *American Journal of Roentgenology* 1 (October 1906).

99. Prince, *Roentgen Technique*, 129–30,

100. Board of Managers, May 5, 1913. Other hospitals had similar rules. For example, *Rules for the Internal Government of the Hospital of the Protestant Episcopal Church in Philadelphia* (1905) notes that "all plates are the property of the hospital."

101. Lange, "Present Status of the Roentgen Ray."

102. E. H. Skinner, "The Ownership of X-ray Plates: Patient and Medical Attendant Entitled to Radiologist's Opinion, Not the Plate," *Modern Hospital* 1 (1913): 30–31.

103. For example, a patient who had been hospitalized for two years with multiple drug–resistant tuberculosis as well as infection with the human immunodeficiency virus in the 1990s was kind enough to attend a teaching conference for medical students. During the preclass preparation, when a slide of his complex chest x ray was flashed on the screen, he was able both to identify it as his own and to interpret it far

more rapidly than either the pulmonary or the infectious diseases specialists who were present. University of Michigan, M2 Multidisciplinary Conference, September 10, 1993.

104. Richard Harrison Shryock, *Medical Licensing in America, 1650–1965* (Baltimore: Johns Hopkins Press, 1967).

105. Walter I. Wardwell, "Chiropractors: Evolution to Acceptance," in *Other Healers: Unorthodox Medicine in America*, edited by Norman Gevitz, 157–91 (Baltimore: Johns Hopkins University Press, 1988).

106. Steven C. Martin, "Chiropractic and the Social Context of Medical Technology, 1895–1925." MS. I am grateful to Dr. Martin for his thoughts on the subject and for allowing me to review the manuscript.

107. William G. Rothstein, *American Physicians in the Nineteenth Century: From Sects to Science* (Baltimore: Johns Hopkins University Press, 1972), 345.

108. William H. Dieffenbach, "A Brief Historical Review and the Present Status of Roentgenotherapy," *Hahnemannian Monthly* 58 (1923): 711–20.

109. See Rollin H. Stevens, "The Coolidge Tube in Roentgen Therapy," *American Institute of Homeopathy Journal* 8 (1915–16): 409–18. Stevens was a former president of the association and liked the tube because it gave constant, reproducible results. In the discussion Dieffenbach noted that "it is not the X-ray that does the curing": "It is the reaction of the patient's organism to these rays that produce changes. A dose of the Coolidge tube radiation will produce remedial changes by means of *curative fibrosis* which we look for."

110. Martin Kaufman, *Homeopathy in America: The Rise and Fall of a Medical Heresy* (Baltimore: Johns Hopkins Press, 1971).

111. Regina Morantz-Sanchez, "So Honored, So Loved? The Women's Medical Movement in Decline," in *"Send Us a Lady Physician": Women Doctors in America, 1835–1920*, edited by Ruth J. Abrams, 231–45 (New York: W. W. Norton, 1985); Mary Roth Walsh, *"Doctors Wanted, No Women Need Apply": Sexual Barriers in the Medical Profession, 1835–1975* (New Haven: Yale University Press, 1977), 186.

112. Robert Herrick, "In the Doctor's Office," *Scribner's Magazine* 42, January 1908, 105–15.

113. There are a disproportionate number of men among the leadership positions. The absolute numbers of female physicians are certainly changing, however. See Regina Morantz-Sanchez, *Sympathy and Science: Women Physicians in American Medicine* (New York: Oxford University Press, 1985), for a discussion of whether there are clear practice differences between male and female physicians.

114. On Sloan, see Peter Morse, *John Sloan's Prints: A Catalogue Raissoné of the Etchings, Lithographs, and Posters* (New Haven: Yale University Press, 1969); and Rowland Elzea and Elizabeth Hawkes, *John Sloan: Spectator of Life* (Wilmington: Delaware Art Museum, 1988). Alternate

titles for the work were "Fluoroscope" and "Department of the Interior." I am grateful to Rebecca Zurier for sharing her insights into John Sloan as well as her thoughts about this etching.

115. Diane R. Karp, *Ars Medica: Art, Medicine, and the Human Condition* (Philadelphia: Philadelphia Museum of Art, 1985), pl. 45, p. 184.

116. Samuel Osherson and Lorna Amara Singham, "The Machine Metaphor in Medicine," in *Social Contexts of Health, Illness, and Patient Care,* Elliot G. Mishler, Lorna Amara Singham, Stuart Hanser, Samuel Osherson, Nancy E. Waxler, and Ramsey Liem (Cambridge: Cambridge University Press, 1981).

117. Stafford, *Body Criticism;* also Henderson, "X Rays and the Quest for Invisible Reality"; and "Francis Picabia."

118. Lana F. Rakow, "Gendered Technology, Gendered Practice," *Critical Studies in Mass Communication* 5 (1988): 68.

119. Jonathan M. Liebenau, "Medicine and Technology," *Perspectives in Biology and Medicine* 27 (1983): 76–92.

120. Diego Rivera used radium as a major theme in some of his other work.

121. I am indebted to participants in a December 1992 seminar at Yale University for insights into this artwork.

122. Evelyn Fox Keller and Christine R. Grontkowski, "The Mind's Eye," in *Discovering Reality: Feminist Perspectives on Epistemology, Metaphysics, Methodology and the Philosophy of Science,* edited by Sandra Harding and Merrill B. Hintikka, 207–24 (Dordrecht: Reidel, 1983); Annette Kuhn, *Women's Pictures: Feminism and Cinema* (London: Routledge and Kegan Paul, 1982), 60–65. Kuhn argues that one cannot understand cinema without also understanding the conditions of reception of each film. One can take a similar perspective with respect to x-ray films. Laura Mulvey, "Visual Pleasure and Narrative Cinema," *Screen* 16 (1975): 6–18; E. A. Kaplan, "Is the Gaze Male?" in *Powers of Desire,* edited by Ann Snitow, Christine Stansell, and Sharon Thompson, 309–27 (New York: Monthly Review Press, 1983).

CHAPTER 6: BLOOD AND BLOOD COUNTS

1. A. Schierbeek, *Measuring the Invisible World: The Life and Times of Antoni van Leeuwenhoek* (London: Abelard-Schuman, 1959), 109.

2. *Medical News* (Philadelphia) 56 (1890): 399.

3. Andrew H. Smith, "Prognosis in Pneumonia," *Medical Record* 49 (1896): 649–51. Willson [sic] O. Bridges, "The Significance of Blood Examinations in Disease," *Western Medical Review* 1 (1896): 26–29. A buffy coat was also said to be present in patients with chlorosis, "on account of the deficiency in the number of white corpuscles." Thomas L. Stedman, *A Dictionary of Medical Science* by Robley Dunglison, 23d ed. (Philadelphia: Lea Brothers, 1903), 284. For an earlier description, see Austin Flint, *A Treatise on the Principles and Practice of*

Medicine, 3d ed. (Philadelphia: Henry C. Lea, 1868), 74. Thus, although we now define the buffy coat as the presence of excessive numbers of white corpuscles, it had a very different meaning before the blood was routinely examined.

4. G. Andral, *An Essay on Blood in Disease,* (Philadelphia: Lea and Blanchard, 1844). For a general discussion of some pioneers in looking at blood, see Camille Dreyfus, *Some Milestones in the History of Hematology* (New York: Grune and Stratton, 1957). Also highly recommended as a unique essay is A.H.T.R.S. (presumably A. H. T. Robb-Smith), "The History of the Hedgehog's Rosary," *St. Bartholomew's Hospital Journal* 40 (1933): 149–52, 166–68, 211–16, 238–40; and 41 (1933): 13–15.

5. The method, although slow, yielded results similar to those we now accept as normal. His 1851 estimation of 5,174,400 red blood cells per cubic millimeter of (his own) blood may be favorably compared to today's accepted normal range for adult men of 4,300,000 to 5,900,000. For more on Vierordt, see W. D. Foster, *A Short History of Clinical Pathology* (Edinburgh and London: E. and S. Livingstone, 1961), 95; W. H. Major, "Karl Vierordt," *Annals of Medical History* n.s. 10 (1938): 463–73.

6. Gowers was best known for his interest in the nervous system. In addition to his work on techniques for counting blood corpuscles, Gowers enjoyed constructing other devices, such as a "safety hypodermic syringe" to prevent overdosage and a magnifying otoscope to look into the ear. M. L. Verso, "Some Nineteenth-Century Pioneers of Haemotology," *Medical History* 15 (1971): 55–67; "The Evolution of Blood-Counting Techniques," *Medical History* 8 (1964): 149–58; Macdonald Critchley, *Sir William Gowers, 1845–1915: A Biographical Appreciation* (London: William Heinemann, 1949).

7. E. Buchanan Baxter and Frederick Willcocks, "Contribution to Clinical Haemometry," *Lancet* 1 (1880): 361–62, 397–99, 439–41.

8. George Dock, "Clinical Pathology in the Eighties and Nineties," *American Journal of Clinical Pathology* 16 (1946): 671–80.

9. See Horace Gray, "Cell-Counting Technic: A Study of Priority," *American Journal of the Medical Sciences* 162 (1921): 526–55; Maxwell M. Wintrobe, *Hematology: The Blossoming of a Science* (Philadelphia: Lea and Febiger, 1985). Gowers's instrument was said to be used more often in England but to be less accurate than other techniques. Alfred C. Coles, *The Blood: How to Examine and Diagnose Its Diseases* (London: J. and A. Churchill, 1898), 1.

10. We now think of the much more numerous red blood cells as having the primary purpose of carrying oxygen throughout the body. The cells contain hemoglobin, which makes them red. The white blood cells are divided into several different varieties. Their primary purpose is to help ward off infection.

11. Significant numbers of immature forms of the red cell are found in the blood only in some pathological conditions.

12. P. Ehrlich and A. Lazarus, *Histology of the Blood: Normal and Pathological* (Cambridge: Cambridge University Press, 1900), 69.
13. Richard C. Cabot, "The Diagnostic and Prognostic Importance of Leucocytosis," *Boston Medical and Surgical Journal* 130 (1894): 277–82.
14. Gordon R. Ward, *Bedside Haematology: An Introduction to the Clinical Study of the So-called Blood Diseases and of Allied Disorders* (Philadelphia and London: W. B. Saunders, 1914), 336.
15. Edwin A. Locke, "The Clinical Value of the Iodine Reaction in the Leucocytes of the Blood," *Boston Medical and Surgical Journal* 147 (1902): 289-96.
16. Richard C. Cabot, *A Guide to the Clinical Examination of the Blood,* 5th ed. (New York: William Wood, 1904), 258.
17. Ralph W. Webster, *Diagnostic Methods: Chemical, Bacteriological, and Microscopic,* 6th ed. (Philadelphia: P. Blakiston's Son, 1920), 565–66.
18. Richard C. Cabot, "The Diagnostic and Prognostic Importance of Leucocytosis," *Boston Medical and Surgical Journal* 130 (1894): 277–82; Jean Captain Sabine, "A History of the Classification of Human Blood Corpuscles," *Bulletin of the History of Medicine* 8 (1940): 696–720, 785–805. The biographical literature on Ehrlich is large, but a useful place to start is Claude E. Dolman, "Paul Ehrlich," in *Dictionary of Scientific Biography,* edited by Charles Coulston Gillispie, 3:295–305 (New York: Charles Scribners Sons, 1981).
19. Although the specific stain was replaced by Giemsa's, Jenner's, and finally Wright's stains. Dock, "Clinical Pathology," 678.
20. Thomas S. Southworth, "The Technique and Diagnostic Value of Ehrlich's Method of Staining the White Blood-Corpuscles," *New York Medical Journal* 57 (1893): 2–7.
21. Frederic E. Sondern, "The Present Status of Blood Examination in Surgical Diagnosis," *Medical Record* 67 (1905): 452–55; both remarked on at length in Charles O. Cooke, "The Value of the Differential Leucocyte Count in Acute Surgical Disease," *Yale Medical Journal* 14 (1907): 12–29.
22. Charles L. Gibson, "The Value of the Differential Leucocyte Count in Acute Surgical Diseases," *Annals of Surgery* (Philadelphia) 43 (1906): 485–99.
23. Cooke, "Value of the Differential Leucocyte Count," 23. This article shows a Gibson-like chart as used by the Rhode Island Hospital for cases of appendicitis.
24. For an example of the *vade mecum* literature, see Ira S. Wile, *Blood Examination in Surgical Diagnosis* (New York: Surgery Publishing Company, 1908), 83. The Massachusetts Homeopathic Hospital used the charts as well; see Helmuth Ulrich, "The Value of Differential Leucocyte Counts, and a New Chart for Recording the Same," *New England Medical Gazette* 48 (1913): 113–16. The author notes Gibson's charts as the basis for his innovation and suggests some minor modifications.

25. T. H. Dexter, "The Interpretation of a Differential Leucocyte Count," *New York State Medical Journal* 10 (1910): 127–28.

26. A. L. Benedict, "Blood Examinations," *Medical Times* (N.Y.) 27 (1899): 321–24.

27. While simultaneously setting up clinical laboratories to do the same thing. Keith Wailoo, " 'A Disease *Sui Generis*': The Origins of Sickle Cell Anemia and the Emergence of Modern Clinical Research, 1904–1924," *Bulletin of the History of Medicine* 65 (1991): 185–208.

28. George Dock, "Laboratory and Clinical Examinations," *Journal of Laboratory and Clinical Medicine* 1 (1915): 22–25.

29. Charles P. Emerson, "The Accuracy of Certain Clinical Methods," *Johns Hopkins Hospital Bulletin* 14, no. 142 (January 1903): 9–18.

30. Ross C. Whitman, "The Technique of Blood-Examinations," *Chicago Medical Recorder* 26 (1904): 24–37.

31. F. W. Higgins, "Blood Examination from the Standpoint of the General Practitioner," *JAMA* 38 (1902): 233–35; William N. Berkeley, "Some Practical Remarks on Clinical Examination of the Blood," *New York Medical Journal* 71 (1900): 599–601; Henry L. Elsner, "On the Value to the Physician of Modern Methods of Diagnosis," *Boston Medical and Surgical Journal* 146 (1902): 101–8.

32. Louis Waldstein, "A New Method of Preparing the Blood for Clinical Purposes," *Proceedings of the New York Pathological Society: 1896* (1897): 67–72.

33. Higgins, "Blood Examination."

34. W. K. West, "The Value of the Examination of the Blood to the General Practitioner," *Journal of the Michigan State Medical Society, Detroit* 1 (1902–3): 43–49.

35. O. H. Perry-Pepper, "Recent Advances in Diagnostic Blood Examination," *Pennsylvania Medical Journal* 17 (1913–14): 431–34.

36. Sterling Bunnell, "Two Aids in Making Blood Counts," *JAMA* 55 (1910): 596.

37. Joel D. Howell, "Early Perceptions of the Electrocardiogram: From Arrhythmia to Infarction," *Bulletin of the History of Medicine* 58 (1984): 83–98.

38. Gordon William, "The Practical Value of Blood Counts," *Bristol Medico-Chirurgical Journal* 21 (1903): 234–45.

39. Charles P. Emerson, "Some Clinical Aspects of Chemistry," *JAMA* 38 (1902): 1359–62.

40. Gordon Wilson, "Discussion," to George Dock, "Correlation of Laboratory and Clinical Teaching," *Southern Medical Journal* 10 (1917): 189.

41. J. Watson Martingdale, "The Value of the Leucocyte Count as a Diagnostic Aid," *Journal of the Medical Society of New Jersey* 4 (1907–8): 329–32.

42. Discussion at the AMA section on diseases of children (*JAMA* 35 [1900]:1321).

43. F. W. Higgins, "Blood Examination."

44. H. E. Monroe, "The Leucocytes and Their Diagnostic Significance," *Illinois Medical Journal* 7 (1905): 268–70.

45. R. E. Colman, "Clinical Records, the Laboratory, and the General Practitioner," *Northwest Medicine* 20 (1921): 254–57.

46. Stanley Joel Reiser, *Medicine and the Reign of Technology* (Cambridge: Cambridge University Press, 1978).

47. "The Effect of Heat upon the Red Blood-Corpuscles," *Medical News* 56 (1890): 399.

48. For discussion of Osler's use of the microscope in general, see Alvin Eli Rodin and Jack D. Key, "Osler the Microscopist: Teaching, Research, and Practice, Part 1: The Canadian Years," *Annals of the Royal College of Physicians and Surgeons of Canada (RCPSC)* 25 (1992): 363–67; Alvin Eli Rodin and Jack D. Key, "Osler the Microscopist: Teaching, Research, and Practice; Part 2: Philadelphia and Baltimore," *Annals of the RCPSC* 25 (1992): 457–59.

49. William Osler, "The Effect of Heat upon the Red Blood Corpuscles," *Medical News* 56 (1890): 435.

50. Christopher Lawrence, "Incommunicable Knowledge: Science, Technology, and the Clinical Art in Britain, 1850–1914," *Journal of Contemporary History* 20 (1985): 503–20.

51. Quoted in Jon Darius, *Beyond Vision* (New York: Oxford University Press, 1984), 14–15. On Foucault, see Harold L. Burstyn, "Jean Bernard Léon Foucault," in *Dictionary of Scientific Biography*, edited by Charles Coulston Gillispie, 5:84–87 (New York: Charles Scribners Sons, 1981).

52. Richard C. Cabot, "The Blood Stream as a Public Highway," *Yale Medical Journal* 10 (1903): 41–44.

53. Although the title was a translation from the German, the choice of words is no less meaningful as an index to contemporary attitudes. Ehrlich and Lazarus, *Histology of the Blood*. The same title was used when the work was used for *Diseases of the Blood*, edited by Alfred Stengel (Philadelphia: W. B. Saunders, 1905), and was little modified for the second edition of the book, *Normal and Pathological Histology of the Blood* (New York: Rebman, 1910).

54. A section heading in Russell C. Maulitz, "The Pathological Tradition," in *Companion Encyclopedia to the History of Medicine*, edited by W. F. Bynum and Roy Porter, 1:169–91 (London: Routledge, 1993).

55. Russell C. Maulitz, "The Whole Company of Pathology," in *History of Pathology*, edited by Teizo Ogawa, 139–61 (Tokyo: Taniguchi Foundation, 1983).

56. Norman Bridge, "The New Science of Medicine," *JAMA* 2 (1884): 309–15.

57. George Dock, "Some Points in the Examination of the Blood in Diagnosis," *Transactions of the Michigan State Medical Society* 17 (1893): 95–101. Dock claimed that, under his supervision at the University of Michigan, "all patients were given complete urine and blood tests on admission." Dock headed the Department of Medicine there from 1891 to 1908. Were this claim true, it would indeed be remarkable, given the

practice at other teaching hospitals. Unfortunately, I have been unable to locate the hospital records for this period which could confirm or deny the claim. See Dock, "Clinical Pathology," 673. On Dock, see Horace W. Davenport, "George Dock at Michigan, 1891–1908," in *Medical Lives and Scientific Medicine at Michigan, 1891–1969*, edited by Joel D. Howell, 29–44 (Ann Arbor: University of Michigan Press, 1993).

58. For two of many examples, see the eminently practical and portable *Clinical Manual: A Guide to the Practical Examination of the Excretions, Secretions, and the Blood, for the Use of Physicians and Students*, by Andrew MacFarlane (New York: G. P. Putnam's Sons, 1894); and G. Klemperer, *The Elements of Clinical Diagnosis* (New York: Macmillan, 1904).

59. Discussion at the AMA section on diseases of children. *JAMA* 35 (1900): 1321.

60. West, "Value of the Examination of the Blood," 43–49.

61. "Death of President McKinley," *JAMA* 37 (1901): 779–86. The count was done five days after the president was shot, leaving a wound from which he did not recover.

62. For examples of blood counts in the academic world of the 1910s, see Oglesby Paul, *The Caring Physician: The Life of Dr. Francis W. Peabody* (Boston: Francis A. Countway Library, 1991), 79–81.

63. T. H. Dexter, "The Interpretation of a Differential Leucocyte Count," *New York State Medical Journal* 10 (1910): 127–28.

64. Daniel Fox, *Health Policies, Health Politics: The British and American Experience, 1911–1965* (Princeton: Princeton University Press, 1986).

65. Bridges, "Significance of Blood Examinations," 26–29.

66. The precise numbers are, for the New York Hospital, 3.91 percent in 1900 and 29.09 percent in 1920; for the Pennsylvania Hospital, 5.22 percent in 1900 and 27.89 percent in 1920.

67. These means were calculated with outliers, defined as lags greater than fifty-five days, omitted from the calculations. With the outliers included the mean number of days changes only in that the value for Pennsylvania Hospital in 1900 is 16.6 days.

68. Berkeley, "Some Practical remarks," 599–601.

69. H. Miller Galt, "On the Value of the Blood Count as an Aid to Diagnosis in Obscure Bacterial and Other Infections," *British Medical Journal* 2 (1913): 1367–69.

70. The amount of pain no doubt had a lot to do with the quality of the available needles.

71. William G. Savage, "Leucocyte Enumeration for Routine Work," *Lancet* 2 (1902): 866.

72. Galt, "On the Value of the Blood Count."

73. For a "pro-finger" perspective, see John C. Da Costa, Jr., *Clinical Hematology* (Philadelphia: P. Blakiston's, 1902), 34. Not everyone agreed. See Albert S. Morrow, *Diagnostic and Therapeutic Technic*, 2d ed. (Philadelphia: W. B. Saunders, 1915), 245–46.

74. Cabot, *Guide to Clinical Examination*, 8.
75. Webster, *Diagnostic Methods*, 415.
76. "Founded by Muhlenburg: Characteristic Features of St. Luke's Hospital," *New York Times*, December 21, 1891, 10.
77. Christopher Crenner, "Professional Measurement: Quantification of Health and Disease in American Medical Practice, 1880–1920" (Ph.D. diss., Harvard University, 1993), 149–52.
78. Whitman, "Technique of Blood-Examinations," 24–37.
79. Dexter, "Interpretation of a Differential Leucocyte Count."

CHAPTER 7: BLOOD AND DISEASES

1. Presentation at the Michigan Historical Collections, Ann Arbor, Michigan, February 6, 1992.
2. W. K. West, "The Value of the Examination of the Blood to the General Practitioner," *Journal of the Michigan State Medical Society* 1 (1902–3): 43–49.
3. E. Maxey, "The Clinical Importance of the Examination of the Blood," *Medical Sentinel* 8 (1900): 355–62.
4. F. W. Higgins, "Blood Examination from the Standpoint of the General Practitioner," *Journal of the American Medical Association* (*JAMA*) 38 (1902): 233–35.
5. H. Miller Galt, "On the Value of the Blood Count as an Aid to Diagnosis in Obscure Bacterial and Other Infections," *British Medical Journal* (*BMJ*) 2 (1913): 1367–69.
6. It is interesting that one sees little reference to menstrual bleeding as a cause of anemia in women. One does, of course, see enormous amounts about another typically female disease, chlorosis, which has been the subject of much historical attention.
7. New York Hospital Case Records (NYHCR) 27 (1900): 3628.
8. Pennsylvania Hospital Case Records (PHCR) 82 (1900): 3520.
9. PHCR 85 (1900): 627. The precision of the examiners was perhaps a little off. On June 1, 1900, her hemoglobin is noted to be 30 percent, with a red blood count (RBC) of 3,410,000. On June 13, her hemoglobin is 52.5 percent, with an RBC of 3,680,000. From the perspective of the 1990s one doubts that her hemoglobin would have changed so much with relatively little change in the RBC count. For additional discussion of error in laboratory tests in this period, see Stanley Joel Reiser, *Medicine and the Reign of Technology* (Cambridge: Cambridge University Press, 1978).
10. PHCR 936 (1925): 3844.
11. In the quantitative sample on which this book is based there was one case at the New York Hospital and three cases at the Pennsylvania Hospital.

12. Much of the history of blood tests has treated them only with specific reference to diseases of the blood, as, for example, Maxwell M. Wintrobe, *Blood, Pure and Eloquent: A Story of Discoveries, of People, and of Ideas* (New York: McGraw-Hill, 1980). Such an approach implicitly assigns their use to a limited group of patients and is of limited help when trying to understand the more general use of such laboratory tests.

13. Malaria was by no means confined to the southern United States. It was one of Cabot's "three continued fevers of New England."

14. Or so it was claimed. *Western Medical Review* 1 (1896): 26–29.

15. In the sample of case records selected for this study there were thirty-seven cases of pneumonia at the New York Hospital and eighty-two at the Pennsylvania Hospital; sixty-three cases of typhoid fever at the Pennsylvania Hospital and twenty at the New York Hospital; and seventy-three cases of appendicitis at the Pennsylvania Hospital and seventy-six at the New York Hospital.

16. William Osler, *The Principles and Practice of Medicine*, 4th ed. (New York: D. Appleton, 1901), 108.

17. Lloyd G. Stevenson, "Exemplary Disease: The Typhoid Pattern," *Journal of the History of Medicine* (1982): 159–81.

18. William Osler, *The Principles and Practice of Medicine* (New York: D. Appleton, 1892), 511; 4th ed. (1901), 131.

19. The difference in the estimates is not altogether unexpected. Osler gave no citations for his estimate (as he did not for most of the quantitative data), so there is no way to readily know the source of his information. The number, however, might well have included all types of hospitals. The two hospitals considered here were urban, were located in northern climes, and may have seen a sicker patient population than the norm, accounting for the somewhat higher percentage of people admitted with pneumonia.

20. The death rate given, 202.2 deaths per 100,000 population, is for "influenza and pneumonia." Most of these deaths in 1900 were probably caused by pneumonia, with deaths from influenza not playing a major role until the influenza epidemic of 1917–18, when the rate reached 588.5 deaths per 100,000 population. *Historical Statistics of the United States: Colonial Times to 1970* (Washington, D.C.: Government Printing Office, 1975), pt. 1, 58. The diagnosis of pneumonia, of course, took a different meaning in this period than it did later (as is the case for any diagnosis). Nonetheless, the point remains that physicians and the general public considered pneumonia to be a serious illness and a common cause of death.

21. William Osler, "On the Study of Pneumonia," *St. Paul Medical Journal* 1 (1899): 5–9. For a brief précis of Osler's ideas, see chapter 3, "Pneumonia," in W. R. Bett, *Osler: The Man and the Legend* (London: William Heinemann, 1951.)

22. William Osler, "A Review of the Cases Studied by the Third and Fourth Year Classes, Johns Hopkins Hospital, Session of 1896–1897," *National Medical Review* 7 (1897): 177–80.

23. Noted in Wesley W. Spink, *Infectious Diseases: Prevention and Treatment in the Nineteenth and Twentieth Centuries* (Minneapolis: University of Minnesota Press, 1978), 209.

24. Richard C. Cabot, "Leucocytosis as an Element in the Prognosis of Pneumonia," *Boston Medical and Surgical Journal* 129 (1893): 117–18. For a better understanding of Cabot, I am indebted to Thomas Andrew Dodds for sharing with me his unpublished 1980 manuscript, "Opening the Windows: Richard Cabot and the Care of the Patient during America's Progressive Era, 1890–1920," some of which has been published as "Richard Cabot: Medical Reformer during the Progressive Era (1890–1920)," *Annals of Internal Medicine* 119 (1993): 417–22.

25. Richard C. Cabot, "The Diagnostic and Prognostic Importance of Leucocytosis," *Boston Medical and Surgical Journal* 130 (1894): 277–82. The perceived wisdom that pneumonia and typhoid were the two diseases in which blood counts were the most useful continued for decades. See C. M. Siever, "The Prognostic Value of the Blood Count," *Texas State Medical Journal* 4 (1908–1909): 259–60.

26. James Ewing, "A Study of the Leucocytosis of Lobar Pneumonia," *New York Medical Journal* 58 (1893): 713–18. For biography, see J. A. del Regato, "James Ewing," *International Journal of Radiation Oncology* 2 (1977): 185–98; and appreciations and biographical data, including a list of Ewing's publications, in the volume edited by Lewis Stephen Pilcher and Frank E. Adair, "International Contributions to the Study of Cancer in Honor of James Ewing," *Annals of Surgery* 31 (1931). The most useful source of biographical material is in the library of the Memorial Sloan-Kettering Cancer Center, New York City. A diary of Ewing's collegiate days at Amherst is in the Amherst College Archives.

27. Edward T. Morman, "Clinical Pathology in America, 1895–1915: Philadelphia as a Test Case," *Bulletin of the History of Medicine* 58 (1984): 198–214.

28. Hayes Martin Collection: James Ewing, "Personal History," record group 500, box 4, folder 66, transcript of interview with J. Stone on January 17, 1944. Library, Memorial Sloan-Kettering Cancer Canter, New York City. Hereinafter referred to as Hayes Martin Collection.

29. His first paper had been a report on "The Syms Operating Room of the Roosevelt Hospital" (*Pittsburgh Medical Review* 6 [1892]: 362–63).

30. James Ewing, Testimonial Dinner, January 31, 1931. Hayes Martin Collection, folder 72.

31. James Ewing, "The Leucocytosis of Diphtheria under the Influence of Serum Therapy," *New York Medical Journal* 62 (1895): 161–68, 196–203.

32. As, for example, his next major work, *Studies on Ganglion Cells* (Utica, N.Y.: State Hospitals Press, 1899).

33. James Ewing, *Clinical Pathology of the Blood* (Philadelphia: Lea Brothers, 1901). A second edition was published in 1903.

34. Osler, "Review of the Cases." Also quoted by T. B. Futcher, "The Blood in Pneumonia," *National Medical Review* 7 (1897): 180–82.

35. Futcher, "Blood in Pneumonia," 181. The East Coast studies on the significance of leucocytosis in pneumonia found their way into more removed parts of the country. See, for example, Willson Bridges [sic], "The Significance of Blood Examinations in Disease," *Western Medical Review* 1 (1896); 26–29.

36. Alfred C. Coles, *The Blood: How to Examine and Diagnose Its Diseases* (London: J. and A. Churchill, 1898), 211. His observation appears to have been correct, as almost all of the authors who take a general overview of the value of blood counts mention pneumonia as a prominent example.

37. Smith, "Prognosis in Pneumonia."

38. Siever, "Prognostic Value of the Blood Count." The organism most commonly the cause of pneumonia was the pneumococcus, and much attention was paid to distinguishing the various types of pneumococci. That subject will not be considered here but is covered well in the massive compilation on the state of the art, Roderick Heffron, *Pneumonia: With Special Reference to Pneumococcus Lobar Pneumonia* (New York: Commonwealth Fund, 1939). Pneumococcal pneumonia was treated with serum therapy. For more discussion, see Harry F. Dowling, *Fighting Infection: Conquests of the Twentieth Century* (Cambridge, Mass.: Harvard University Press, 1977).

39. Smith reported a 31.2 percent death rate at Presbyterian Hospital in 1896. Smith, "Prognosis in Pneumonia." In 1993 the in-hospital death rate was reported as 16 percent. F. L. Brancati, J. W. Chow, M. M. Wagener, S. J. Vacarello, and V. L. Yu, "Is Pneumonia Really the Old Man's Friend? Two-Year Prognosis after Community-Acquired Pneumonia," *Lancet* 342 (1993): 30–33.

40. PHCR 556 (1920): 5216.

41. PHCR 556 (1920): 5264.

42. Spink, *Infectious Diseases*, 242.

43. *Historical Statistics*, 58. The diagnosis of typhoid fever was usually made on clinical grounds, and one cannot be sure that the diagnoses recorded are the same ones that we would make in the late twentieth century. Nonetheless, what is clear is that contemporaries perceived a sharp drop in the disease prevalence. See also Arthur L. Bloomfield, *A Bibliography of Internal Medicine: Communicable Diseases* (Chicago: University of Chicago Press, 1958); Dowling, *Fighting Infection*; and Michael P. McCarthy, *Typhoid and the Politics of Public Health in Nineteenth-Century Philadelphia* (Philadelphia: American Philosophical Society, 1987).

44. Bett, *Osler*, 18.

45. Frederick P. Gay, *Typhoid Fever Considered as a Problem of Scientific Medicine* (New York: Macmillan, 1918). Despite changes in scientific

thought, typhoid fever continued to be seen within a broader social context. Judith Walzer Leavitt, " 'Typhoid Mary' Strikes Back: Bacteriological Theory and Practice in Early-Twentieth Century Public Health," *ISIS* 83 (1992): 608–29. The disease also attracted a good deal of attention in the press. Terra Ziporyn, *Disease in the Popular American Press: The Case of Diphtheria, Typhoid Fever, and Syphilis, 1870–1920* (New York: Greenwood Press, 1988).

46. On complications, see the classic pair of books written by authors from Jefferson Medical College, Hobart Amory Hare, *The Medical Complications, Accidents and Sequelae of Typhoid or Enteric Fever* (Philadelphia: Lea Brothers, 1899); and William W. Keen, *The Surgical Complications and Sequels of Typhoid Fever* (Philadelphia: W. B. Saunders, 1898).

47. Horace W. Davenport, *Doctor Dock: Teaching and Learning Medicine at the Turn of the Century* (New Brunswick: Rutgers University Press, 1987), 238.

48. D. J. Milton Miller, "Report of a Case of Perforation in Typhoid Fever Closed by an Adherent Tag of Omentum, Followed by a Relapse, Second Perforation, and Death," *Boston Medical and Surgical Journal* (May 25, 1899). That the surgical approach to perforation was new in 1900, see "The Past Year's Advances in Medicine and Surgery," *Medical News* January 6, 1900: 25. Abdominal pain in typhoid fever was a common concern. For another type of discussion, see Russell Sturgis Rowland, "Acute Abdominal Symptoms in Typhoid Fever from Inflamed Mesenteric Glands," *JAMA* 46 (1906): 507–8.

49. M. Howard Fusell, "Specific Infections: Typhoid Fever," in *Handbook of Medical Treatment*, edited by John C. Da Costa, Jr., 1:3-27 (Philadelphia: F. A. Davis, 1918).

50. Davenport, *Doctor Dock*, 190.

51. J. Watson Martingdale, "The Value of the Leucocyte Count as a Diagnostic Aid," *Journal of the Medical Society of New Jersey* 4 (1907–8): 329–32. Similar cases are found in many other publications, though not always with such a telling comment. For example, E. S. Van Duyn, "Influence of the Leucocyte Count in the Decision for or against Immediate Operation," *Transactions of the Medical Association of Central New York* 10 (1903): 32–40.

52. Gay, *Typhoid Fever*, 89.

53. Julius Friedenwald, "The Diazo Reaction of Ehrlich," *New York Medical Journal* 58 (1893): 745–48.

54. Davenport, *Doctor Dock*, 195.

55. Yet just how widely remains a matter for conjecture, unless we have more evidence from patient case records. Although it was indeed discussed widely, and probably applied widely as well, at least one general practitioner, who was a proponent of blood tests in general, commented in reference to Widal tests that "the country practitioner cannot do them" and that he used a commercial laboratory. He did not indicate

why the country practitioner could do a blood count and not a Widal test. Nor do we know just how easy it was to find a laboratory to do a Widal test. J. S. Turbeville, "Discussion" (of John A. Lanford, "Value and Limitations of Blood Examinations"), *Transactions of the Medical Association of Alabama* (1917): 299–302.

56. Charles Lyman Greene, "The Serum Test of Widal and the Possibility of Its Application without Microscopic Examination, with a Report of Cases and Demonstration of Method," reprinted from the *Medical Record* of December 5, 1896.

57. W. H. Welch et al., "Summary of Views Expressed at the Discussion on Serum Diagnosis at the Meeting of the American Medical Association in Philadelphia," *JAMA* 29 (1897): 314–15. See also the several papers presented and published in the same issue of *JAMA*, and particularly the discussion for examples of tensions between a self-described "country doctor" and the "college professors and makers of text-books."

58. Davenport, *Doctor Dock*, 194.

59. Erna Lesky, "Viennese Serological Research about the Year 1900: Its Contribution to the Development of Clinical Medicine," *Bulletin of the New York Academy of Medicine* 49 (1973): 100–111. Another marker of how the test was accepted comes from the increasing attention Cabot gave it in the editions of his book on blood.

60. Wm. H. Bailey, "The Laboratory Specialist as a Clinical Consultant," *Journal of Laboratory and Clinical Medicine* 7 (1921–22): 410–16.

61. Davenport, *Doctor Dock*, 194.

62. PHCR 157 (1909): 407.

63. For example, PHCR 85 (1900): 455.

64. PHCR 96 (1902): 3290; 157 (1909): 307.

65. As has been ably demonstrated by Dale C. Smith, "A Historical Overview of the Recognition of Appendicitis," *New York State Journal of Medicine* 86 (1986): 571–83, 639–47. For an example of viewing the Fitz presentation as having an "electrifying effect in clearing the atmosphere of the confusion which had existed since the teaching of Dupuytren," see Hyman Morrison, "The Chapter on Appendicitis in a Biography of Reginald Heber Fitz," *Bulletin of the History of Medicine* 20 (1946): 259–69. See also Stewart M. Brooks, *McBurney's Point: The Story of Appendicitis* (South Brunswick: A. S. Barnes, 1969); and Sir Zachary Cope, "The Evolution of the Operative Treatment of Appendicitis," *A History of the Acute Abdomen* (London: Oxford University Press, 1965), 32–46. A succinct account by someone who played a major role in the disease (as is detailed shortly in this chapter) is provided by John M. Deaver, "Appendicitis Then and Now," MS read to the Jefferson Medical College, May 5, 1920, in the Deaver papers at the College of Physicians of Philadelphia, box 1, ser. 1, folder 40. For an account of a musical composition dedicated in 1896 to a surgeon who operated for appendicitis, see E. Lee Strohl and Willis G. Diffenbaugh, "The Appendicitis

Two Step by Felix Mendelssohn," *Surgery, Gynecology and Obstetrics* 127 (1968): 842–46.

66. Homer Gage, "Appendicitis: Some Impressions Derived from an Experience of Forty-four Cases," *Boston Medical and Surgical Journal* 130 (1894): 508–13.
67. For biographical information, see obituary in *JAMA* 74 (1920): 1414; and Howard A. Kelly and Walter L. Burrage, *Dictionary of American Medical Biography* (New York: D. Appleton, 1928). This John Chalmers Da Costa, Jr. (1871–1920) (although the "Jr." is omitted in the aforementioned Kelly and Burrage *Dictionary*), should be carefully distinguished from his father, John Chalmers Da Costa (1834–1910), who graduated from Jefferson in 1878 and served there as a gynecologist, and his uncle, also named John Chalmers Da Costa (1863–1933), a noted surgeon who graduated from Jefferson in 1885 and returned there to occupy the first Samuel D. Gross Chair as Professor of Surgery. This Da Costa family appears not to be related to Jacob Mendes Da Costa (1833–1900), another noted Jefferson faculty member who specialized in internal medicine in a slightly earlier era.
68. John Chalmers Da Costa, Jr., *Clinical Hematology* (Philadelphia: P. Blakiston's Son, 1902); "The Clinical Value of Blood Examinations in Appendicitis: A Study Based on the Examination of One Hundred and Eighteen Cases in the German Hospital, Philadelphia," *Transactions of the American Surgical Association* 19 (1901): 60–71. It is worth noting that Da Costa's cases came from the surgical service of John Deaver, who, as will be discussed momentarily, vigorously disagreed with Da Costa's message.
69. In 1911, nearing his peak of national fame as operative surgeon, Deaver was appointed professor of clinical surgery at Penn; later a Practice of Surgery was designated specifically for him. He was senior chair of surgery for four years, from 1918. Known for his dramatic clinical teaching, Deaver didn't leave much to the house staff. He encouraged his young surgeons to "study the physiological sciences underlying modern surgical diagnosis and treatment, which he himself had not had the ability to learn." He expressed contempt for pathology, "seeming to doubt a science of disease." Isador S. Ravdin, "John B. Deaver, Master Surgeon," *Philadelphia Medicine* 56 (1960): 741–49; A. P. C. Ashurst, "Memoir of John Deaver, M.D.," *Annals of Surgery* 95 (1932): 637–40; Damon B. Pfeiffer, "Memoir of John B. Deaver, M.D.," *Transactions and Studies of the College of Physicians of Philadelphia*, 3d ser. 54 (1932): lxxxvii–lxxxix; William A. Damon, "A Brief History of the John Rhea Barton Chair of Surgery," *Transactions and Studies of the College of Physicians of Philadelphia*, 4th ser. 23 (1955): 94–104; Robert H. Ivy, "Personal Recollections of Holders of the John Rhea Barton Professorship of Surgery at the University of Pennsylvania School of Medicine," 42 (1975): 239–62. Surgeons remember Deaver particularly for the Deaver incision, in which medial displacement of the rectus muscle

follows an incision into the right lower abdominal quadrant. Ira M. Rutkow, *The History of Surgery in the United States, 1775–1900* (San Francisco: Norman Publishing, 1988), 1:121.

70. Deaver also once used his regular operating room to operate on his dog. Priscilla Deaver Kelley, MS reminiscences, handwritten, in the Mutter Museum of the College of Physicians of Philadelphia.

71. Ashhurst, "Memoir of John Deaver"; Pfeiffer, "Memoir of John B. Deaver"; Loyal Davis, *Fellowship of Surgeons: A History of the American College of Surgeons* (Chicago: American College of Surgeons, 1960), 50–51.

72. Deaver, "Reminiscences," 3.

73. Pfeiffer, "Memoir of John B. Deaver," lxxxviii.

74. Ivy, "Personal Recollections," 250.

75. He also created the phrase "an inch and a half, a minute and a half, a week and a half," to indicate the length of the incision, the duration of the operation, and the stay of the patient in hospital when early operation was employed." Ashurst, "Memoir of John Deaver," 638.

76. By 1897 Herman Mynter had concluded that "surgical treatment [of appendicitis] must be considered the conservative treatment." *Appendicitis and Its Surgical Treatment with a Report of Seventy-Five Operated Cases* (Philadelphia: J. B. Lippincott, 1897), 3.

77. *Transactions of the American Surgical Association* (Philadelphia) 19 (1901): 115–22; see also *Philadelphia Medical Journal* 7 (1901): 1055–57.

78. This idea, that a scientific physician tended to have a narrow outlook, can be found in many other sources, such as stated by another distinguished surgeon, Charles H. Mayo ("Problems in Medical Education," Dedication on the Montgomery Ward Memorial Building, Northwestern University Medical School [Chicago: Northwestern University Press, 1929], 91–97).

79. Richard C. Cabot, "The Ideal of Accuracy in Clinical Work: Its Importance, Its Limitation," *Boston Medical and Surgical Journal* 151 (1904): 557–60; G. Russell, "The Use and Limitations of Blood Counting," *Guy's Hospital Gazette* 17 (1903); 515–25; Frederick E. Sondern, "The Present Status of Blood Examination in Surgical Diagnosis," *Medical Record* 67 (1905): 452–55; H. A. Fairbairn, "The Clinical Significance of the Blood Count as Exemplified by a Series of Hospital Histories," *Long Island Medical Journal* 12 (1908): 231–34. Deaver continued to attract attention for some time (see, e.g., Asher Yaguda, "Studies on Schilling Count in Appendicitis," *American Journal of Clinical Pathology* 1 [1931]: 39–50).

80. After all, the study was done on John Deaver's service at the German Hospital. The fact that Deaver and Da Costa were able to use the same groups of patients for very different conclusions bespeaks an underlying congeniality between the two which was sometimes belied by their public statements.

81. For direct quotations against Deaver, see Cabot, "Ideal of Accuracy;" Fairbairn, "The Clinical Significance of the Blood Count;" and Frederick E. Sondern, "The Present Status of Blood Examination."

82. John B. Deaver, "The Acute Abdomen" (paper delivered to the Tri-County Medical Society in Lancaster, Pa., June 26, 1925), John B. Deaver papers of the College of Physicians of Philadelphia, box 3, ser. 1, folder 104.

83. John B. Deaver, "The Romance of Surgery" (paper delivered to the Iowa State Medical Society, Des Moines, May 13, 1926), John B. Deaver papers of the College of Physicians of Philadelphia, box 3, ser. 1, folder 111.

84. C. M. Siever, "The Prognostic Value of the Blood Count," *Texas State Medical Journal* 4 (1908–9): 259–60.

85. See Thomas A. Shallow, Memoir of Dr. John Chalmers DaCosta, *Transactions of the College of Physicians of Philadelphia*, ser. 4, 1, (1933): lxx–lxxvi.

86. John Chalmers Da Costa, *A Manual of Modern Surgery* (Philadelphia: W. B. Saunders, 1894). Da Costa first published an enormously influential textbook of surgery in 1894 and had in 1900 seen the third edition of that text (of what were to be a total of ten) appear in local bookstores. For many decades the book was one of the most popular surgical texts, reaching a level of popularity for surgeons similar to the success of William Osler's *Principles and Practice of Medicine*. Rutkow, *History of Surgery*, 1:115.

87. G. E. Erikson, "William Williams Keen, Jr.," in *Dictionary of American Medical Biography*, edited by Martin Kaufman, Stuart Galishoff, and Todd Savitt, 1:406–7 (Westport, Conn.: Greenwood Press, 1984). John Chalmers DaCosta, "Surgical Tuberculosis," in *Surgery: Its Principles and Practice*, edited by William Williams Keen, 1:593–661 (Philadelphia: W. B. Saunders, 1906). John Chalmers Da Costa also wrote chapters in other volumes on "Surgery among the Insane and Surgery of Insanity" (2:788–815), perhaps as a result of his earlier time as physician in a mental institution; and on "Surgery of the Tongue" (3:655–701). Deaver, together with Damon B. Pfeiffer, wrote a chapter on "Appendicitis" in the 1921 edition (8:434–50).

88. "Examination of the Blood," 1:110–44.

89. John B. Deaver, *A Treatise on Appendicitis* (Philadelphia: P. Blakiston's Son, 1896).

90. John B. Deaver, "Reminiscences" (paper delivered to the Hippocrates-Galen Medical Society of Washington, D.C., December 8, 1927), John B. Deaver papers of the College of Physicians of Philadelphia, box 4, ser. 1, folder 129.

91. John B. Deaver, "What Attributes Go to Make a Surgeon?" (paper delivered to the College of Physicians of Philadelphia Section on Medical History, December 18, 1928), John B. Deaver papers of the College of Physicians of Philadelphia, box 4, ser. 1, folder 138.

92. Some 1,008 appendices are noted to have been received "on deposit" by the Mütter Museum. See the annual report of the Mütter Museum, April 1, 1905. The specimens were occasionally used for demonstrations; see A. O. J. Kelly (the pathologist at the German Hospital), to John H. Brinton, chairman of the Committee on the Mütter Museum of the College of Physicians, November 2, 1905, in the Collection of the College of Physicians of Philadelphia. The cards remain at the Mütter Museum; the fate of the appendices themselves is unknown, although they were probably discarded.

93. "The Radical Treatment of Hernia," *American Journal of the Medical Sciences* n.s. 109 (1895): 660–65; *Appendicitis*, listed in the *Surgeon General's Index Catalog* as being published in Philadelphia by E. W. Eckel in 1895. The same material was published in slightly different form in the *Journal of the American Medical Association* 25 (1895): 46–50; and *Richmond Journal of Practice* 9 (1895): 254–63.

94. This omission may have attracted the attention of contemporaries; in the preface to the second edition (1900) Deaver states, "I have not been unmindful of, nor have I neglected to refer to, the excellent work already done and still being done . . ." (vi). Indeed, the book included a bibliography, which is inexplicably gone by the time of the fourth edition.

95. For one of many examples, see J. B. Deaver and I. S. Ravdin, "Carcinoma of the Duodenum," *American Journal of the Medical Sciences* 159 (1920): 469–77.

96. "Routine Duties of the Surgical Poop" (for Professor John B. Deaver), MS, 22. In the Deaver file of the Mütter Museum of the College of Physicians of Philadelphia.

97. It is interesting that this is the first instance in which he is willing to make an exception to his general conclusion about the uselessness of blood counts. One might speculate that this change is the result of having too many surgical deaths in people who were extremely ill.

98. Deaver, "Appendicitis," 13.

99. Van Duyn, "Influence of the Leucocyte Count."

100. James T. R. Davison, "The Examination of Blood in Disease," *Liverpool Medico-Chirurgical Journal* 2 (1882): 283–87.

101. J. C. Hubbard, "The Practical Value of the White Blood Cell Count in Surgical Cases," *Boston Medical and Surgical Journal* 142 (1900): 409–11.

102. William Coleman, "Experimental Physiology and Statistical Inference: The Therapeutic Trial in Nineteenth-Century Germany," in *The Probabilistic Revolution*, vol. 2: *Ideas in the Sciences*, edited by Lorenz Kruger, Gerd Gigerenzer, and Mary S. Morgan, 201–26 (Cambridge, Mass.: MIT Press, 1987). Most discussion of statistical and numerical attitudes among physicians has centered on therapeutic trials, rather than prognostic indicators. For a traditional and some-

what less subtle reading of the history of numerical studies in clinical trials, see J. P. Bull, "The Historical Development of Clinical Therapeutic Trials," *Journal of Chronic Diseases* 10 (1959): 218–48.

103. For a cogent discussion of the politics of variation, with particular reference to anesthesia, see Martin Pernick, "From the Universal to the Particular: Professionalism, Anesthesia, and Human Individuality," in *A Calculus of Suffering: Pain, Professionalism, and Anesthesia in Nineteenth-Century America* (New York: Columbia University Press, 1985), 125–47.

104. John B. Deaver, "Address to the Graduating Class of St. Louis University," ca. May 22, 1909, John B. Deaver papers of the College of Physicians of Philadelphia, box 1, ser. 1, folder 2. Also in the same address, Deaver noted that the "subordinate place of the laboratory in the active battle with disease [should be] well understood."

105. Deaver, "When to Open and When Not to Open the Abdomen in Acute Surgical Conditions" (paper delivered to the Long Island College Hospital Association, Brooklyn, November 2, 1928), John B. Deaver papers of the College of Physicians of Philadelphia, box 4, ser. 1, folder 136.

106. Deaver, "When to Open," 20–21. Many lectures in this archive express similar thoughts.

107. See the several papers on "The Treatment of Appendicitis," *Boston Medical and Surgical Journal* 152 (1905): 325–51. The treatment of a more generalized infection of the peritoneal cavity—that is, peritonitis—was somewhat more controversial.

108. On the impact of the automobile for patients and physicians, see Peter J. Ling, *America and the Automobile: Technology, Reform, and Social Change, 1893–1923* (New York: St. Martin's Press, 1990), 26–29. Problems of transportation and the shift to an office-based practice are also discussed in George Rosen, *The Structure of American Medical Practice, 1875–1941* (Philadelphia: University of Pennsylvania Press, 1983).

109. Owen Tully Stratton, *Medicine Man* (Norman: University of Oklahoma Press, 1989), 167–68.

110. Davenport, *Doctor Dock*, 164–65.

111. Maurice H. Richardson, "Remarks on Appendicitis," *Boston Medical and Surgical Journal* 152 (1905): 334–39.

112. John B. Deaver, "Some Atypical Cases of Appendicitis" (paper delivered to the Academy of Medicine of Northern New Jersey [an audience composed mostly of general practitioners], April 23, 1929), John B. Deaver papers of the College of Physicians Philadelphia, box 4, ser. 1, folder 142.

113. R. H. Fitz, "Some Observations on Appendicitis," *Boston Medical and Surgical Journal* 152 (1905): 339–41.

114. Davenport, *Doctor Dock*, 164.

115. W. K. West, "The Value of the Examination of the Blood to the General Practitioner," *Journal of the Michigan State Medical Society* 1 (1902–3): 43–49.

116. John M. Wyeth, "The Value of Clinical Microscopy, Bacteriology, and Chemistry in Surgical Practice," *Boston Medical and Surgical Journal* 144 (1901): 541–47; Henry L. Elsner, "On the Value to the Physician of Modern Methods of Diagnosis."

117. Cabot, "Ideal of Accuracy," 557–60.

118. Harry Gauss, "The Evolution of Clinical Pathology," *Journal of Laboratory and Clinical Medicine* 8 (1923): 703–19.

119. Kenneth M. Lynch, "Pathological Anatomy as the Keystone of the Practice of Clinical Pathology," *American Journal of Clinical Pathology* 1 (1931): 277–84.

120. Harry P. Smith, "Clinical Pathology: Its Creators and Practitioners," *American Journal of Clinical Pathology* 31 (1959): 238–93; Bailey, "Laboratory Specialist."

121. Or, perhaps, reflecting patients who were less sick. The available data make it very hard to say. One source cites a fatality rate in 1925 of 13.9 percent, but without indicating the source of the data. Brooks, *McBurney's Point*, 130.

122. Frederic W. Bancroft, "Acute Appendicitis: A Review of Five Hundred and Eighty-four Consecutive Cases," *JAMA* 75 (1920): 1635–38.

123. NYHCR 43 (1910): 9569.

124. NYHCR 9 (1920): 831.

125. NYHCR 35 (1920): 162; 41 (1920): 100.

126. NYHCR 14 (1920): 780.

127. The 95 percent confidence interval at the Pennsylvania Hospital is 10–16 percent; at the New York Hospital, 85–93 percent. In addition to being statistically significant differences, this data probably understates the magnitude of the difference between the two hospitals. The New York Hospital data extends only to 1920, the Pennsylvania Hospital data to 1925. One would expect to see even more differential counts done at the New York Hospital by 1925, which would increase the (already dramatic) difference between the two institutions.

128. They appeared to be better equipped than some other, less prestigious hospitals, where, as late as 1910, physicians complained that there was simply not any apparatus available with which to do differential counts. Minutes of the Medical Board of the Willard Parker and Riverside Hospital, March 10, 1910, on loan to the New York Academy of Medicine.

129. Francis R. Packard, *Some Account of the Pennsylvania Hospital of Philadelphia from 1751 to 1938* (Philadelphia: Eagle Press, 1938), 108–9; Morman, "Clinical Pathology."

130. For example, the very first article, Warfield T. Longcope, "On the Pathological Histology of Hodgkin's Disease, with a Report of a Series

of Cases," *Ayer Clinical Laboratory Bulletin* 1 (1903): 5–76. Also Longcope, "A Study of the Bone-Marrow in Typhoid Fever and Other Acute Infections," *Ayer Clinical Laboratory Bulletin* 2 (1905): 1–28.

131. Simon Flexner, "Announcement," *Ayer Laboratory Clinical Bulletin* 1 (1903): 1. Contrary to his assertions, the occasional study did deal with practical, routine matters. One study of the diagnosis of typhoid fever noted that bacilli can be isolated several days before the Widal reaction, in a study of "the practical value of blood cultures in the routine procedures of medical diagnosis." Louis M. Warfield, "The Report of a Series of Blood Cultures in Typhoid Fever, *Ayer Clinical Laboratory Bulletin* 1 (1903): 77–80.

132. The reports in the *Ayer Clinical Laboratory Bulletin* are at first numerous and original—that is, there is no indication that they have been published elsewhere. By the end of the first series most of the major articles are reprinted from other medical journals. The bulletin ceased publication with the 1906 number and did not resume until 1922, without substantive comment on the reasons for the interruption. The republication of articles from other journals was still evidently controversial, as the bulletin did not do so for several issues, and when it again started to republish articles a note advised readers of the change in policy and assured them that original articles would continue to be published. "Forward," *Ayer Clinical Laboratory Bulletin* 11 (1928): 5–6.

133. John R. Powell, to the Pennsylvania Hospital Board of Managers, June 1, 1926.

134. Minutes of the Medical Board, April 29, 1897. General background is provided by Charles T. Olcott, "Pathology at the New York Hospital, 1810–1932," *Bulletin of the History of Medicine* 34 (1960): 137–47.

135. Annual report 1915.

136. He received an A.B. degree from Harvard in 1886 and an M.D. degree in 1889. He took an internship at St. Luke's from 1890 to 1892 and then studied abroad, at Heidelberg and Vienna. Biographical information from manuscripts in the biographical file, New York Hospital Archives.

137. Charles L. Gibson, "A Surgical 'Follow-up' System," *Annals of Surgery* 64 (1916): 349–52; "An Analysis of the Results of a Six Year Follow-up System in a Hospital Surgical Service," *Annals of Surgery* 70 (1919): 661–94; "The Results of Operations for Chronic Appendicitis: A Study of 555 Cases," *American Journal of the Medical Sciences* 159 (1920): 654–63; "The Results of Operations for Chronic Appendicitis (2d ser.)," *American Journal of the Medical Sciences* 163 (1924) 807–12.

138. Eugene H. Pool and Frederick W. Bancroft, "Systematization of a Surgical Service," *JAMA* 69 (1917): 1599–1602.

139. Ralph G. Stillman, "A Criticism of Hospital Laboratory Examinations," *JAMA* 76 (1921): 1816–17.

140. *Western Medical Review* (Lincoln, Nebr.) 1 (1896): 26–29.

141. West, "Value of the Examination of the Blood."
142. Elsner, "Value to the Physician," 108.

CHAPTER 8: MACHINES AND MEDICINE

1. Seymour Perry, review of *The Changing Economics of Medical Technology* ed. Annetine C. Gelijns and Ethan Halm and *Technology and Health Care in a Era of Limits*, ed. Annetine C. Gelijns, *New England Journal of Medicine* 329 (1993): 1748–49.
2. On the importance of context in a broad sense, see Burton A. Weisbrod on the role of insurance coverage in determining technology in "The Health Care Quadrilemma: An Essay on Technological Change, Insurance, Quality of Care, and Cost Containment," *Journal of Economic Literature* 29 (1991): 523–52; or, on the importance of specific reimbursement mechanisms, Nancy M. Kane and Paul D. Manoukian, "The Effect of the Medicare Prospective Payment System on the Adoption of New Technology: The Case of Cochlear Implants," *New England Journal of Medicine* 321 (1989): 1378–83.
3. Donald MacKenzie and Judy Wajcman, "Introductory Essay," in *The Social Shaping of Technology: How the Refrigerator Got Its Hum*, edited by MacKenzie and Wajcman, 2–25 (Philadelphia: Milton Keynes, 1985).
4. For more on the social context of technology, see Sandra Harding, "Knowledge, Technology, and Social Relations," *Journal of Medicine and Philosophy* 3 (1978): 346–58.
5. Joel D. Howell, "Diagnostic Technologies: X-rays, Electrocardiograms, and CAT Scans," *Southern California Law Review* 65 (1991): 529–64.
6. Thomas P. Hughes makes a related point in "Machines and Medicine: A Projection of Analogies between Electric Power Systems and Health Care Systems," *International Journal of Technology Assessment* 2 (1986): 285–95. In this article Hughes examines how hospitals may be understood as part of the larger universe of the health care system.
7. One of the classic discussions of the ways that workers in another field took control of a new technology is David Noble, *Forces of Production: A Social History of Industrial Automation* (New York: Alfred A. Knopf, 1984).
8. Christopher Lawrence examines how the electrocardiogram only gradually came to be seen as a defining technology for coronary thrombosis in " 'Definite and Material': Coronary Thrombosis and Cardiologists in the 1920," in *Framing Disease: Studies in Cultural History*, edited by Charles E. Rosenberg and Janet Golden, 50–82 (New Brunswick: Rutgers University Press, 1992).
9. Jeffrey P. Baker, "The Incubator Controversy: Pediatricians and the Origins of Premature Infant Technology in the United States, 1890 to 1910," *Pediatrics* 87 (1991): 654–62.

10. Obviously, if the patient and caregiver are the same person, this argument is reduced to a discussion of whether a person can, or should, serve in both capacities at once, a discussion that falls beyond the purview of this book.

11. Although he uses a different set of terminology and explores a different set of subjects, Charles Bosk's "quasi-normative error" clearly reflects a similar type of local culture. Bosk defines the term in the context of a study of medical mistakes: the error takes place when a subordinate fails to follow the practice patterns of his or her superior, even when there is no clear reason to believe that one choice or another is correct. Bosk uses the error to explain why some house officers fail to succeed in their training programs. But it also reflects the explicit power of a few people to shape the practice patterns of many others around them, which is part of what constitutes a local culture. Charles L. Bosk, *Forgive and Remember: Managing Medical Failure* (Chicago: University of Chicago Press, 1979).

12. Kaveh T. Safavi and Rodney A. Hayward, "Choosing between Apples and Apples: Physicians' Choices of Prescription Drugs That Have Similar Side Effects and Efficacies," *Journal of General Internal Medicine* 7 (1992): 32–37.

13. For a discussion of more recent differences in technology adoption among different hospitals, see Louise Russell, *Technology in Hospitals: Medical Advances and Their Diffusion* (Washington, D.C.: Brookings Institution, 1979).

14. For a cogent discussion of the risks and benefits of drawing conclusions from a single case study, see Terrence J. McDonald, *The Parameters of Urban Fiscal Policy: Socioeconomic Change and Political Culture in San Francisco, 1860–1906* (Berkeley: University of California Press, 1986), esp. 262ff.

15. Charles E. Rosenberg, "The Therapeutic Revolution," in *The Therapeutic Revolution: Essays in the Social History of American Medicine,* edited by Morris J. Vogel and Charles E. Rosenberg, 3–25 (Philadelphia: University of Pennsylvania Press, 1979).

16. The term *little-ticket technology* came into common use in the 1970s, as part of discussions about technology utilization and cost containment. Attention at first focused on the "big-ticket" items that were easy to see and price, items such as the CAT scanner. It soon became apparent, however, that a good deal of time and money was being spent on other, smaller, less-visible technologies, such as blood tests and urine tests, which have come to be known as "little-ticket" technologies. See Thomas W. Moloney and David Rogers, "Medical Technology—A Different View of the Contentious Debate over Costs," *New England Journal of Medicine* 301 (1979): 1413–19.

17. For the inappropriate use of two common tests used to study how fast blood clots, one estimate was a cost of over $60,000 per year for the medical service of a single hospital. Stephen B. Erban, Judith L. Kinman,

and J. Sanford Schwartz, "Routine Use of the Prothrombin and Partial Thromboplastin Times," *JAMA* 262 (1989): 2428–32.

18. On the importance of a systems approach, although one more in the "macro" perspective, see Hughes, "Machines and Medicine."

19. Barbara Duden, *Disembodying Women: Perspectives on Pregnancy and the Unborn*, translated by Lee Hoinacki (Cambridge, Mass.: Harvard University Press, 1993), 75–78.

20. Hughes, "Machines and Medicine."

21. For example, John C. Fletcher and Mark I. Evans, "Maternal Bonding in Early Fetal Ultrasound Examination," *New England Journal of Medicine* 308 (1983): 392–93. For analysis of the historical and technological creation of the "fetus," a topic of great contemporary interest, see Duden, *Disembodying Women.*

22. Mary Roth Walsh, *"Doctors Wanted, No Women Need Apply": Sexual Barriers in the Medical Profession, 1835–1975* (New Haven: Yale University Press, 1977), 186; Regina Morantz-Sanchez, "So Honored, So Loved? The Women's Medical Movement in Decline," in *"Send Us a Lady Physician": Women Doctors in America, 1835–1920,* edited by Ruth J. Abrams, 231–45 (New York: W. W. Norton, 1985).

23. For an example of such a study, see Regina Markell Morantz and Sue Zschoche, "Professionalism, Feminism, and Gender Roles: A Comparative Study of Nineteenth-Century Medical Therapeutics," *Journal of American History* 67 (1980): 568–88. Recent studies suggest that female physicians are more likely than male physicians to request some forms of screening tests for women. See Nicole Lurie, Jonathan Slater, Paul McGovern, Jaqueline Ekstrum, Louis Quam, and Karen Margolis, "Preventive Care for Women: Does the Sex of the Physician Matter?" *New England Journal of Medicine* 329 (1993): 478–82.

24. Virginia Berridge, "Introduction: AIDS and Contemporary History," in *AIDS and Contemporary History,* edited by Virginia Berridge and Philip Strong, 1–14 (Cambridge: Cambridge University Press, 1993).

25. Although difficult to define precisely, this movement is related to Continuous Quality Improvement (which often goes by its own three-letter acronym, CQI). Many of the ideas come from the work of W. Edwards Deming, who helped change industrial practices, first in post–World War II Japan and later in the United States. Deming, *Out of the Crisis* (Cambridge, Mass.: MIT Press, 1986).

26. Glenn L. Laffel and Donald M. Berwick, "Quality Health Care," *JAMA* 270 (1993): 254–55.

27. Donald M. Berwick, "The Clinical Process and the Quality Process," *Quality Management in Health Care* 1 (1992): 1–8.

28. See, for example, Henry J. Aaron and William Schwartz, *The Painful Prescription: Rationing Health Care* (Washington, D.C.: Brookings, 1984); "Rationing Health Care: The Choice before Us," *Science* 247 (1990): 418–22; Stuart H. Altman and Robert Blendon, eds., *Medical Technology: The Culprit behind Health Care Costs?* (Washington, D.C.:

Government Printing Office, 1979); Christopher Anderson, "Research and Health Care Costs," *Science* 261 (1993): 416–18; J. K. Inglehart, "Opinion Polls on Health Care," *New England Journal of Medicine* 310 (1984): 1616–20; Ronald Dworkin, "Will Clinton's Plan Be Fair?" *New York Review of Books* 41 (January 13, 1994): 20–25; and Jonathan A. Showstack, Stephen A. Schroeder, and Michael F. Matsumoto, "Changes in the Use of Medical Technologies, 1972–1977: A Study of Ten Inpatient Diagnoses," *New England Journal of Medicine* 306 (1982): 706–12.

29. For cautions against seeing technology as necessarily cost enhancing, see Victor R. Fuchs, "The Health Sector's Share of the Gross National Product," *Science* 247 (1990): 534–38 and Eli Ginzberg, "High-Tech Medicine and Rising Health Care Costs," *JAMA* 263 (1990): 1820–22.

30. For a general overview of ways to change physicians' behavior, see Peter J. Greco and John M. Eisenberg, "Changing Physicians' Practices," *New England Journal of Medicine* 329 (1993): 1271–74.

31. Joel D. Howell and Catherine G. McLaughlin, "Regional Variation in 1917 Health Care Expenditures," *Medical Care* 27 (1989): 772–88.

32. Rosenberg and Golden, *Framing Disease*. For more recent disease construction, see Lynn Payer, *Medicine and Culture: Varieties of Treatment in the United States, England, West Germany, and France* (New York: Henry Holt, 1988).

33. Two recent examples from the Agency for Health Care Policy and Research are *Clinical Practice Guideline: Acute Pain Management: Operative or Medical Procedures or Trauma* (Washington, D.C.: U.S. Department of Health and Human Services, 1992); and *Clinical Practice Guideline: Urinary Incontinence in Adults* (Washington, D.C.: U.S. Department of Health and Human Services, 1992). See also Robert H. Brook, "Practice Guidelines and Practicing Medicine: Are They Compatible?" *JAMA* 26, no. 2 (1989): 3027–30.

34. Clement J. McDonald and J. Marc Overhage, "Guidelines You Can Follow and Can Trust: An Ideal and an Example," *JAMA* 271 (1994): 872–73.

35. Sean R. Tunis, Robert S. A. Hayward, Mark C. Wilson, Haya R. Rubin, Eric B. Brass, Mary Johnston, and Earl P. Steinberg, "Internists' Attitudes about Clinical Practice Guidelines," *Annals of Internal Medicine* 120 (1994): 956–63; Sandra J. Tanenbaum, "What Physicians Know," *New England Journal of Medicine* 329 (1993): 1268–71.

36. An overview may be found in the theme issue "Making Good on the Promise: Disseminating and Implementing Practice Guidelines," *Quality Review Bulletin* 18 (December 1992).

37. I. S. Udvarhelyi, C. Gatsonis, A. Epstein, et al., "Acute Myocardial Infarction in the Medicare Population: Process of Care and Clinical Outcomes," *JAMA* 268 (1992): 2530–36.

38. Many of these studies have revolved around the decisions about whether to admit people with chest pain to a coronary care unit, a common problem in the emergency department of most hospitals.

Admitting people who do not need to be admitted is extremely expensive; not admitting people who need to be admitted can be fatal. See M. W. Pozen, R. B. D'Agostino, H. P. Selker, P. A.Sytkowski, and W. B. Hood, Jr., "A Predictive Instrument to Improve Coronary-Care-Unit Admission Practices in Acute Ischemic Disease: A Prospective Multicenter Clinical Trial," *New England Journal of Medicine* 310 (1984): 1273–78; H. P. Selker, J. L. Griffith, and R. B. D'Agostino, "A Time-Insensitive Predictive Instrument for Acute Myocardial Infarction Mortality: A Multicenter Study," *Medical Care* 29 (1991): 1196–1211.

39. Rosemary Stevens, *In Sickness and in Wealth: American Hospitals in the Twentieth Century* (New York: Basic Books, 1989).

40. The chart in E. A. Codman, *A Study in Hospital Efficiency as Demonstrated by the Case Report of the First Five Years of a Private Hospital* (Boston: Th. Todd, 1918), was so large that it was inserted as a "fold-out" in a pocket in the back of the book, and it still would hardly suffice for even a moderate-size hospital.

41. James W. Cortada, *Before the Computer: IBM, NCR, Burroughs, and Remington Rand and the Industry They Created, 1865–1956* (Princeton: Princeton University Press, 1993).

42. On the potential problems with such an approach, see Noralou P. Roos, Leslie L. Roos, Jana Mossy, and Betty Havens, "Using Administrative Data to Predict Important Health Outcomes: Entry to Hospital, Nursing Home, and Death," *Medical Care* 26 (1988): 221–39.

43. Martin Tolchin, "White House Planning ID for Health Care," *New York Times*, August 28, 1993, 1:7. The proposal faces opposition on the grounds that it could infringe on people's privacy.

44. R. Listernick, L. Frisone, and B. L. Silverman, "Delayed Diagnosis of Infants with Abnormal Neonatal Screens," *JAMA* 267 (1992): 1095–99.

APPENDIX

1. Portions of the pilot study were reported as Joel D. Howell, "Early Use of X-ray Machines and Electrocardiographs at the Pennsylvania Hospital: 1897–1927," *Journal of the American Medical Association (JAMA)* 255 (1986): 2320–23; "Machines and Medicine: Technology Transforms the American Hospital," in *The American General Hospital: Communities and Social Contexts*, edited by Diana Elizabeth Long and Janet Golden, 109–34 (Ithaca: Cornell University Press, 1989); "Diagnostic Technologies: X-rays, Electrocardiograms, and CAT Scans," *Southern California Law Review* 65 (1991): 529–64.

2. Leslie Kish, *Survey Sampling* (New York: John Wiley, 1965); Graham Kalton, *Introduction to Survey Sampling* (Beverly Hills: Sage Publications, 1983).

3. For a detailed discussion of the practicalities of selecting records to be sampled from hospital archives, see Joel D. Howell, "Preserving Patient

Records to Support Health Care Delivery, Teaching, and Research" in *Designing Archival Programs to Advance Knowledge in the Health Fields*, edited by Nancy McCall and Lisa A. Mix (Baltimore: Johns Hopkins University Press, 1995).

4. *Classification of Diseases, as Adopted by the Massachusetts General Hospital, Boston City Hospital, Carney Hospital, Peter Bent Brigham Hospital, Massachusetts Homeopathic Hospital, and Others,* 7th ed. (Boston: Griffith-Stillings Press, 1926).

5. Available from Computing Resource Center, Santa Monica, Calif.

INDEX

Library of Congress Cataloging-in-Publication Data

Howell, Joel D.
  Technology in the hospital : transforming patient care in the
early twentieth century / Joel D. Howell.
    p. cm.
  Includes bibliographical references and index.
  ISBN 0-8018-5020-7 (hc : alk. paper)
  1. Hospitals—United States—Diagnostic services—History—20th
century. 2. Medical technology—United States—History—20th
century. 3. Hospital care—United States—History—20th century.
I. Title
  [DNLM: 1. Technology, Medical—history—United States. 2. History
of Medicine, 20th Cent.—United States. 3. Equipment and Supplies,
Hospital—history—United States. WZ 70 AA1 H8t 1995]
RA975.5.D47H68 1995
610'.28—dc20
DNLM/DLC
for Library of Congress   94-38601